Third Edition

Oncology Nurse Navigation
Delivering Patient-Centered Care
Across the Continuum

Edited by
Deborah M. Christensen, MSN, APRN, AOCNS®
Cynthia Cantril, MPH, RN, OCN®-Emeritus

Oncology Nursing Society
Pittsburgh, Pennsylvania

ONS Publications Department
Publisher and Director of Publications: Lynn Nace, BA
Acquisitions Editor: Dave Burns, BA
Staff Editor II: Andrew Petyak, BA, PMP
Design and Production Administrator: Dany Sjoen

Copyright © 2025 by Oncology Nursing Society. All rights reserved. No part of the material protected by this copyright may be reproduced or utilized in any form, electronic or mechanical, including photocopying, recording, or by an information storage and retrieval system, without written permission from the copyright owner. For information, visit www.ons.org/publications-journals/permissions-archives, or send an email to pubpermissions@ons.org.

Library of Congress Cataloging-in-Publication Data
Names: Christensen, Deborah M. editor | Cantril, Cynthia editor
Title: Oncology nurse navigation : delivering patient-centered care across the continuum / edited by Deborah M. Christensen, MSN, APRN, AOCNS, and Cynthia Cantril, MPH, RN, OCN.
Description: Third edition. | Pittsburgh, Pennsylvania : Oncology Nursing Society, [2025] | Includes bibliographical references and index. |
Identifiers: LCCN 2025016698 | ISBN 9781635930689 paperback | ISBN 9781635930696 ebook
Subjects: LCSH: Cancer--Nursing
Classification: LCC RC266 .O52 2025 | DDC 616.99/40231--dc23/eng/20250616
LC record available at https://lccn.loc.gov/2025016698

Publisher's Note

This book is published by the Oncology Nursing Society (ONS). ONS neither represents nor guarantees that the practices described herein will, if followed, ensure safe and effective patient care. The recommendations contained in this book reflect ONS's judgment regarding the state of general knowledge and practice in the field as of the date of publication. The recommendations may not be appropriate for use in all circumstances. Those who use this book should make their own determinations regarding specific safe and appropriate patient care practices, taking into account the personnel, equipment, and practices available at the hospital or other facility at which they are located. The editors and publisher cannot be held responsible for any liability incurred as a consequence from the use or application of any of the contents of this book. Figures and tables are used as examples only. They are not meant to be all-inclusive, nor do they represent endorsement of any particular institution by ONS. Mention of specific products and opinions related to those products do not indicate or imply endorsement by ONS. Websites mentioned are provided for information only; the hosts are responsible for their own content and availability. Unless otherwise indicated, dollar amounts reflect U.S. dollars.

ONS publications are originally published in English. Publishers wishing to translate ONS publications must contact ONS about licensing arrangements. ONS publications cannot be translated without obtaining written permission from ONS. (Individual tables and figures that are reprinted or adapted require additional permission from the original source.) Because translations from English may not always be accurate or precise, ONS disclaims any responsibility for inaccuracies in words or meaning that may occur as a result of the translation. Readers relying on precise information should check the original English version.

Printed in the United States of America

Innovation • Excellence • Advocacy • Inclusivity

Contributors

Editors

Deborah M. Christensen, MSN, APRN, AOCNS®
Independent Consultant
Cancer Help Desk
Burlingame, California
Chapter 1. Current and Future State of Navigation; Chapter 5. Models of Oncology Navigation; Chapter 9. Personalized Communication Across the Cancer Care Continuum; Chapter 10. Navigating Each Phase of the Patient Journey; Chapter 12. Personalized Medicine and Novel Therapies

Cynthia Cantril, MPH, RN, OCN®-Emeritus
Owner
Cantril Cancer Recovery and Resources
Chapter 1. Current and Future State of Navigation

Authors

Stephanie Bonfilio, MSN, RN, OCN®, ONN-CG
Oncology Navigation Manager
St. Elizabeth Healthcare
Edgewood, Kentucky
Chapter 7. Measuring Nurse-Led Patient Outcomes

Rachel Brody, PhD(c), MSN, RN
Assistant Director of Nursing
Age Friendly Project Director
Montefiore Medical Center
Bronx, New York
Chapter 11. Unique Navigation Issues

Amanda Bruffy, MBAHM, BSN, RN, CNRN, OCN®
Director of Radiation Oncology and Oncology Nurse Navigation
Centra Alan B. Pearson Regional Cancer Center
Lynchburg, Virginia
Chapter 5. Models of Oncology Navigation

Darcy Burbage, DNP, RN, AOCN®, CBCN®
Oncology Clinical Nurse Specialist/Consultant
Newark, Delaware
Chapter 14. Survivorship Navigation

Katie L. Fanslau, DNP, RN
Penn Cancer Network Administrator
Penn Medicine
Philadelphia, Pennsylvania
Chapter 13. Spiritual Considerations

Kristin Ferguson, DNP, MBA, RN, OCN®
Senior Director, Strategic Operations: Bone Marrow Transplant and Cell Therapy
MedStar Georgetown University Hospital
Washington, DC
Chapter 6. Determining Community and Program Needs

Lauren V. Ghazal, PhD, FNP-BC
Assistant Professor, School of Nursing
University of Rochester
Rochester, New York
Chapter 17. Pediatrics, Adolescents, and Young Adults

Chris Gosselin, MBA, BSN, RN
Chapter 7. Measuring Nurse-Led Patient Outcomes

Sarah H. Kagan, PhD, RN, AOCN®, GCNS-BC, FAAN, FGSA
Lucy Walker Honorary Professor of Gerontological Nursing, School of Nursing
Gerontology Clinical Nurse Specialist, Abramson Cancer Center at Pennsylvania Hospital, Penn Medicine
University of Pennsylvania
Philadelphia, Pennsylvania
Chapter 16. Gero-Oncology Considerations

Lisa Lampton, MSN, MBA, RN, CBCN®, OCN®
Breast Nurse Navigation Manager
Memorial Hermann Health System
Houston, Texas
Chapter 4. Oncology Nurse Navigator Role and Competencies

Helen Meldrum, EdD
Associate Professor of Psychology
Bentley University
Waltham, Massachusetts
Chapter 15. Mental Health Issues

Claudia T. Miller, BSN, RN, OCN®, ONN-CG
Thoracic Oncology Nurse Navigator
Medical University of South Carolina
Hollings Cancer Center
Charleston, South Carolina
Chapter 10. Navigating Each Phase of the Patient Journey

Jacqueline Miller, MSN, RN, OCN®
Director of Oncology Navigation
Jefferson Health
Philadelphia, Pennsylvania
Chapter 3. Understanding the Business of Navigation

Bonny Morris, PhD, MSPH, RN
Vice President, Navigation
Patient Navigation
American Cancer Society
Chapter 1. Current and Future State of Navigation

Dan Sherman, MA, LPC
Financial Navigator
Trinity Health, St. Mary's
Grand Rapids, Michigan
Chapter 8. Interventions Addressing Financial Toxicity

Tricia Strusowski, MS, RN
CEO and Cofounder
TurnKey Oncology
Bear, Delaware
Chapter 7. Measuring Nurse-Led Patient Outcomes

Tara Sweeney, BSN, RN, CHPN, OCN®
Lead Oncology Nurse Navigator
Main Line Health
Bryn Mawr, Pennsylvania
Chapter 14. Survivorship Navigation

Marybeth Tetlow, MSN, RN, BMTCN®, OCN®
RN Hematology Oncology Nurse Coordinator
Duke Blood Cancer Center
Duke University Hospital
Durham, North Carolina
Chapter 17. Pediatrics, Adolescents, and Young Adults

Kathleen Wiley, MSN, RN, AOCNS®
Director of Oncology Nursing Practice
Oncology Nursing Society
Pittsburgh, Pennsylvania
Chapter 2. Access to Care

Disclosure

Editors and authors of books and guidelines provided by the Oncology Nursing Society are expected to disclose to the readers any significant financial interest or other relationships with the manufacturer(s) of any commercial products.

A vested interest may be considered to exist if a contributor is affiliated with or has a financial interest in commercial organizations that may have a direct or indirect interest in the subject matter. A "financial interest" may include, but is not limited to, being a shareholder in the organization; being an employee of the commercial organization; serving on an organization's speakers bureau; or receiving research funding from the organization. An "affiliation" may be holding a position on an advisory board or some other role of benefit to the commercial organization. Vested interest statements appear in the front matter for each publication.

Contributors are expected to disclose any unlabeled or investigational use of products discussed in their content. This information is acknowledged solely for the information of the readers.

The contributors provided the following disclosure and vested interest information:

Cynthia Cantril, MPH, RN, OCN®-Emeritus: Cancer Help Desk, consultant or advisory role

Stephanie Bonfilio, MSN, RN, OCN®, ONN-CG: Amplity, consultant or advisory role; Academy of Oncology Nurse and Patient Navigators, Oncology Nursing Society, other remuneration

Amanda Bruffy, MBAHM, BSN, RN, CNRN, OCN®: Oncology Nursing Society, honoraria, other remuneration

Darcy Burbage, DNP, RN, AOCN®, CBCN®: Oncology Nursing Society, employment of leadership position; Cancer Care Connection, Patient Navigation Conference, honoraria

Katie L. Fanslau, DNP, RN: Association of Cancer Care Centers, consultant or advisory role, other remuneration

Kristin Ferguson, DNP, MBA, RN, OCN®: Advanced Practice Providers Oncology Summit, honoraria

Helen Meldrum, EdD: Pfizer, honoraria, other remuneration

Claudia T. Miller, BSN, RN, OCN®, ONN-CG: American Cancer Society, consultant or advisory role, honoraria, other remuneration

Dan Sherman, MA, LPC: NaVectis Group, Pink Fund, employment or leadership position; TailorMed, consultant or advisory role; Memorial Sloan Kettering, research funding

Tricia Strusowski, MS, RN: Academy of Oncology Nurse and Patient Navigators, employment or leadership position; Blueprint Navigation, SHARE Cancer Support, consultant or advisory role; Academy of Oncology Nurse and Patient Navigators, honoraria, expert testimony

Marybeth Tetlow, MSN, RN, BMTCN®, OCN®: Nursing and Patient Care Innovations, employment or leadership position, stock ownership

Licensing Opportunities

The Oncology Nursing Society (ONS) produces some of the most highly respected educational resources in the field of oncology nursing, including ONS's award-winning journals, books, online courses, evidence-based resources, core competencies, videos, and information available on the ONS website at www.ons.org. ONS welcomes opportunities to license reuse of these intellectual properties to other organizations.

Licensing opportunities include the following:

- **Reprints**—Purchase high-quality reprints of ONS journal articles, book chapters, and other content directly from ONS, or obtain permission to produce your own reprints.
- **Translations**—Translate and then resell or share ONS resources internationally.
- **Integration**—Purchase a license to incorporate ONS's oncology-specific telephone triage protocols or other resources into your institution's EMR or EHR system.
- **Cobranding**—Display your company's logo on ONS resources for distribution to your organization's employees or customers.
- **Educational reuse**—Supplement your staff or student educational programs using ONS resources.
- **Customization**—Customize ONS intellectual property for inclusion in your own products or services.
- **Bulk purchases**—Buy ONS books and online courses in high quantities to receive great savings compared to regular pricing.

As you read through the pages of this book, think about whether any of these opportunities are the right fit for you as you consider reusing ONS content—and the contents of this book—for your organization.

Contact licensing@ons.org with your licensing questions or requests.

Table of Contents

Acknowledgments xi

Section I. Current and Future States of Oncology Patient Navigation 1

Chapter 1. Current and Future State of Navigation 3
Overview 3
Nurse Navigation: A Strategy to Optimize the Experiences of Patients With Cancer and Their Families 4
A Brief History of Navigation 5
Barriers Limiting or Preventing Access to Cancer Care 7
Using Patient Navigation to Bolster the Oncology Workforce 7
Summary 15
References 15

Chapter 2. Access to Care 19
Overview 19
Barriers to Care 20
Summary 24
References 24

Section II. Steps for Implementing, Growing, and Sustaining Oncology Navigation 27

Chapter 3. Understanding the Business of Navigation 29
Overview 29
Building a Navigation Program Step by Step ... 29
Summary 38
References 38

Chapter 4. Oncology Nurse Navigator Role and Competencies 41
Overview 41
Role Definitions 41
Oncology Nurse Navigator Competencies 43
Application of Competencies to Practice 44

Summary 45
References 46

Chapter 5. Models of Oncology Navigation 49
Overview 49
Oncology Navigation Roles 49
Staff Selection Strategies 51
Customary Navigation Models 51
Specialized Navigation Models 53
Setting-Specific Navigation 54
Summary 56
References 57

Chapter 6. Determining Community and Program Needs 59
Overview 59
Cancer Program Accreditations and Requirements 60
Determining Program Needs 61
External Community Assessment 61
Internal Community Assessment 64
Needs Assessment Data and Program Monitoring 67
Examples of Best Practices in Navigation Processes 68
Summary 73
References 73

Chapter 7. Measuring Nurse-Led Patient Outcomes 77
Overview 77
Establishing Navigation Metrics 78
Centers for Medicare and Medicaid Principal Illness Navigation Billing Codes 81
Continued Development and Application of Navigation Metrics 81
Summary 89
References 89

Chapter 8. Interventions Addressing Financial Toxicity 91
Overview 91

Impact of Financial Toxicity 91
Financial Navigation Considerations 93
Financial Resources 97
Insurance Optimization 100
Summary 108
References 109

Section III. Noteworthy Navigation Topics From the Experts 113

Chapter 9. Personalized Communication Across the Cancer Care Continuum 115
Overview 115
Prediagnosis to Diagnosis: Navigating Uncertainty 116
Treatment: Supporting Informed Decision-Making.. 117
Cancer Survivorship: Fostering Resilience 119
Cancer Recurrence: Renewing Dialogue........ 119
Hospice and End of Life: Ensuring Peace and Comfort 120
Age-Related Communication Considerations 121
Communication Strategies in Action.............. 124
Summary 125
References 126

Chapter 10. Navigating Each Phase of the Patient Journey 129
Overview 129
Prevention and Screening 130
Diagnosis 131
Treatment... 133
Survivorship 135
Advanced, Metastatic, and Recurrent Disease.. 137
End of Life 138
Summary 140
References 141

Chapter 11. Unique Navigation Issues.......... 145
Overview 145
Navigating Diverse Environments 145
Case Studies Depicting Unique Navigation Issues.. 146
Summary 152
References 153

Chapter 12. Personalized Medicine and Novel Therapies 155
Overview 155
Targeting the Hallmarks of Cancer Development.. 156
Diagnostic and Biomarker Testing Techniques ... 157

Cancer Biomarker Identification and Application 158
Targeted Cancer Therapy.............................. 159
Overcoming Challenges in Providing Precision Oncology 163
Summary 166
References 167

Chapter 13. Spiritual Considerations 171
Overview 171
Spirituality Versus Religion 171
Nursing Care and Spirituality......................... 173
Spiritual Care Training................................... 175
Spiritual Care Assessment Tools and Frameworks... 178
Oncology Nurse Navigation and Spiritual Care... 179
Workplace Well-Being and Spirituality 181
Summary 183
References 184

Section IV. Personalized Care for Unique Populations 187

Chapter 14. Survivorship Navigation 189
Overview 189
Stages of Survivorship 190
Components of Survivorship Care 190
Long-Term and Late Effects of Treatment....... 192
Symptom Clusters 193
Physical Needs 195
Immune-Related Adverse Effects.................. 197
Psychosocial Needs....................................... 197
Sexual Health: Intimacy, Sexuality, and Fertility 199
Financial and Time Toxicity 200
The Role of the Oncology Nurse Navigator in Survivorship Care 200
Resources to Assist in the Care of Survivors . 204
Program Development 205
Future Opportunities in Survivorship Navigation.. 206
Summary 207
References 207

Chapter 15. Mental Health Issues................ 211
Overview 211
Addressing Mental Health and Cancer.......... 212
Patients With Severe Mental Illness and Impairment 213
Patients With Anxiety and Panic Disorders 214
Patients With Suicidal Depression................. 217
Patients With Psychosis 220

Patients Using Chemical Coping................... 224
When Patients Are Peers.............................. 228
The Navigator's Wellness in the Post-
    Pandemic Years....................................... 228
Summary 232
References 234

Chapter 16. Gero-Oncology Considerations ... 241
Overview 241
Foundations of Age-Friendly Oncology
    Care.. 242
The M's of Age-Friendly Oncology Nurse
    Navigation.. 244
Summary 251
References 253

**Chapter 17. Pediatrics, Adolescents, and
Young Adults 261**
Overview 261
Trends, Transitions, and the Role of the
    Oncology Nurse Navigator...................... 262
Challenges Faced by Adolescents and
    Young Adults With Cancer 263
Psychosocial Interventions........................... 271
Recommended Supportive Care Resources.... 273
Summary 275
References 275

Chapter 18. Navigation Resources 285

Index 289

Acknowledgments

The year 2025 marks the 50th anniversary of the Oncology Nursing (ONS), representing half a century of development in oncology nursing as a distinct nursing specialty. This milestone coincides with the publication of the third edition of this comprehensive work on oncology nurse navigation, covering the entire cancer care continuum and reflecting the progress made since the initial role delineation study.

The editors express their gratitude to each other and their loved ones who have supported this endeavor. Special thanks to Brenda M. Nevidjon, MSN, RN, FAAN, for her national support of nurse navigation and Pamela J. Haylock, PhD, RN, FAAN, who co-created the first stand-alone nurse navigator job description for Montana and has been a constant guide to the editors. The clinical team at ONS and Kathleen Wiley, MSN, RN, AOCNS®, leading the new competency work, were essential content guides.

The authors who contributed their time and expertise to this timely body of work have played a crucial role in advancing the field of oncology nurse navigation. Looking forward, oncology nurse navigation will continue to be profoundly important in providing comprehensive care for patients with cancer. As the field evolves, the work presented in this edition will serve as a valuable resource for both current and future oncology nurse navigators, supporting their critical role in patient care and outcomes.

SECTION I
Current and Future States of Oncology Patient Navigation

Chapter 1. Current and Future State of Navigation
Chapter 2. Access to Care

CHAPTER 1

Current and Future State of Navigation

Cynthia Cantril, MPH, RN, OCN®-Emeritus, Deborah M. Christensen, MSN, APRN, AOCNS®, and Bonny Morris, PhD, MSPH, RN

> **KEY TOPICS**
> nurse navigation history and evolution, competencies, position statement

Access to comprehensive healthcare services is a precursor to equitable, quality health care. Nurses are uniquely qualified to help improve the quality of health care by helping people navigate the healthcare system, providing close monitoring and follow-up across the care continuum, focusing care on the whole person, and providing care that is culturally respectful and appropriate. Nurses can help overcome barriers to quality care, including structural inequities and implicit bias, through care management, person-centered care, and cultural humility. (Wakefield et al., 2021, p. 111)

Overview

This third edition of *Oncology Nurse Navigation: Delivering Patient-Centered Care Across the Continuum* reflects the evolution and growth of the oncology nurse navigator (ONN) role and the application of ONN competencies throughout the cancer trajectory. Pertinent and timely chapter topics include planning, implementing, and sustaining navigation programs, professional standards, competencies, programmatic metrics, financial challenges, the mental health of patients, models of care, and personalized care for unique populations.

This introductory chapter will detail milestones and policy-related initiatives that have shaped navigation as it exists today. It also will review anticipated challenges, directions, and sustainability considerations around navigation as an essential element of cancer care. Further, it will highlight select initiatives responsible for shaping oncology nurse navigation standards and competencies. Collaborative models and thoughts regarding the future of the professional navigator role, challenges, and sustainability of navigation programs will also be addressed.

Nurse Navigation: A Strategy to Optimize the Experiences of Patients With Cancer and Their Families

As a professional organization committed to advancing oncology nursing, providing quality cancer care, and reducing disparities in cancer care outcomes, the Oncology Nursing Society (ONS) plays a critical role in supplying resources and support for professional nurses providing navigation services as a strategy to optimize the experiences of patients with cancer and their families. It also advocates for the advancement of the navigation role.

Care coordination has long been recognized as a traditional strength of the nursing profession regardless of the care setting. Nurses have a well-documented capacity for problem-solving, innovation, and adaptability, as well as their engagement in multiple levels and settings throughout the healthcare system. Care coordination is "the deliberate organization of patient care activities between two or more participants (including the patient) involved in a patient's care to facilitate the appropriate delivery of health care services" (McDonald et al., 2007, p. 5). It is needed to increase access to the healthcare system and overcome obstacles such as fragmentation, communication, and costs (McDonald et al., 2007).

In the United States, care coordination is a vital strategy to improve the quality and value of healthcare services (Lamb & Newhouse, 2018). Oncology nurses with various job titles have provided these services for decades. Harold Freeman's work in the early 1990s fostered the emergence of the ONN role. At this time, nurses in navigation roles assumed facility-specific titles, job descriptions, and responsibilities. Many members of ONS assumed ONN roles and sought support from their professional organizations. The *2017 Oncology Nurse Navigator Core Competencies* defined the ONN role as:

> A professional RN with oncology-specific clinical knowledge who offers individualized assistance to patients, families, and caregivers to help overcome healthcare system barriers. Using the nursing process, an ONN provides education and resources to facilitate informed decision-making and timely access to quality health and psychosocial care throughout all phases of the cancer care continuum. (ONS, 2017, p. 4)

In October 2024, ONS and the Oncology Nursing Certification Corporation (ONCC) further demonstrated commitment to navigation by publishing the *Oncology Nurse Navigator Competencies*. The process of developing competencies and models was comprehensive and rigorous, resulting in 194 statements in 13 domains. The competencies were articulated for adoption in a multitude of practice areas, recognizing the diversity of interprofessional teams. Resources differed depending on the practice setting. The ONN competencies "define the foundation of this specialty role and how the nurse navigator implements necessary skills and abilities, regardless of the patient population or practice setting" (ONS & ONCC, 2024, p. 4). The ONN competency model framework identifies the critical pillars involved in care coordination and management, including interprofessional collaboration (see Figure 1-1). For additional details on competencies, see Chapter 4.

A Brief History of Navigation

In 1989, the American Cancer Society's (ACS's) *National Hearings on Cancer and the Poor* and the resulting *Report to the Nation: Cancer in the Poor* revealed that economically disadvantaged individuals encountered significant obstacles to accessing cancer care. These findings led to the concept of patient navigation, a significant component of cancer care worldwide (Chen et al., 2024; Freeman & Rodriguez, 2011; Knudsen et al., 2022; Vargas et al., 2008).

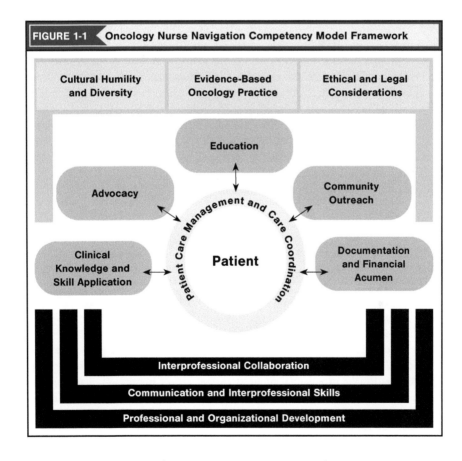

FIGURE 1-1. Oncology Nurse Navigation Competency Model Framework

Progressing into the 1990s, ACS funded Freeman to devise, test, and publish the outcomes of a navigation model at Harlem Hospital, located in the Harlem neighborhood of New York City (Freeman, 2012). He viewed patient navigation, then performed by community health workers, as a strategy to reduce disparities in the diagnosis and treatment of breast cancer in a marginalized population.

The strides made by Freeman occurred in the context of several previous decades of new cancer initiatives. For example, the National Cancer Act of 1971, signed into law by President Richard Nixon, gave the director of the National Cancer Institute (NCI) the ability to guide the National Cancer Program. This law also allowed for the creation of the President's Cancer Panel (2023), which still provides oversight to the National Cancer Program. Freeman's impact on this program was significant, evidenced by the focus of the 2001 President's Cancer Panel Report, *Voices of a Broken System: Real People, Real Problems*, in finding "what is happening to real people" (Freeman & Reuben, 2001, p. ii). In a year-long process during which seven regional meetings were held throughout the United States, panel members heard "firsthand from people with cancer, their families, and the health professionals, administrators, advocates, and volunteers who serve them" (Freeman & Reuben, 2001, p. i). A moral tenet echoed throughout these hearings and captured the essence of the panel's findings and its subsequent recommendation that "no person in America with cancer should go untreated, experience insurance-related diagnosis or treatment delays that jeopardize survival, or be bankrupted by a cancer diagnosis" (Freeman & Reuben, 2001, p. i). Freeman and Reuben (2001) also identified barriers, such as financial, physical, cultural, and educational, that limit or prevent access to cancer care, persist in the modern day, and continue to inform the direction of navigation programs and services.

The President's Cancer Panel has since focused on leveraging the benefits of navigation to decrease cancer outcome inequities. In 2023, it held a public, three-meeting series, *Reducing Cancer Care Inequities: Leveraging Technology to Enhance Patient Navigation*, to address the interplay between the power and opportunity of technology in patient care and the need to apply it with deep thought to avoid unintended consequences, including exacerbation of inequities. Focusing on technology supports two National Cancer Plan goals around eliminating inequities and delivering optimal care (President's Cancer Panel, 2024b). Separately, in 2024, the President's Cancer Panel held a public, two-day virtual meeting, *Developing and Retaining a Robust and Diverse Cancer Workforce: Challenges and Opportunities Across the National Cancer Program*, to assess and identify approaches to building a sustainable and diverse oncology workforce despite staff shortages, burnout, and other current-day realities experienced by many oncology professions, including navigation (President's Cancer Panel, 2024a).

The meetings were informed by the National Cancer Plan, released by NCI in 2023 (Association of Cancer Care Centers, 2023). The goals of this plan were to align with the Cancer Moonshot, an initiative established in 2016 by then–Vice President Joe Biden to make exponential progress around cancer prevention, diagnosis, and treatment (NCI, 2023). These national structures and initiatives, Freeman's seminal work around navigation, and the contributions of countless others have led to the current scope of navigation.

Barriers Limiting or Preventing Access to Cancer Care

The scope of navigation programs and services reflects the cancer care trajectory and includes prevention, early detection, diagnosis, treatment, palliation, survivorship, and end of life (Freeman & Rodriguez, 2011; ONS, 2021). More recently acknowledged barriers to quality care and optimal outcomes include complexity, access, and affordability of the U.S. health system, as well as racism, ageism, and social determinants of health, including but not limited to educational achievement, rurality, income, marital status, literacy, and health literacy (Fleary & Ettienne, 2019; Iheduru-Anderson & Wahi, 2022; Levitt & Altman, 2023; Nora et al., 2021; Stowell et al., 2024). The process of navigation continues to be challenged by what Freeman described as the "discovery–delivery disconnect," the lack of uniform access to quality cancer care among vulnerable populations (Freeman, 2012, p. 1614). Table 1-1 outlines historical milestones in the ongoing evolution of oncology nurse and patient navigation.

Using Patient Navigation to Bolster the Oncology Workforce

In describing what is widely viewed as "the global burden of cancer," epidemiologists reported that two million new cancer cases and 61,200 cancer deaths occur annually in the United States alone (Siegel et al., 2024). Cancer was expected to exceed 20 million new cases and cause nearly 10 million cancer-related deaths worldwide in 2022, the most recent projection available at the time of publication (Bray et al., 2024). The World Health Organization (2024) projected that new cancer cases will exceed 27 million by 2040 and 35 million by 2050 (Bray et al., 2024). Advances in cancer care have resulted in improved survival after diagnosis and treatment but have also contributed to the rapid growth in the number of patients needing cancer care services (Takvorian et al., 2020). It is estimated that the global economic cost of cancer from 2020–2050 will be $25.2 trillion (international dollars) based on 2017 price numbers (Chen et al., 2023).

Given these projections, it is essential to prepare expert oncology healthcare workers, as they provide direct care and services and also understand and devise cost-effective measures and strategies. Unfortunately, the increase in cancer survivors far outpaces the number of experts and practicing oncology clinicians. Oncologists and oncology nurses active during the 1970s are at or beyond retirement age. In some geographic areas, this disparity is exacerbated by the known maldistribution of oncologists, with more significant shortages observed in rural areas (Shulman et al., 2020).

Expansion of the oncology workforce to include patient navigation programs and services throughout the cancer care trajectory provides a host of documented benefits (Chan et al., 2023; Strusowski et al., 2024). Effective navigation processes and well-prepared navigators improve access to care, enhance care integration, and advance health outcomes for individuals and families affected by cancer (Budde et

TABLE 1-1. Historical Timeline of Navigation

Year	Event or Publication
1989	The American Cancer Society (ACS) holds the *National Hearings on Cancer and the Poor* and publishes the *Report to the Nation: Cancer in the Poor* (National Cancer Navigation Roundtable [NNRT], n.d.).
1990	ACS funds Harold Freeman's navigation pilot at Harlem Hospital (NNRT, n.d.).
1997	President Bill Clinton names Freeman the Member and Chair of the President's Cancer Panel (Wooley & Peters, n.d.).
2004	A study by Freeman in *Oncology Issues* demonstrates the effectiveness of patient navigation in reducing diagnostic delays and enhancing access to timely care for disadvantaged populations (Freeman, 2004).
2005	President George W. Bush signs the Patient Navigator Outreach and Chronic Disease Prevention Act, providing funding to the Health Resources and Services Administration for demonstration projects and research on patient navigation (NNRT, n.d.).
2005	ACS launches the Patient Navigation Program in Cancer Care, establishing navigation programs in healthcare systems across the country (NNRT, n.d.).
2007	The Harold P. Freeman Patient Navigation Institute launches the first navigation training course (NNRT, n.d.).
2008	The Oncology Nursing Society (ONS) establishes the Navigation Focus Group.
2009	The Academy of Oncology Nurse and Patient Navigators is founded to provide a network for all professionals involved and interested in patient navigation and survivorship care services (NNRT, n.d.).
2010	The Association of Oncology Social Work, National Association of Social Workers, and ONS issue their *Joint Position on the Role of Oncology Nursing and Oncology Social Work in Patient Navigation* (NNRT, n.d.).
2010	The Patient Protection and Affordable Care Act was passed and included navigation (NNRT, n.d.).
2012	ONS publishes the *Oncology Nurse Navigation Role Delineation Study* (Brown et al., 2012).
2012	The American College of Surgeons Commission on Cancer includes navigation as a required component for program accreditation (Freeman, 2012).
2013	ONS publishes the *Oncology Nurse Navigator Core Competencies* (NNRT, n.d.).
2014	The first edition of ONS's *Oncology Nurse Navigation: Delivering Patient-Centered Care Across the Continuum* is published.
2017	ACS's National Navigation Roundtable is established as a coalition of public, private, and voluntary organizations to address issues around patient navigation and to disseminate best practices (NNRT, n.d.).

(Continued on next page)

TABLE 1-1	Historical Timeline of Navigation *(Continued)*
Year	Event or Publication
2017	ONS publishes the *2017 Oncology Nurse Navigator Core Competencies* (ONS, 2017).
2017	ACS's Global Navigation Program is launched (ACS, n.d.-b).
2018	ONS and the Oncology Nursing Certification Corporation publish the results of the 2016 role delineation study, a follow-up to the 2012 study (Baileys et al., 2018).
2020	ONS publishes the second edition of *Oncology Nurse Navigation: Delivering Patient-Centered Care Across the Continuum*.
2021	ONS publishes a revised position statement *Role of the Oncology Nurse Navigator Throughout the Cancer Trajectory* (ONS, 2021).
2022	The Professional Oncology Navigation Task Force, a voice of professional organizations with the goal of solidifying and standardizing definitions, scopes, and roles of navigators, publishes *Oncology Navigation Standards of Professional Practice* (NNRT, n.d.).
2023	The Centers for Medicare and Medicaid Services decides to offer reimbursement for some level of patient navigation services for patients with cancer (NNRT, n.d.).
2024	ONS publishes an update to *Oncology Nurse Navigator Competencies* (ONS & Oncology Nursing Certification Corporation, 2024).

al., 2022). Realizing the importance of navigation by disparity in personnel, a collaboration of the International Society of Nurses in Cancer Care, Queensland University of Technology, European Oncology Nursing Society, Cyprus University of Technology, and ONS produced the position statement *Cancer Nursing's Potential to Reduce the Growing Burden of Cancer Across the World* (Yates et al., 2021). The statement contends that the worldwide nursing workforce, consisting of more than 20 million nurses and midwives, has unrealized potential to reduce the burden of cancer across the cancer trajectory through education, prevention, screening and early detection, treatment, palliative care, survivorship, and research. The position asserts the following (Yates et al., 2021, pp. 3436–3437):

- Nurses are essential to the success of reducing cancer incidence, improving survival and quality of life, and providing better palliative care.
- Well-prepared cancer nurses demonstrate wide-ranging impacts across the spectrum of cancer care in many high-income countries. To benefit from this expertise, substantial efforts to build nursing workforce capacity are required in low-, middle-, and high-income countries where the nursing workforce does not have access to adequate education.
- The role of the cancer nurse needs to be formally recognized as a key part of global cancer control efforts, and appropriate resources should be mandated within all cancer control programs.

- Government and nongovernmental organizations must optimize the substantial resources of nurses to ensure the burden of cancer is reduced worldwide.

The following section details the components needed to build patient navigation capabilities across the cancer care continuum.

Collaboration on Standards

Several national credentialing organizations, including the American College of Surgeons Commission on Cancer and the National Accreditation Program for Breast Centers, mandate navigation as part of accreditation standards in recognition of its effect on program quality and outcomes. In 2012, the American College of Surgeons Commission on Cancer required navigation as a component of program accreditation (Green, 2012). A language revision expanded "patient navigation" to "addressing barriers to care," acknowledging navigation as a critical component (American College of Surgeons, 2024). Although some credentialing and certifying organizations include navigation as a qualifying criterion, uniform definitions of navigation roles and programs, role preparation, and qualifications are evolving.

In 2020, a collaboration among the Professional Oncology Navigation Task Force, the Academy of Oncology Nurse and Patient Navigators (AONN+), the Association of Oncology Social Work (AOSW), the Association of Pediatric Hematology/Oncology Nurses, and ONS crafted *Oncology Navigation Standards of Professional Practice* (Franklin et al., 2022). This document offers guidance for best practices in navigation to clinical ONNs, social work navigators, and patient navigators. These standards describe the knowledge and skills that all professional navigators should possess to deliver high-quality, competent, and ethical services to people affected by cancer. Helpful features include suggested benchmarks for healthcare employers, as well as information for policymakers and decision-makers, healthcare professionals, and the public, aimed at advancing understanding of the role of professional oncology navigators.

Role Delineation and Competencies

Defining and refining the roles and skills required for ONN practice have been among ONS's priorities since the publication of the first role delineation study (Brown et al., 2012). A second role delineation study conducted in 2016 aimed to redefine the role and determine the need for an ONN certification examination under the auspices of ONCC and identify task domains associated with nurse navigation (Lubejko et al., 2017). However, it did not find adequate differences in knowledge and responsibilities of the ONN and other certifications granted to clinical and staff oncology nursing roles. Nevertheless, these role delineation study efforts guide education and preparation for the ONN role and identify contemporary and impending ONN core competencies. Such findings and recommendations led to the revision of the 2013 *Oncology Nurse Navigator Core Competencies* and the ONS position statement on the *Role of the Oncology Nurse Navigator Throughout the Cancer Trajectory* (ONS, 2017, 2021) (see Figure 1-2).

Program Design

Even with standardization, healthcare systems must plan and adapt navigation models and approaches based on changing and emerging service areas, patient population needs, and available resources. Navigation models in place include numerous roles and titles and a variety of staff expectations, competencies, and responsibilities. Navigation services often employ clinical navigators, patient navigators, community health workers, navigation support staff, and combinations thereof (Franklin et al., 2022).

A U.S. survey conducted by Wells et al. (2022) compared differences between clinical and non-clinical oncology navigators, including differences in services provided, engagement in the cancer care continuum, and personal and program characteristics. Most participants were more likely to have a bachelor's degree or higher, were funded by operational budgets, and were less likely to work in community-based or nonprofit organizations. Clinical navigators (licensed as either social workers or nurses) were more likely to perform basic navigation, care coordination, treatment and related support, clinical trial support, and peer support and engage in end-of-life and palliative care navigation. Findings demonstrated the different work settings and functions of these two roles, and it was hypothesized that non-clinical navigators are more likely to face job insecurity because they are more likely to work in nonprofit organizations and are primarily funded by grants. As navigation services become more reimbursable

FIGURE 1-2 Oncology Nursing Society Position Statement on the Role of the Oncology Nurse Navigator Throughout the Cancer Trajectory

- Navigation services should begin with prevention and screening activities and facilitate care transitions through diagnosis, treatment, survivorship, and end-of-life care.
- The oncology nurse navigator (ONN) should practice in accordance with the Oncology Nursing Society (ONS) *Oncology Nurse Navigator Core Competencies* as applicable to their practice. The core competencies of the ONN role include coordination of care, communication, education, and professional role.
- The ONN role can be tailored to meet the needs of patients in each care environment but should fulfill the tenets of the ONS-defined competencies.
- Nurses in ONN roles should possess comprehensive oncology expertise, as evidenced by certification through the Oncology Nursing Certification Corporation or other oncology nursing certification accredited by the National Commission for Certifying Agencies.
- The ONN advocates for adherence to evidence-based clinical practice guidelines and pathways and participates in the collection and analysis of patient outcome data to optimize patient and organizational outcomes.
- Determination of ONN workload and allocation of resources should be based upon data from reliable and valid metrics, including health system standards and measures sensitive to the ONN contribution to the navigation process.

through the Centers for Medicare and Medicaid Services (CMS), navigation programs may attain a greater level of financial sustainability.

Navigator Education and Preparation

As navigation programs and services continue to develop, efforts to standardize roles, responsibilities, and processes call for standardized preparation. One training and credentialing program is targeted to clinical (licensed) navigators as well as those without a clinical license and is produced by the ACS Leadership in Oncology Navigation (ACS LION) program. The curriculum meets CMS requirements for Principal Illness Navigation (PIN) reimbursement, is based on the Professional Oncology Navigation Task Force's *Oncology Navigation Standards of Professional Practice*, and supports role delineation among clinical and patient navigators (Morris et al., 2024).

Other training programs for professionals without a clinical license are also available, including the Patient Navigation and Community Health Worker Training by the Colorado Patient Navigator Training Collaborative, the Susan G. Komen Patient Navigation Training Program, and the Triage Cancer Insurance and Financial Intensive Training for Health Care. The Oncology Patient Navigator Training: The Fundamentals, developed and offered by George Washington University School of Medicine and Health Sciences, was the first competency-based program to be designed and was primarily implemented for navigators who do not hold clinical licenses (Kashima et al., 2018).

Nurses who wish to demonstrate mastery of navigation domains can sit for an examination offered through AONN+ to become certified as an Oncology Nurse Navigator–Certified Generalist (AONN+ Foundation for Learning, n.d.). Testing is available in person, typically at an AONN+ annual conference.

Financial Considerations

How funding is provided for navigation programs, staffing, and research has a unique history. The Patient Navigator and Chronic Disease and Prevention Act (2005), signed into law by President George W. Bush, provided funding to Health Resources and Services Administration demonstration projects and research on patient navigation. The Biden Cancer Moonshot Initiative, created in 2016 under President Barack Obama and led by then–Vice President Joe Biden, included navigation-related challenges as an area of focus, resulting in crucial navigation-related developments (ACS Cancer Action Network, 2024). Over the past two decades, research and policies have been supported by national organizations such as CMS, NCI, and the Centers for Disease Control and Prevention (ACS Action Network, 2023; Centers for Disease Control and Prevention, 2024; CMS, n.d.; NCI, 2006).

Navigation has historically relied on a combination of cyclic grants, individual system support, philanthropy, and operational funding, making programmatic long-term planning, staffing, and expansion of services an almost impossible challenge. A step forward for financial stability occurred in January 2024, when CMS established coding and payment for navigation services as a measure that could improve health equity among patients with serious conditions, including cancer (CMS, 2024). These codes (e.g., PIN) and those for principal care management (PCM) may be leveraged to reimburse navigation services. In a brief review of what this reimbursement could mean for oncology nurses, Fischer-Cartlidge and Graham (2024) noted that the CMS rule for PIN outlines requirements for navigation providers that are already standard components of nursing education. The authors cautioned that "the CMS rule's language largely skews toward non-clinical navigators, which leaves questions for nurses providing navigation services" (Fischer-Cartlidge & Graham, 2024, para. 5). However, nurse navigators do provide non-clinical navigation services reimbursable through PIN, and PCM remains a viable mechanism for reimbursement for clinical navigation. Beginning in 2024, ACS LION provided support for oncology program leaders and navigation teams to incorporate these codes from the CMS Physician Fee Schedule and develop sustainable navigation programs. ACS LION offerings include boot camps, learning collaboratives, and webinar series in collaboration with organizations such as ONS and the American Society for Clinical Oncology (ASCO) to help programs take advantage of this new revenue opportunity.

Navigation program leaders seeking to build or expand navigation programs through developing effective navigation business plans may take advantage of educational and informational resources developed through the collaborative efforts of ACS, AONN+, ASCO, and other organizations. These programs guide participating organizations through the use of a navigation business case tool kit found on the ACS Leadership in Oncology Navigation website (ACS, n.d.-c).

Focus on the Future

Role Integration

Programmatic assessment and evaluation are fundamental to establishing and expanding navigation programs. Further research in role integration is necessary to fulfill the promises of navigation and navigators in the oncology workforce. A study from Belgium highlighted a lack of role clarity, interprofessional team dynamics, and the presence or absence of guidance or coaching as the challenges to role integration of ONNs and advanced practice nurses within oncology teams (Van Hecke et al., 2023). The authors proposed a mentorship program process with experts and managers to improve integration.

Trapani et al. (2024) performed a systematic review of international literature evaluating strategies for capacity building and scaling up of the oncology care workforce. They concluded that improving and sustaining the oncology workforce is not merely an issue of increasing the number of oncology professionals but must also include capacity and infrastructure to support the workforce and patients.

Role Integrity

The recognition, inclusion, evolution, and standardization of oncology navigation over the past decades should be celebrated. As advocacy for the role continues, healthcare professionals must take care not to dilute or diffuse the value of the role by trying to include it in more places. In an effort toward expanding the reach of navigation, it would be easy for the healthcare system to label more and more people and roles as *navigators* until the term begins to lose its meaning. Clinical nurse navigators should adhere to ONS's 2021 position statement, most notably the position that ONNs should be certified oncology nurses through ONCC (ONS, 2021).

Technology-Driven Navigation

Rapid advancements in technology, such as artificial intelligence (AI), telehealth, and digital health platforms, can improve healthcare system efficiency and enhance patient outcomes and access to care (Donmez et al., 2024). However, technology also poses potential threats, such as inadequate application (app) training and the loss of human connection when technology solutions are used as substitutes. ONNs must know the benefits and risks of incorporating these solutions into their nursing practice.

Telehealth may be beneficial in reducing disparities in rural cancer outcomes; however, many rural residents do not have technology available because of geographic barriers. Telehealth platforms, including videoconferencing and mobile apps, have been used by ONNs to connect patients living in rural areas with resources and to consolidate appointments when they must travel (Morris, 2021). Mobile apps are being developed and adapted to help patients report and monitor symptoms, receive reminders, and access educational resources (Rowett & Christensen, 2020). For example, in 2023, ACS launched a patient- and caregiver-facing app that navigators can use to provide digital navigation. It is available in English and Spanish (with additional languages forthcoming) and downloadable from the iOS and Android app stores (ACS, n.d.-a).

The widespread availability of AI, such as OpenAI, presents opportunities. Driven by machine learning's natural language processing, AI technologies have significantly but indirectly affected patients. For example, clinician-facing technologies have been incorporated into daily practice, including machine-learning instruments that identify disease patterns and forecast treatment results (Kelkar et al., 2024).

A relatively new field with enormous therapeutic potential but limited safety measures is patient-facing AI (PF-AI) apps that directly interact with patients. Although PF-AI can address patient questions, simplify educational assets, and provide resources, overreliance on this technology could compromise patient dignity and the quality of therapeutic interactions and lead to impersonal care (Kelkar et al., 2024). Research exploring nursing professionals' perspectives on the future of apps demonstrates nurses' excitement for this technology; however, it also highlights the significance of maintaining ethical standards and preserving the human element in patient care (Rony et al., 2024). A challenge for current and future ONNs will be leveraging PF-AI to enhance practice without compromising the personal touch that is the essence of nursing and patient care.

Summary

In the context of an increasingly complex U.S. healthcare system, the ONN role has stayed true to Freeman's goals and purpose while deepening, broadening, and evolving its ability to reduce barriers to timely diagnosis, treatment, and follow-up in the management of cancer. Many common barriers to care identified in the 1990s remain relevant, but further identification and understanding of them have grown amidst an ever-changing healthcare environment. Beneficial outcomes linked to navigation in cancer care settings are identified across various phases of the continuum, from screening and diagnosis to treatment, survivorship, end-of-life care, and patient and family satisfaction. Improved outcomes are linked to navigation services across populations often associated with poorer outcomes, such as racial and ethnic minorities, low-income individuals, rural residents, those with limited English proficiency, and pediatric, adolescent, young adult, and older adult populations. In a rapidly evolving healthcare landscape, implementing patient navigation programs has emerged as a pivotal strategy to enhance patient care, improve health outcomes, and increase healthcare system efficiency.

References

Academy of Oncology Nurse and Patient Navigators Foundation for Learning. (n.d.). *Certification: Become a certified oncology navigator through AONN+ Foundation for Learning.* https://aonnffl.org

American Cancer Society. (n.d.-a). *ACS CARES™.* https://www.cancer.org/support-programs-and-services/acs-cares.html

American Cancer Society. (n.d.-b). *Global patient support.* https://www.cancer.org/about-us/our-global-health-work/cancer-care-patient-support.html#:~:text=Starting%20in%202016%2C%20ACS%20began,other%20parts%20of%20the%20world

American Cancer Society. (n.d.-c). *Leadership in oncology navigation.* https://www.cancer.org/health-care-professionals/resources-for-professionals/patient-navigator-training.html

American Cancer Society Cancer Action Network. (2023, November 2). *New Medicare reimbursement strategy for patient navigation services will better serve patients with cancer and other serious illnesses* [Press release]. https://www.fightcancer.org/releases/new-medicare-reimbursement-strategy-patient-navigation-services-will-better-serve-patients

American Cancer Society Cancer Action Network. (2024, March 8). *Biden Cancer Moonshot announced expanded coverage for patient navigation in private health plans* [Press release]. https://www.fightcancer.org/releases/biden-cancer-moonshot-announces-expanded-coverage-patient-navigation-private-health-plans-0

American College of Surgeons. (2024). *Optimal resources for cancer care: 2020 standards.* https://www.facs.org/quality-programs/cancer-programs/commission-on-cancer/standards-and-resources/2020

Association of Cancer Care Centers. (2023, October 12). *Highlights from the President's Cancer Panel: Building a strong legacy.* ACCCBuzz Blog. https://www.accc-cancer.org/acccbuzz/blog-post-template/accc-buzz/2023/10/12/highlights-from-the-president-s-cancer-panel-building-on-a-strong-legacy

Baileys, K., McMullen, L., Lubejko, B., Christensen, D., Haylock, P.J., Rose, T., ... Srdanovic, D. (2018). Nurse navigator core competencies: An update to reflect the evolution of the role. *Clinical Journal of Oncology Nursing, 22*(3), 272–281. https://doi.org/10.1188/18.CJON.272-281

Bray, F., Laversanne, M., Sung, H., Ferlay, J., Siegel, R.L., Soerjomataram, I., & Jemal, A. (2024). Global cancer statistics 2022: GLOBOCAN estimates of incidence and mortality worldwide for 36 cancers in 185 countries. *CA: A Cancer Journal for Clinicians, 74*(3), 229–263. https://doi.org/10.3322/caac.21834

Brown, C.G., Cantril, C., McMullen, L., Barkley, D.L., Dietz, M., Murphy, C.M., & Fabrey, L.J. (2012). Oncology nurse navigator role delineation study. *Clinical Journal of Oncology Nursing, 16*(6), 581–585. https://doi.org/10.1188/12.CJON.581-585

Budde, H., Williams, G.A., Scarpetti, G., Kroezen, M., & Maier, C.B. (2022). *What are patient navigators and how can they improve integration of care* [Policy brief]. World Health Organization. European Observatory on Health Systems and Policies. https://www.ncbi.nlm.nih.gov/books/NBK577640

Centers for Disease Control and Prevention. (2024). *Patient navigation*. https://www.cdc.gov/cancer/php/interventions/patient-navigation.html

Centers for Medicare and Medicaid Services. (n.d.). *Principal illness navigation services*. https://www.medicare.gov/coverage/principal-illness-navigation-services

Centers for Medicare and Medicaid Services. (2024). *Health equity services in the 2024 physician fee schedule final rule*. https://www.cms.gov/files/document/mln9201074-health-equity-services-2024-physician-fee-schedule-final-rule.pdf-0

Chan, R.J., Milch, V.E., Crawford-Williams, F., Agbejule, O.A., Joseph, R., Johal, J., ... Hart, N.H. (2023). Patient navigation across the cancer care continuum: An overview of systematic reviews and emerging literature. *CA: A Cancer Journal for Clinicians, 73*(6), 565–589. https://doi.org/10.3322/caac.21788

Chen, M., Wu, V.S., Falk, D., Cheatham, C., Cullen, J., & Hoehn, R. (2024). Patient navigation in cancer treatment: A systematic review. *Current Oncology Reports, 26*(5), 504–537. https://link.springer.com/article/10.1007/s11912-024-01514-9

Chen, S., Cao, Z., Prettner, K., Kuhn, M., Yang, J., Jiao, L., ... Wang, C. (2023). Estimates and projections of the global economic cost of 29 cancers in 204 countries and territories from 2020 to 2050. *JAMA Oncology, 9*(4), 465–472. http://doi.org/10.1001/jamaoncol.2022.7826

Donmez, E., Kilic, B., Dulger, Z., & Ozdas, T. (2024). Innovative cancer follow-up with telehealth: A new method for oncology nurses. *Seminars in Oncology Nursing, 40*(3), 151649. https://doi.org/10.1016/j.soncn.2024.151649

Fischer-Cartlidge, E., & Graham, E.L. (2024). What the new CMS reimbursement for principal illness navigation means for oncology nurses. *ONS Voice*. https://www.ons.org/publications-research/voice/advocacy/what-new-cms-reimbursement-principal-illness-navigation-means

Fleary, S.A., & Ettienne, R. (2019). Social disparities in health literacy in the United States. *Health Literacy Research and Practice, 3*, e47–e52. https://doi.org/10.3928/24748307-20190131-01

Franklin, E.F., Dean, M.S., Johnston, D.M., Nevidjon, B.M., Burke, S.L., & Simms Booth, L.M. (2022). Solidifying roles, responsibilities, and the process of navigation across the continuum of cancer care: The Professional Oncology Navigation Task Force. *Cancer, 128*(S13), 2669–2672. https://doi.org/10.1002/cncr.34095

Freeman, H.P. (2004). A model patient navigation program: Breaking down barriers to ensure that all individuals with cancer receive timely diagnosis and treatment. *Oncology Issues, 19*(5), 44–46. https://doi.org/10.1080/10463356.2004.11884227

Freeman, H.P. (2012). The origin, evolution, and principles of patient navigation. *Cancer Epidemiology, Biomarkers and Prevention, 21*(10), 1614–1617. https://web.archive.org/web/20190223094008id_/http://pdfs.semanticscholar.org/4558/da236acd1aa80fe7edbe2a150c87072427ab.pdf

Freeman, H.P., & Reuben, S.H. (2001). *Voices of a broken system: Real people, real problems*. President's Cancer Panel Report of the Chairman: 2000–2001. https://deainfo.nci.nih.gov/advisory/pcp/archive/pcp00-01rpt/pcpvideo/voices_files/pdffiles/pcpbook.pdf

Freeman, H.P., & Rodriguez, R.L. (2011). History and principles of patient navigation. *Cancer, 117*(Suppl. 15), 3537–3540. https://doi.org/10.1002/cncr.26262

Green, L.M. (2012, October 8). *Opportunity knocks: New ACoS standard requires navigation process in place by 2015* [Conference]. OncLive. https://www.onclive.com/view/opportunity-knocks-new-acs-standard-requires-navigation-process-in-place-by-2015

Iheduru-Anderson, K.C., & Wahi, M.M. (2022). Race and racism discourse in U.S. nursing: Challenging the silence. *Online Journal of Issues in Nursing, 27*, 1. https://doi.org/10.3912/ojin.vol27no01man01

Kashima, K., Phillips, S., Harvey, A., Van Kirk Villalobos, A., & Pratt-Chapman, M. (2018). Efficacy of the competency-based oncology patient navigator training. *Journal of Oncology Navigation and Survivorship, 9*(12), 519–524. https://pmc.ncbi.nlm.nih.gov/articles/PMC6879008

Kelkar, A.H., Hantel, A., Koranteng, E., Cutler, C.S., Hammer, M.J., & Abel, G.A. (2024). Digital health to patient-facing artificial intelligence: Ethical implications and threats to dignity for patients with cancer. *JCO Oncology Practice, 20*(3), 314–317. https://doi.org/10.1200/OP.23.00412

Knudsen, K.E., Wiatrek, D.E., Greenwald, J., McComb, K., & Sharpe, K. (2022). The American Cancer Society and patient navigation: Past and future perspectives. *Cancer, 128*(Suppl. 13), 2673–2677. https://doi.org/10.1002/cncr.34206

Lamb, G., & Newhouse, R. (2018). *Care coordination: A blueprint for action for RNs*. American Nurses Association. https://www.nursingworld.org/nurses-books/care-coordination-blueprint-for-action-for-rns/?sr sltid=AfmBOopTQXTGlIX8quzgecPIy-npXbHBSydBvyM8MEzr7svAdogT-eo7

Levitt, L., & Altman, D. (2023). Complexity in the US health care system is the enemy of access and affordability. *JAMA Health Forum, 4*(10), e234430. https://doi.org/10.1001/jamahealthforum.2023.4430

Lubejko, B.G., Bellfield, S., Kahn, E., Lee, C., Peterson, N., Rose, T., ... McCorkle, M. (2017). Oncology nurse navigation. *Clinical Journal of Oncology Nursing, 21*(1), 43–50. https://doi.org/10.1188/17.CJON.43 -50

McDonald, K.M., Sundaram, V., Bravata, D.M., Lewis, R., Lin, N., Kraft, S.A., ... Owens, D.K. (2007). Definitions of care coordination and related terms. In *Closing the quality gap: A critical analysis of quality improvement strategies* (Vol. 7: Care coordination). Agency for Healthcare Research and Quality. https://www.ncbi.nlm.nih.gov/books/NBK44015

Morris, B. (2021). *A multilevel mixed methods examination of treatment nonadherence among rural cancer survivors* [Doctoral dissertation, Virginia Commonwealth University] https://doi.org/10.25829 /2THB-ET72

Morris, B., Kamal, A., Franklin, E., Calhoun, E., Balistreri, J., & Sivendran, S. (2024). Development of a professional oncology navigation training and credentialing program: ACS Leadership in Oncology Navigation (ACS LION) [Meeting abstract]. *Journal of Clinical Oncology, 42*(16, Suppl.), 9045. https://doi.org/10.1200/JCO.2024.42.16 suppl.90

National Cancer Institute. (2006). *Patient navigator research program projects* [Brochure]. https://www .cancer.gov/pnrp-brochure.pdf

National Cancer Institute. (2023). *History of the Cancer Moonshot*. https://www.cancer.gov/research/key-initiatives/moonshot-cancer-initiative/history

National Cancer Navigation Roundtable. (n.d.). History of patient navigation. *American Cancer Society*. https://navigationroundtable.org/patient-navigation/history-of-patient-navigation/

Nora, A.E., McDonald, M.E., Syrop, C.H., & Haugsdal, M.L. (2021). Upstream oncology: Identifying social determinants of health in a gynecologic oncology population. *Proceedings in Obstetrics and Gynecology, 10*(2), 1–13. https://doi.org/10.17077/2154-4751.1507

Oncology Nursing Society. (2013). *Oncology Nursing Society oncology nurse navigator core competencies*. https://www.georgiacancerinfo.org/articleImages/articlePDF_335.pdf

Oncology Nursing Society. (2017). *2017 oncology nurse navigator core competencies*. https://www.ons.org /sites/default/files/2017-05/2017_Oncology_Nurse_Navigator_Competencies.pdf

Oncology Nursing Society. (2021). *Role of the oncology nurse navigator throughout the cancer trajectory* [Position statement]. https://www.ons.org/make-difference/advocacy-and-policy/position-statements/ONN

Oncology Nursing Society & Oncology Nursing Certification Corporation. (2024). *Oncology nurse navigator competencies*. https://www.ons.org/oncology-nurse-navigator-competencies

President's Cancer Panel. (2023). *What is the National Cancer Program?* National Institutes of Health. https://prescancerpanel.cancer.gov/about/blogs/national-cancer-program/

President's Cancer Panel. (2024a). *Developing and retaining a robust and diverse cancer workforce: Challenges and opportunities across the National Cancer Program*. National Institutes of Health. https:// prescancerpanel-prod.cancer.gov/ncp/meetings/2024-09-12

President's Cancer Panel. (2024b). *Reducing cancer care inequities: Leveraging technology to enhance patient navigation*. National Institutes of Health. https://prescancerpanel.cancer.gov/reports/2023/inequities

Rony, M.K.K., Kayesh, I., Das Bala, S., Akter, F., & Parvin, M.R. (2024). Artificial intelligence in future nursing care: Exploring perspectives of nursing professionals—A descriptive qualitative study. *Heliyon, 10*(4), e25718. https://doi.org/10.1016/j.heliyon.2024.e25718

Rowett, K.E., & Christensen, D. (2020). Oncology nurse navigation expansion of the navigator role through telehealth. *Clinical Journal of Oncology Nursing, 24*(3), 24–31. https://doi.org/10.1188/20.CJON.S1.24-31

Shulman, L.N., Sheldon, L.K., & Benz, E.J. (2020). The future of cancer care in the United States—overcoming workforce capacity limitations. *JAMA Oncology, 6*(3), 327–328. http://doi.org/10.1001/jamaoncol.2019.5358

Siegel, R.L., Giaquinto, A.N., & Jemal, A. (2024). Cancer statistics, 2024. *CA: A Cancer Journal for Clinicians, 74*(1), 12–49. https://doi.org/10.3322/caac.21820

Stowell, M., Spiers, G.F., Kunonga, P., Beyer, F., Richmond, C., Craig, D., & Hanratty, B. (2024). Caring for older people as a social determinant of health: findings from a scoping review of observational studies. *Journal of Long-Term Care, 2024*, 28–41. http://doi.org/10.31389/jltc.207

Strusowski, T., Johnston, D., & Nevidjon, B. (2024). AONN+ navigation metrics that support the oncology navigation standards of professional practice. *Seminars in Oncology Nursing, 40*(2), 151589. https://doi.org/10.1016/j.soncn.2024.151589

Takvorian, S.U., Balogh, E., Nass, S., Valentin, V.L., Hoffman-Hogg, L., Oyer, R.A., ... Shulman, L.N. (2020). Developing and sustaining an effective and resilient oncology careforce: Opportunities for action. *Journal of the National Cancer Institute, 112*(7), 663–670. https://doi.org/10.1093/jnci/djz239

Trapani, D., Murthy, S.S., Hammad, N., Casolino, R., Moreira, D.C., Roitberg, F., ... Ilbawi, A.M. (2024). Policy strategies for capacity building and scale up of the workforce for comprehensive cancer care: A systematic review. *ESMO Open, 9*(4), 102946. https://doi.org/10.1016/j.esmoop.2024.102946

Van Hecke, A., Vlerick, I., Akhayad, S., Daem, M., Decoene, E., & Kinnaer, L.-M. (2023). Dynamics and processes influencing role integration of advanced practice nurses and nurse navigators in oncology teams. *European Journal of Oncology Nursing, 62*, 102257. https://doi.org/10.1016/j.ejon.2022.102257

Vargas, R.B., Ryan, G.W., Jackson, C.A., Rodriguez, R., & Freeman, H.P. (2008). Characteristics of the original patient navigation programs to reduce disparities in the diagnosis and treatment of breast cancer. *Cancer, 113*(2), 426–433. https://doi.org/10.1002/cncr.23547

Wakefield, M.K., Williams, D.R., Le Menestrel, S., & Flaubert, J.L. (Eds.). (2021). *The future of nursing 2020–2030: Charting a path to achieve health equity*. National Academy of Medicine. https://doi.org/10.17226/25982

Wells, K.J., Wightman, P., Cobian Aguilar, R., Dwyer, A.J., Garcia-Alcaraz, C., Saavedra Ferrer, E.L., ... Calhoun, E. (2022). Comparing clinical and nonclinical cancer patient navigators: A national study in the United States. *Cancer, 128*(Suppl. 13), 2601–2609. https://doi.org/10.1002/cncr.33880

Wooley, J., & Peters, G. (n.d.). William J. Clinton: Digest of other White House announcements. *The American Presidency Project*. https://www.presidency.ucsb.edu/documents/digest-other-white-house-announcements-136

World Health Organization. (2024, February 1). *Global cancer burden growing, amidst mounting need for services*. https://www.who.int/news/item/01-02-2024-global-cancer-burden-growing--amidst-mounting-need-for-services

Yates, P., Charalambous, A., Fennimore, L., So, W.K.W., Suh, E.E., Woodford, E., & Young, A. (2020). Cancer nursing's potential to reduce the growing burden of cancer across the world. *Oncology Nursing Forum, 47*(6), 625–627. https://doi.org/10.1188/20.ONF.625-627

CHAPTER 2

Access to Care

Kathleen Wiley, MSN, RN, AOCNS®

> **KEY TOPICS**
> barriers to care, access, social determinants of health

Overview

The healthcare system is especially complex for patients with cancer and their caregivers, often requiring them to navigate multiple appointments, procedures, tests, care settings, providers, and specialists—all for the management of a disease that relies on very timely care. Barriers can arise at all points along the cancer trajectory, from screening and diagnosis to survivorship. One of the primary purposes of navigation is to identify and remove these barriers (Chan et al., 2023; Chen et al., 2024; Freund et al., 2014). Ensuring patients with cancer achieve and maintain access to care is critically important to improve outcomes, cost of care, and quality of life and to close the gap in health disparities. Oncology nurse navigators (ONNs) are uniquely positioned to provide consistent support to patients and caregivers throughout the cancer continuum. ONNs assess potential barriers and address them before access to care is negatively affected. A significant challenge for ONNs is that barriers to care vary from patient to patient and are greatly influenced by social determinants of health, diagnoses, goals of care, and phases of treatment within the cancer care continuum (Korn et al., 2022). Research suggests that as navigators employ interventions tailored to the specific needs of patients and their caregivers, time from diagnosis to initiation of treatment and statistically significant reductions in treatment delays occur (Chan et al., 2023; Chen et al., 2024; Freund et al., 2014). ONNs are charged with carefully assessing the needs of patients and their caregivers throughout the cancer continuum and working with patients, families, and the healthcare team to optimize outcomes.

This chapter will review common barriers to care through the lens of social determinants of health. It will also cover individual experiences with these barriers and how they may manifest within the healthcare system. Awareness of these issues will help ONNs ask appropriate questions of patients, identify patients at high risk for barriers, and individualize approaches to care.

Barriers to Care

Establishing and maintaining access to healthcare providers, services, and treatments is necessary to achieve optimal patient outcomes. As an essential member of the healthcare team, ONNs assess for barriers to care that may lead to poor patient outcomes, exacerbate disparities, and put a strain on the healthcare system. Left unmanaged, barriers to quality care affect access to cancer screening, lead to a later diagnosis, and potentially limit one's ability to complete prescribed treatment regimens (Tucker-Seeley et al., 2024). Navigators have the unique challenge of identifying and mitigating barriers to care throughout the care continuum.

The National Academies of Sciences, Engineering, and Medicine (2019) outlined a multipronged approach to mitigating barriers to access that included awareness, adjustment, assistance, alignment, and advocacy (see Table 2-1). Using this framework, ONNs can approach barriers through these tenets to develop a patient-centered, individualized plan to ensure access to care. The framework aptly demonstrates that, although multiple patients may experience the same barrier, no two patients experience them in the same way. The underlying cause and resulting mitigation strategies will differ from patient to patient. Using a framework that considers each barrier to accessing care through the lens of social determinants of health and individualized strategies optimizes the practice of nurse navigators and improves patient care.

Transportation

A reliable means of transportation to care services is critical for patients to receive timely cancer care. Transportation insecurity prevents access to care in situations in

TABLE 2-1   5 A's Framework for Access to Care

Framework Tenet	Example in Practice
Awareness—identifying the risks of limited access to care	Screening for insurance status, providing access to transportation and high-speed internet, assessing health literacy
Adjustment—alteration of care to accommodate barriers to care	Moving visits to remote when possible (in the setting of transportation barriers)
Assistance—activities that connect patients with resources	Providing transportation vouchers or medical translators
Alignment—activities that connect communities with resources	Creating partnerships with healthcare systems and community programs (e.g., food assistance programs)
Advocacy—efforts by health systems to influence accessibility to community resources	Advocating for lower medical costs or improved transportation infrastructure

Note. Based on National Academies of Sciences, Engineering, and Medicine, 2019.

which patients lack the material, economic, or social resources necessary to secure transportation to and from healthcare-related appointments (Graboyes et al., 2022). An estimated 3.6 million people in the United States do not obtain medical care because of transportation insecurity (Wolfe et al., 2020). In a study evaluating the impact of navigation services on lung cancer screening, lack of transportation or challenges in paying for transportation and parking costs were commonly cited as barriers to accessing screening services (Craddock Lee et al., 2023). Transportation challenges disproportionately affect individuals with low socioeconomic status, those with chronic conditions, the uninsured and underinsured, people of color, the less educated, and older patients (Wolfe et al., 2020). Common transportation barriers may include but are not limited to long distances and lengthy travel times to reach needed services, transportation costs, lack of vehicle access, or inadequate infrastructure (Hallgren et al., 2023; Wolfe et al., 2020). Lack of vehicle access is especially problematic when patients are traveling from a rural area for care, as public transportation is less available in those areas. Preventive care and healthcare services also are less available. As such, those residing in a rural area have significantly decreased cancer prevention services, more diagnoses at an advanced stage, and higher mortality rates than their urban counterparts. Furthermore, patients residing in rural areas are less likely to enroll in clinical trials or maintain survivorship care (Wercholuk et al., 2022).

Transportation barriers leave patients with limited options other than missed or postponed appointments with providers and scheduled treatments. Implications of missed appointments and treatments jeopardize care outcomes and put an economic strain on the cost of cancer care for individual and global healthcare systems (Graboyes et al., 2022). When transportation barriers are identified, patients should be offered assistance through transportation vouchers or the use of telehealth when available and appropriate.

High-Speed Internet

Advances in web-based technologies have transformed the way health care is delivered. In the cancer setting, patients use high-speed internet to access patient portals, review laboratory and radiology results, send direct messages to providers, schedule appointments, request refills, attend telehealth appointments, and research medical information. Additionally, the use of electronic patient-reported outcomes and other digital healthcare tools streamlines communication with providers, enhances patient autonomy and involvement with care, optimizes symptom management and early warning sign recognition, and allows for home-based care (Pritchett et al., 2023). However, the potential benefits of telehealth and digital health tools cannot be realized if patients encounter barriers to obtaining high-speed internet. Up to one-quarter of Americans have limited digital access or lack access entirely (Early & Hernandez, 2021). A research study determining the extent of access issues demonstrated that up to 41.4% of Medicare beneficiaries lacked a computer with a high-speed internet connection, and 40.9% lacked a smartphone with wireless functionality. This barrier is known as the *digital divide* and disproportionately affects rural and tribal areas and those with an annual income of less than $30,000 (Pritchett et al., 2023). The COVID-19 pandemic amplified the impact of the lack of high-speed internet and helped to prioritize addressing this issue as a social determinant of health.

Healthy People 2030 is a federal public health priority outlining initiatives to improve individual, organizational, and community health. One initiative is to increase the number of individuals who can view, send, and download electronic health records and who report positive engagement with their electronic health records (Early & Hernandez, 2021).

As a means of promoting clinical trial enrollment and participation, researchers are exploring the effects of using digital technologies to enroll and communicate with research participants (Kasahara et al., 2024). Should these strategies prove ideal for clinical trial enrollment, ONNs should be prepared to advocate on behalf of patients with limited access to high-speed internet. Patients with a lack of reliable high-speed internet may find themselves at additional disadvantages should these strategies prove ideal for clinical trial enrollment.

When developing plans for how providers will share results and update treatment plans and how patients will communicate with the healthcare team, ONNs should assess patients' digital capabilities and digital literacy to determine if accommodations are needed.

Insurance Status

Access to adequate health insurance minimizes unexpected and high medical costs for patients with cancer. It is well documented that inadequate or lack of medical insurance is one of the most significant barriers to care and ultimately can lead to negative impacts on health. Research suggests that lack of medical coverage is associated with poor cancer care outcomes, including diagnosis at later stages. Those without insurance are also less likely to receive evidence-based care throughout the continuum, including a lack of preventive services. Gaps in coverage for even one month can delay patients seeking care (Yabroff et al., 2020; Zhao et al., 2020). Yabroff et al. (2020) saw a correlation between gaps in medical coverage and a decreased likelihood of receiving various preventive services, including mammograms, Pap testing, and human papillomavirus vaccination.

Cancer care costs and the healthcare insurance infrastructure are complex and challenging for most consumers to understand. The Patient Protection and Affordable Care Act of 2010 transformed healthcare coverage in the United States and increased the number of citizens with healthcare coverage. The Medicaid Expansion arm of the act improved access to the most vulnerable and disadvantaged populations (Zhao et al., 2020). However, cancer care remains one of the most expensive drivers of healthcare costs, and patients require careful navigation to understand coverage options and cost-sharing responsibilities. ONNs should routinely assess for barriers to health insurance coverage, especially for younger patients, people of color, and those who have a lower socioeconomic status, as these groups are most likely to be uninsured in the United States (Zhao et al., 2020). Those who are uninsured or underinsured are less likely to report complications, seek medical care, and may have complications securing prescription therapies.

Primary Language

Language barriers between healthcare professionals and patients with cancer present an additional level of complexity. Individuals whose primary language is the same as their healthcare providers are shown to have a stronger understanding of their care plan, an ability to engage and navigate the healthcare system, and are more likely to communicate concerns with the healthcare team. Furthermore, therapeutic relationships with providers are more organically formed (Pandey et al., 2021). A language barrier has the potential to influence care negatively and may result in an inability to access needed cancer care services. Historically, on-site interpreters, trained ad hoc hospital personnel, and language line or video interpretation have been used in the healthcare setting to counteract this barrier. It is paramount to ensure that caregivers are not used as medical translators, as information may not be translated as intended, or patients may not want a family member to have their medical information (Pandey et al., 2021).

Best Practices for the Oncology Nurse Navigator

Barriers that affect access to care are unique to each patient with cancer. The primary goal of navigation is to identify potential and actual barriers to care throughout the care trajectory as patient circumstances change. As patients with cancer move through different phases of care, ONNs ensure a seamless transition between each phase by recognizing common barriers that can arise in their specific specialty area and geographic location. Doing so will allow ONNs to anticipate needs and potential barriers before access to care is negatively influenced. Issues are unique to each patient, and despite two patients being prescribed the same treatment plan, their experience and ease of adhering to the plan will not be mirrored. ONNs need to remember that each patient is an individual with unique needs.

In 2024, the Oncology Nursing Society and the Oncology Nursing Certification Corporation released the updated *Oncology Nurse Navigator Competencies* as the framework for ONNs to guide patients through their unique cancer journeys. These competencies underscore the importance of ONNs in identifying and addressing barriers to care and establishing a trusting relationship between patients and their healthcare team. Barriers to care will evolve throughout the care trajectory and may depend on the phase of treatment and goals of care. For example, a patient diagnosed with breast cancer who lives in a rural area may not initially experience a transportation barrier for intermittent consultations and postoperative visits. However, if daily radiation therapy is part of their treatment plan, a transportation barrier may develop because of the distance traveled and high fuel costs. By assessing potential barriers to care initially and during each transition of care, ONNs can ensure that the plan to address barriers evolves with the circumstances.

Summary

Barriers negatively affecting access to care are often systemically rooted. ONNs and their associated organizations have the opportunity to advocate for the needed policy changes to address deeply rooted barriers that exacerbate disparities in care. Healthcare clinicians cannot assume unlimited access to resources and should work with local and federal policymakers to remove barriers to cancer care throughout the continuum. Using a framework to assess for barriers, account for social determinants of health, and individualize interventions for patients, ONNs have the unique ability to advocate for patients and improve outcomes.

References

Chan, R.J., Milch, V.E., Crawford-Williams, F., Agbejule, O.A., Joseph, R., Johal, J., ... Hart, N.H. (2023). Patient navigation across the cancer care continuum: An overview of systematic reviews and emerging literature. *CA: A Cancer Journal for Clinicians, 73*(6), 565–589. https://doi.org/10.3322/caac.21788

Chen, M., Wu, V.S., Falk, D., Cheatham, C., Cullen, J., & Hoehn, R. (2024). Patient navigation in cancer treatment: A systematic review. *Current Oncology Reports, 26*(5), 504–537. https://doi.org/10.1007/s11912-024-01514-9

Craddock Lee, S.J., Lee, J., Zhu, H., Chen, P.M., Wahid, U., Hamann, H.A., ... Gerber, D.E. (2023). Assessing barriers and facilitators to lung cancer screening: Initial findings from a patient navigation intervention. *Population Health Management, 26*(3), 177–184. https://doi.org/10.1089/pop.2023.0053

Early, J., & Hernandez, A. (2021). Digital disenfranchisement and COVID-19: broadband internet access as a social determinant of health. *Health Promotion Practice, 22*(5), 605–610. https://doi.org/10.1177/15248399211014490

Freund, K.M., Battaglia, T.A., Calhoun, E., Darnell, J.S., Dudley, D.J., Fiscella, K., ... Paskett, E.D. (2014). Impact of patient navigation on timely cancer care: The Patient Navigation Research Program. *Journal of the National Cancer Institute, 106*(6), 1–9. https://doi.org/10.1093/jnci/dju115

Graboyes, E.M., Chaiyachati, K.H., Sisto Gall, J., Johnson, W., Krishnan, J.A., McManus, S.S., ... Yabroff, K.R. (2022). Addressing transportation insecurity among patients with cancer. *Journal of the National Cancer Institute, 114*(12), 1593–1600. https://doi.org/10.1093/jnci/djac134

Hallgren, E., Yeary, K.H.K., DelNero, P., Johnson-Wells, B., Purvis, R.S., Moore, R., ... McElfish, P.A. (2023). Barriers, facilitators, and priority needs related to cancer prevention, control, and research in rural, persistent poverty areas. *Cancer Causes and Control, 34*(12), 1145–1155. https://doi.org/10.1007/s10552-023-01756-1

Kasahara, A., Mitchell, J., Yang, J., Cuomo, R.E., McMann, T.J., & Mackey, T.K. (2024). Digital technologies used in clinical trial recruitment and enrollment including application to trial diversity and inclusion: A systematic review. *Digital Health, 10*, 20552076241242390. https://doi.org/10.1177/20552076241242390

Korn, A.R., Walsh-Bailey, C., Pilar, M., Sandler, B., Bhattacharjee, P., Moore, W.T., ... Oh, A.Y. (2022). Social determinants of health and cancer screening implementation and outcomes in the USA: A systematic review protocol. *Systematic Reviews, 11*(1), 117. https://doi.org/10.1186/s13643-022-01995-4

National Academies of Sciences, Engineering, and Medicine. (2019). Five health care sector activities to better integrate social care. In *Integrating social care into the delivery of health care: Moving upstream to improve the nation's health* (pp. 33–58). National Academies Press. https://www.ncbi.nlm.nih.gov/books/NBK552593

Oncology Nursing Society & Oncology Nursing Certification Corporation. (2024). *Oncology nurse navigator competencies*. https://www.ons.org/oncology-nurse-navigator-competencies

Pandey, M., Maina, R.G., Amoyaw, J., Li, Y., Kamrul, R., Michaels, C.R., & Maroof, R. (2021). Impacts of English language proficiency on healthcare access, use, and outcomes among immigrants: A qualitative study. *BMC Health Services Research, 21*, 741. https://doi.org/10.1186/s12913-021-06750-4

Pritchett, J.C., Patt, D., Thanarajasingam, G., Schuster, A., & Snyder, C. (2023). Patient-reported outcomes, digital health, and the quest to improve health equity. *American Society of Clinical Oncology Educational Book, 43*, e390678. https://doi.org/10.1200/edbk_390678

Tucker-Seeley, R., Abu-Khalaf, M., Bona, K., Shastri, S., Johnson, W., Phillips, J., ... Hinyard, L. (2024). Social determinants of health and cancer care: An ASCO policy statement. *JCO Oncology Practice, 20*(5), 621–630. https://doi.org/10.1200/op.23.00810

Wercholuk, A.N., Parikh, A.A., & Snyder, R.A. (2022). The road less traveled: Transportation barriers to cancer care delivery in the rural patient population. *JCO Oncology Practice, 18*(9), 652–662. https://doi.org/10.1200/op.22.00122

Wolfe, M.K., McDonald, N.C., & Holme, G.M. (2020). Transportation barriers to health care in the United States: Findings from the National Interview Survey, 1997–2017. *American Journal of Public Health, 110*(6), 815822. https://doi.org/https://doi.org/10.2105/AJPH.2020.305579.

Yabroff, K.R., Reeder-Hayes, K., Zhao, J., Halpern, M.T., Lopez, A.M., Bernal-Mizrachi, L., ... Patel, M. (2020). Health insurance coverage disruptions and cancer care and outcomes: Systematic review of published research. *Journal of the National Cancer Institute, 112*(7), 671–687. https://doi.org/10.1093/jnci/djaa048

Zhao, J., Mao, Z., Fedewa, S.A., Nogueira, L., Yabroff, K.R., Jemal, A., & Han, X. (2020). The Affordable Care Act and access to care across the cancer control continuum: A review at 10 years. *CA: A Cancer Journal for Clinicians, 70*(3), 165–181. https://doi.org/10.3322/caac.21604

SECTION II
Steps for Implementing, Growing, and Sustaining Oncology Navigation

Chapter 3. Understanding the Business of Navigation
Chapter 4. Oncology Nurse Navigator Role and Competencies
Chapter 5. Models of Oncology Navigation
Chapter 6. Determining Community and Program Needs
Chapter 7. Measuring Nurse-Led Patient Outcomes
Chapter 8. Interventions Addressing Financial Toxicity

CHAPTER 3

Understanding the Business of Navigation

Jacqueline Miller, MSN, RN, OCN®

> **KEY TOPICS**
> business plan, financial plan, sustainability, champions

Overview

Historically, oncology navigation programs have been funded by the operational budgets of healthcare systems or with support from philanthropy and grants. As part of the overhead cost, navigation program leaders are often responsible for supplying metrics, justifying costs, and, wherever possible, offering evidence of a return on investment. These data are critical for the sustainability and growth of all navigation programs.

Patient navigation programs and processes continue to proliferate, and a mounting body of evidence supports the value of navigation and oncology navigation as a nursing role. Navigation in oncology has demonstrated benefits for people at risk for or diagnosed with cancer, such as a shorter time to diagnosis and treatment, increased patient and caregiver knowledge, better adherence to care, and improved quality of life (Chan et al., 2023; Garfield et al., 2022). Institutional return on investment includes increases in patient retention and physician loyalty. Furthermore, decreases in emergency department and hospital visits have been associated with oncology navigation (Kline et al., 2019; Kokorelias et al., 2021). Patients report having increased overall satisfaction and their emotional needs met in institutions providing oncology navigation services (Chan et al., 2023; Kline et al., 2019; Yackzan et al., 2019).

This chapter will explore the business side of oncology navigation for new programs and programs seeking growth and sustainability.

Building a Navigation Program Step by Step

The major steps for building a navigation program mirror those of the nursing process. It begins with assessment and moves to identifying clear, measurable goals based on patient, community, and institutional needs. Next, it establishes a plan and puts it into motion. It finally evaluates, monitors, and reassesses the program at defined intervals.

Assessment: Patient, Community, and Institution

Why is a navigation program needed? When starting a new program, this question will be asked countless times. Team planners need to be prepared with an answer based on a reliable assessment tool. The American College of Surgeons Commission on Cancer *Standard 8.1: Addressing Barriers to Care* offers a list of resources to complete a cancer barrier analysis (American College of Surgeons, 2019). See Chapter 6 of the current publication for details on how to perform a community needs assessment. As identifying and addressing barriers to care are hallmarks of navigation, these resources are an excellent starting point to build a framework for the program.

Identification: Mission, Goals, Champions, and Metrics

Mission and Vision

A mission statement is a short statement defining the purpose of and who will receive a service. Defining the purpose, values, and goals of a program should be completed at its initiation. These serve as a guidepost so leaders and team members remain focused.

All aspects of a program should cascade down from the mission statement. A navigation program vision should be created with quick wins, longer-term goals, and identification of who will be involved, providing stakeholders and readers with the big picture. A vision should also be individualized and made meaningful for the specific organization. The vision for a navigation program in a small rural community hospital will be different than one in an extensive urban academic healthcare system. All team members can contribute to innovative programs. An organization's mission and vision can be cascaded into navigation statements. Engaging navigation champions in the mission, vision, and goal-setting process will significantly boost buy-in.

Goals for the Navigation Service

Before planning processes begin, program planners must fully understand their institution's motivators for implementing a navigation program. In a scoping review of 34 papers, Valaitis et al. (2017) found three major institutional motivators for establishing navigation programs: the need to improve the delivery of health and social services, the need to support and manage specific health needs or specific population needs, and the need to improve the quality of life and well-being of patients. From these findings, the authors suggested that providers working toward initiating patient navigation programs "consider explicitly identifying motivators for them so that benefits may be easily visible to adopters to support implementation" (Valaitis et al., 2017, p. 5).

Navigation program goals should cascade down from organizational and oncology service line goals to reflect uniformity. Goals should be identified early in program planning as a guidepost and referenced throughout development. SMART (specific, measurable, achievable, relevant, and time bound) goals will provide a foundational framework for developing a new program. Sample new navigation program goals may include decreasing the time from positive biopsy to first oncology consultation to five business days by the end of the calendar year or reducing the outmigration of new patients with cancer by 80% by the end of the calendar year.

Navigation Champion and Stakeholder Support

Clinical champions play a critical role in reducing implementation barriers, promoting program development, and establishing peer buy-in (Morena et al., 2022). Champions could be influential, knowledgeable, and respected oncology nurse leaders, physicians, administrators, members of the facility's board of directors, community advocates, and others who support the program. Champions often pave the initial pathway of integrating a new navigation program into existing workflows, as they have access to a network of team members (internal and external). Communication of champion support to this network creates an environment of acceptance and engagement. A formal announcement of champions is critical in starting a new navigation program.

Metrics for Oncology Nurse Navigation

The creators of an oncology navigation program need to decide which metrics they will use to measure its impact. Additionally, the mechanism to collect data will need to be decided. Larger programs may use reports generated from electronic health records, whereas smaller programs could collect data on spreadsheets. Collecting, analyzing, and reporting navigation metrics to champions, team members, and leadership will validate navigation services and build support. Refer to Chapter 7 for more detailed information on these metrics.

Planning: Roles, Operations, and Marketing

Job Descriptions

A business plan begins with the creation of job descriptions. The Oncology Nursing Society and Oncology Nursing Certification Corporation (2024) *Oncology Nurse Navigator Competencies* provide an excellent reference point for job descriptions. The competencies offer measurements and methods for 13 subtopics directly related to the nurse navigator role. Job descriptions for clinical navigators (e.g., oncology nurse navigators, licensed oncology social workers) and non-clinical navigators can be tailored to an institution's specific needs. Role delineation starts with organized job descriptions.

Organizational, Operational, and Financial Plan

The organizational plan provides a thorough view of the navigation team and detailed job descriptions of key team members, qualification profiles, recruitment plans, and organizational relationships. It also includes an organizational chart, showing the hierarchical structure of the program and defining the chain of command and lines of authority, reporting, and links to the healthcare system. External consultants or contractors are identified, and their functions and contributions are described. This section also may include a statement of the program's management philosophy, values, and culture.

The operational plan summarizes operating expenses, such as initial and projected capital expenses, salaries, annual expenses, insurance, communication technologies, building fees, office supplies, signage, and marketing materials. Small programs may create an operational plan on a single spreadsheet. More extensive programs will benefit from additional technology to generate reports and automate processes.

Most navigation services are not traditional revenue generators; the financial metrics presented in the business plan can reflect the potential for return on investment and other outcomes of navigation that have financial and business implications, such as public and private grants and other philanthropic contributions. The financial plan summarizes expenses, including professional and clerical support, technological needs, and other operating expenses. If program planners are requesting additional funding, they should outline funding requirements, clearly explaining their monetary needs over a stated time and intentions for using that funding (U.S. Small Business Administration, 2024). Additionally, the Centers for Medicare and Medicaid Services has approved reimbursement for navigation services. Chapter 7 discusses the nuances related to these billing codes.

Market Share and Competitor Analysis

A market share and competitor analysis outlines competition to the navigation program that currently exists in the facility's defined service area (usually identified by administration and marketing experts). It shows what is currently being offered to patients and users in a similar format and could affect the number of people likely to use the service. The analysis can also state how the program and services differ from those already operating in the area. Qualities of the market should be specifically highlighted—for example, populations known to experience barriers to access and care, patient groups, high-incidence cancers, distance to services and transportation issues, seasonal weather challenges, and age and gender demographics. Online searches for "market share and competitor analysis templates" will result in manual templates as well as automated services if this information is unavailable through the individual institution.

Marketing and Business Strategies

Program planners should collaborate with a facility's marketing experts to devise and produce effective program promotion strategies. They should consider the location of services offered and delivered, benefits for patients, and what might attract them to use the planned services. If such data are available, the projected numbers of patients that would be expected to be served by the facility in a given week,

month, or year should be highlighted. The marketing plan should reflect an understanding of the target population and the professional image of the program and its team members. Various media strategies need to be considered to reach target populations. Marketing strategies must also target at least five distinct key stakeholder groups:
- Oncology physicians in medical and therapeutic radiology, technologists, and office personnel
- Internal departmental professional service physicians, nurses, nutritionists, managers, and staff, such as radiology personnel, laboratory staff, homecare and palliative care providers, rehabilitation staff, library staff, institutional review board personnel, research coordinators, cancer registry personnel, technology and electronic health records experts, and medical records personnel and coordinators
- Primary care physicians in the service area or referral base, advanced practice nurses, physician assistants, and additional office staff in primary care settings
- Personnel in community-based programs, such as faith-based organizations and local American Cancer Society programs that provide resources and patient assistance
- Diverse populations representing patients using navigation services

Implementation: Timing and Deliverables

Development of this section, essentially a timetable, requires careful consideration of all aspects of the program as a whole and what it will take to be up and running. It details the *what*, *how*, and *when* of developing the new or expanded service. Other details include days and hours of operation, resources needed (e.g., equipment, staff, facilities, supplies, technology, finances), planning, and program and policy development. Program planners should consider who the stakeholders are and who needs to be actively involved in planning processes. They should estimate the time required for gathering stakeholders, reaching a consensus around planning, developing policy, addressing operational and organizational issues, and devising a realistic implementation schedule. Attention to common factors influencing the successful implementation and maintenance of navigation programs (see Table 3-1) can provide program planners with valuable guidance during the planning process (Valaitis et al., 2017).

"A good business plan guides you through each stage of starting and managing your business. You'll use your business plan as a roadmap for how to structure, run, and grow your new business. It's a way to think through the key elements of your business" (U.S. Small Business Administration, 2024, para. 1). Creating a business plan is not a solo endeavor; it requires input and cooperation from people involved in planning, implementing, and maintaining the activity.

Many business plan templates exist, and each organization will likely have preferences and specifications for internally prepared business plans (see Figure 3-1). A strong strategy is to use data and recommendations published by other institutions or service lines and programs within the home institution.

TABLE 3-1. Factors Influencing Successful Implementation and Maintenance of Navigation Programs

Factors	Elements Describing Each Factor
1. Patient characteristics	• Complexity of clients and patients • The need to first address the basic needs of clients and patients (e.g., shelter) • Caregivers of clients or patients being patients themselves • Geographic restrictions (e.g., access to services in rural communities) • Language barriers • Respect for cultural values

2. Effective recruitment and training of navigators	• Recruitment of lay navigators supported by word of mouth
	• Maintenance of ongoing training to support:
	  – Growth and development of navigators
	  – Role transitions
	  – Problem-solving for complex cases
	  – Collaboration and mutual support among navigators
	  – Orientation to the needs of the population being served by navigators

3. Role clarity	• Clear boundaries set for navigators (particularly lay navigators) in their role – Clarifying role boundaries with patients or clients as well as physicians • Valuing role clarification • Management of anxiety when taking on a new navigation role to build confidence
4. Effective and clear operational processes	• Careful development of planning processes • Development of policies and procedures to support program activities • Establishment of documentation mechanisms, such as clinical intake forms • Use of consensus decision-making approaches • Provision of clinical supervision and steering committee oversight • Regular communication between agencies for planning purposes • Mechanisms to address scheduling and referral challenges

5. Adequate human, financial, and tangible resources, including technological resources	Provision for:
	• Human resources
	  – Dedicated, committed, engaged, and adequately trained clinical staff
	  – External availability of experts such as attorneys
	• Financial resources
	  – Secured external funding
	• Tangible resources
	  – Appropriate space for the navigator and navigation work

(Continued on next page)

TABLE 3-1. Factors Influencing Successful Implementation and Maintenance of Navigation Programs *(Continued)*

Factors	Elements Describing Each Factor

5. Adequate human, financial, and tangible resources, including technological resources *(Cont.)*	• Technological resources
	  – Internet resources to locate resources and support complex cases
	  – Electronic health records to support documentation of evidence-based care plans and patient assessments
	  – Electronic health records to support access to community resources, coordinate transitions, and promote self-management
	  – Email or phones to support communication with physicians
	• Adequate time to support transitional care and provide comprehensive care to a large caseload

6. Strong inter- and intra-organizational relationships and partnerships	• Encouraging commitment from all professionals involved
	• Establishment of a self-governing team environment in the practice (supports role development)
	• Development of strong relationships with community agencies by:
	  – Development of a community charter
	  – Establishment of a community-based steering committee
	  – Development of communication strategies with partner agencies
	  – Mechanisms to address inter-organizational issues with power differentials and other tensions between agencies

7. Lack of available services in a community	• Addressing the problem of "navigation to nowhere" (inadequate or nonexistent local services)
8. Effective communication between providers	• Encouragement of consistent attendance at regular meetings by staff (monthly) • Sharing updates related to patient/client progress (through electronic health records) regularly • Involvement of physicians in meetings regularly • Communication between all care providers
9. Program uptake and buy-in by end users of the program	• Selling or getting buy-in to the navigation program with consumers • Use of diverse strategies for recruitment to programs – Recruitment strategies are not successful with all population groups (i.e., outreach); they need to be tailored. • Addressing potential stigma in getting participation in mental health navigation programs
10. Valuing of navigators	• Valuing navigators by providing them with opportunities to be recognized and heard

(Continued on next page)

TABLE 3-1	Factors Influencing Successful Implementation and Maintenance of Navigation Programs *(Continued)*
Factors	**Elements Describing Each Factor**

11. Evaluation of navigation programs	• Evaluation of navigation programs
	  – Developing an evaluation plan with the team for ongoing evaluation
	  – Considering community-based participatory research approaches
	  – Focusing on program-related processes (the degree to which mission or goals are met)
	  – Considering using preidentified indicators
	  – Addressing potential problems with lack of access to data, monitoring health status changes over time, and attribution of outcomes to navigation interventions

Note. From "Implementation and Maintenance of Patient Navigation Programs Linking Primary Care With Community-Based Health and Social Services: A Scoping Literature Review," by R.K. Valaitis, N. Carter, A. Lam, J. Nicholl, J. Feather, and L. Cleghorn, 2017, *BMC Health Services Research, 17*, pp. 6–7 (https://doi.org/10.1186/s12913-017-2046-1). Copyright 2017 by the authors, licensed under CC BY 4.0 (https://creativecommons.org/licenses/by/4.0).

FIGURE 3-1 Typical Elements of a Business Plan

- Executive summary
- Introduction: mission, vision, and goals (short and long term)
- Description of the business
- Market share and competition analysis
- Marketing or business strategies
- Development and implementation plan and schedule
- Organizational plan: services, staff requirements, and qualifications profiles
- Operational plan: operating expenses (e.g., salaries, annual expenses, insurance, communication technologies, building fees, office supplies, signage, capital expenses, marketing materials)
- Financial plan: key revenue and expense metrics
- Appendix

Note. Based on information from Hatchett & Coady, 2013; Johnson & Garvin, 2017.

Evaluation: Analysis, Metrics, and Sustainability

Existing navigation programs should be evaluated regularly to ensure that barriers to care are being addressed and that patient needs are met. Role delineation is a priority as the navigation team expands. In 2022, the Professional Oncology Navigation Task Force, comprised of members representing professional organizations relevant to navigation, published the *Oncology Navigation Standards of Professional Practice*. This document provides navigators with "clear information regarding the standards of professional practice" (Professional Oncology Navigation Task Force, 2022, p. E15). Despite increasing focus on standardized pathways, metrics, and sustainability in navigation, the role of the navigator is often determined by individual cancer centers (Ciccarelli et al., 2020). The *Oncology Navigation Standards of Professional Practice* is the first evidence-based navigation framework that offers role delineation between navigation roles.

Analysis and Reengagement

Patient satisfaction surveys, team meetings, and informal huddles offer an opportunity to identify gaps between ideal and current navigation services. Questions may include the following:
- Do all patients, regardless of disease site, receive the same level of navigation services?
- What is the appointment no-show rate and the most common reason?
- Are patients reporting that their needs are being met on the patient satisfaction survey?

This process is more effective initially with smaller groups to avoid information fatigue. Once gaps are identified and prioritized, action plans can be developed to expand or restructure existing services. If a navigation program has been running smoothly for several years, the original navigation champions may have retired, moved, or sought new priorities. Reengaging champions, both original and new, ensures support for navigation programs. It is also much easier to gain new champions for a program that is already successful. Regular meetings and communication strengthen support from existing champions. New champions can expand support networks and are essential to sustaining navigation programs.

Sustainability

The stability and endurance of navigation programs have been measured by reviewing funding mechanisms, length of program existence, and institutional participation in accreditation and alternative funding models, such as the Enhancing Oncology Model (replacing the Oncology Care Model) and Merit-Based Incentive Payment System Alternative Payment Models (MIPS APMs) (Garfield et al., 2022). National Cancer Institute–designated institutions, academic centers, and non-academic clinical settings report operational sources that primarily provide their funding. In contrast, community-based and nonprofit organizations rely on a mix of grants and some operations sources. Research has shown minimal participation in the Enhancing Oncology Model and MIPS APMs programs that require navigation. Similarly, organizations that are forgoing accreditation exhibit less sustainable measures.

The Centers for Medicare and Medicaid Services has approved billing codes for oncology navigation: Principal Care Management (PCM) for clinical navigation and Principal Illness Navigation (PIN) for non-clinical navigation. Although this first step in navigation reimbursement is encouraging, it may not result in a budget-neutral environment.

Summary

Research continues to show how oncology navigation benefits patients, their loved ones, healthcare teams, and institutions. From its beginnings, navigation in oncology has improved timeliness from suspicious findings to diagnosis and treatment. Additional benefits include significant improvement in treatment adherence, reduced hospital and emergency department visits, and satisfied patients and caregivers (Chan et al., 2023; Garfield et al., 2022; Kokorelias et al., 2021). Oncology program leaders acknowledge these benefits as the rationale for developing, growing, and sustaining oncology navigation from the community setting to academic and National Cancer Institute–designated cancer centers. Oncology program administrators must overcome the challenges of inadequate funding, limited internal and external resources, and a lack of institutional champions to realize these benefits for patients.

Building a strong business plan involves assessing the needs of patients, the community, and the program and identifying relevant program goals. From that foundation, the development and implementation of a plan, followed by diligent evaluation and reassessment, will be necessary to sustain the program and meet the needs of patients, organizations, and communities.

The author would like to acknowledge Rosangel Klein, MS, RN, CNS, OCN®, and Pamela J. Haylock, PhD, RN, FAAN, for their contribution to this chapter that remains unchanged from the previous edition of this book.

References

American College of Surgeons. (2019). *Optimal resources for cancer care: 2020 standards.* https://www.facs.org/quality-programs/cancer-programs/commission-on-cancer/standards-and-resources/2020

Chan, R.J., Milch, V.E., Crawford-Williams, F., Agbejule, O.A., Joseph, R., Johal, J., ... Hart, N.H. (2023). Patient navigation across the cancer care continuum: An overview of systematic reviews and emerging literature. *CA: A Cancer Journal for Clinicians, 73*(6), 565–589. https://doi.org/10.3322/caac.21788

Ciccarelli, H., Csik, V.P., Rogers, A., Scheid, K., & Vadseth, C. (2020). Delineating roles in a hybrid nurse and patient navigation model can reduce care variation. *Journal of Oncology Navigation and Survivorship, 11*(1). https://www.jons-online.com/issues/2020/january-2020-vol-11-no-1/2761-delineating-roles-in-a-hybrid-nurse-and-patient-navigation-model-can-reduce-care-variation

Garfield, K.M., Franklin, E.F., Battaglia, T.A., Dwyer, A.J., Freund, K.M., Wightman, P.D., & Rohan, E.A. (2022). Evaluating the sustainability of patient navigation programs in oncology by length of existence, funding, and payment model participation. *Cancer, 128*(Suppl. 13), 2578–2589. https://doi.org/10.1002/cncr.33932

Hatchett, R., & Coady, E. (2013). Writing a business plan to support a cardiac service. *British Journal of Cardiac Nursing, 8*(4), 190–192. https://doi.org/10.12968/bjca.2013.8.4.190

Johnson, J.E., & Garvin, W.S. (2017). Advanced practice nurses: Developing a business plan for an independent ambulatory clinical practice. *Nursing Economics, 35*(3), 126–133. https://library.aaacn.org/p/a/advanced-practice-nurses-developing-a-business-plan-for-an-independent-ambulatory-clinical-practice-12218

Kline, R.M., Rocque, G.B., Rohan, E.A., Blackley, K.A., Cantril, C.A., Pratt-Chapman, M.L., ... Shulman, L.N. (2019). Patient navigation in cancer: The business case to support clinical needs. *Journal of Oncology Practice, 15*(11), 585–590. https://doi.org/10.1200/JOP.19.00230

Kokorelias, K.M., Shiers-Hanley, J.E., Rios, J., Knoepfli, A., & Hitzig, S.L. (2021). Factors influencing the implementation of patient navigation programs for adults with complex needs: A scoping review of the literature. *Health Services Insights, 14,* 11786329211033267. https://doi.org/10.1177/11786329211033267

Morena, A.L., Gaias, L.M., & Larkin, C. (2022). Understanding the role of clinical champions and their impact on clinician behavior change: The need for causal pathway mechanisms. *Frontiers in Health Services, 2,* 896885. https://doi.org/10.3389/frhs.2022.896885

Oncology Nursing Society & Oncology Nursing Certification Corporation. (2024). *Oncology nurse navigator competencies.* https://www.ons.org/oncology-nurse-navigator-competencies

Professional Oncology Navigation Task Force. (2022). Oncology navigation standards of professional practice. *Clinical Journal of Oncology Nursing, 26*(3), E14–E25. https://doi.org/10.1188/22.CJON.E14-E25

U.S. Small Business Administration. (2024, November 1). *Write your business plan.* https://www.sba.gov/business-guide/plan-your-business/write-your-business-plan

Valaitis, R.K., Carter, N., Lam, A., Nicholl, J., Feather, J., & Cleghorn L. (2017). Implementation and maintenance of patient navigation programs linking primary care with community-based health and social services: A scoping literature review. *BMC Health Services Research, 17*(1), 1–14. https://doi.org/10.1186/s12913-017-2046-1

Yackzan, S., Stanifer, S., Barker, S., Blair, B., Glass, A., Weyl, H., & Wheeler, P. (2019). Outcome measurement: Patient satisfaction scores and contact with oncology nurse navigators. *Clinical Journal of Oncology Nursing, 23*(1), 76–81. https://doi.org/10.1188/19.CJON.76-81

CHAPTER 4

Oncology Nurse Navigator Role and Competencies

Lisa Lampton, MSN, MBA, RN, CBCN®, OCN®

> **KEY TOPICS**
> competencies, role definition

Overview

Over the past 30 years, the depth and breadth of the navigator role have changed drastically; however, the overarching concept remains the same—to reduce barriers and improve access to timely, quality health care (Professional Oncology Navigation Task Force [PONT], 2022). Navigation services have expanded to include all phases of the cancer trajectory and have been a mandated standard for cancer programs accredited by the American College of Surgeons Commission on Cancer since 2015 (PONT, 2022).

Entering the navigation world can seem daunting, particularly for those without a clear definition of what it means to be a professional oncology nurse navigator (ONN). Since 2011, numerous publications, journal articles, role delineation studies, and web-based educational courses have been developed on the subject, the bulk of which have come from the Oncology Nursing Society (ONS).

In 2022, PONT published an article providing clear standards of professional practice for both clinical and non-clinical navigators, including ethical boundaries, interprofessional collaboration, psychosocial assessment, and advocacy for survivorship care planning. It also set forth the standard that ONNs should have earned, at minimum, a bachelor's degree.

This chapter will detail the current state of the ONN's scope of practice, role definitions, and core competencies.

Role Definitions

Although many different roles and job titles within an organization can fall under the all-encompassing umbrella of *navigation*, significant differences exist between the scope and responsibilities of clinical and non-clinical navigators. Differences can be further distilled from within the group of clinical navigators, which includes ONNs and oncology social workers (OSWs).

Oncology Nurse Navigators

The definition of an ONN was detailed in Chapter 1. This professional RN role has "oncology-specific clinical knowledge and offers individualized assistance to patients, families, and caregivers to help overcome healthcare system barriers" (ONS, 2017, p. 4).

When evaluating this definition within the context of other available literature, the key characteristics that set the ONN apart from an oncology nurse generalist are the ability to identify and address specific obstacles to care and a broad knowledge of the general cancer treatment landscape as a whole. This second characteristic is counter to a focus on more patient-centric care delivery tasks, such as the administration of antineoplastic treatments or immunotherapy in a clinical setting (Lubejko et al., 2017).

ONNs provide a wide range of navigation services across a multitude of practice settings, each performing a slightly different function. A diagnostic navigator in a breast center, for instance, may assist with care coordination to reduce delays in obtaining imaging and biopsy. In another realm, a treatment navigator can address knowledge gaps and alleviate pre-appointment anxiety for patients scheduled for consultation at a cancer center (Kline et al., 2019; Wang et al., 2021).

Non-Clinical Navigators

Historically called lay navigators, the title has evolved to non-clinical or patient navigators with the publication of the PONT standards. Depending on the organization and workflow, the non-clinical navigator can help reduce the workload of ONNs by managing tasks and efforts that do not require a nursing license, such as providing emotional support, coordinating appointments, or detailing financial assistance resources. This team member can also escalate any clinical concerns to the registered nurse, such as treatment-related side effects, the need for clinical education, or an acute mental health crisis (Anderson et al., 2021).

Community health workers can provide another layer of emotional and social support to patients and caregivers. These non-clinical individuals typically work and reside in underserved urban or rural communities and help reduce health disparities by providing culturally appropriate education, promoting communication between community members and the local health system, and advocating for the needs of the population they represent (National Heart, Lung, and Blood Institute, 2014).

The role of the financial navigator is also being incorporated into cancer programs and institutions to assist patients with mitigating the cost of treatments and other expenses. These professionals can guide patients and their families or caregivers through complex insurance policies, determine what assistance programs may be available for their disease or treatment regimen, and provide early intervention for patients at risk for financial toxicity associated with cancer care (Sherman & Fessele, 2019). Although comprehensive financial navigation programs may not yet be available at every institution or practice that treats patients with cancer, a growing body of literature describes the value of making these services a standard facet of high-quality oncology care (Smith et al., 2022; Watabayashi et al., 2020).

Oncology Social Workers

OSWs provide a unique perspective on the social and emotional health needs of individuals with cancer and their families to the interprofessional care team. The scope of practice for the OSW, set forth by the Association of Oncology Social Work (2024), comprises having knowledge of various oncologic diseases and their treatment courses, providing psychosocial support along all phases of the cancer continuum, ensuring community services and assistance programs are available to meet the needs of survivors, and serving as advocates for patients and caregivers to help them access quality care. OSWs are licensed practitioners with a master's degree in social work. They may obtain special certification (OSW-C™) by submitting documentation of at least 4,000 hours of direct work experience and a portfolio of three demonstrated practice activities specific to oncology to their accrediting body (Board of Oncology Social Work Certification, 2022).

Case Managers

Case managers are healthcare professionals who typically serve as liaisons among patients, the healthcare team, and insurance providers to ensure optimal resource utilization and value for the delivery of services and care (Case Management Society of America, n.d.). When employed by hospitals or other healthcare facilities, case managers play an integral role in the discharge planning process. They are responsible for ensuring that an individual has the appropriate resources to safely return home or assist with transfers to other levels of care as indicated.

Oncology case managers are in a unique position to lend their specialty expertise to insurance providers or health organizations, as they are equipped with the knowledge and skills to help patients navigate their cancer care and understand the coverage benefits specific to oncology (Robbins & DeMeyer, 2022). Studies have shown that when case management is directly involved in the care coordination and follow-up monitoring of individuals with complex hematologic conditions, the rates of hospital readmission and unplanned emergency department visits are reduced (Garnett et al., 2020).

Oncology Nurse Navigator Competencies

ONS developed the initial *ONN Core Competencies* in 2013, releasing updated versions in 2017 and 2024. These updates were to ensure that competencies reflected the evolving nature of the role and healthcare environment. Within the 2024 revision, *Oncology Nurse Navigator Competencies*, are 13 domains with statements related to the knowledge, skills, and abilities of ONNs, with the recognition that additional competencies may apply depending on the ONN's role (ONS & Oncology Nursing Certification Corporation, 2024, p. 4).

- **Ethical and Legal Considerations** addresses legal and ethical standards, regulatory requirements, and upholding professional integrity.
- **Cultural Humility and Diversity** ensures that care promotes the principles of equity, inclusion, and justice.
- **Interprofessional Team Collaboration** addresses the need to create and optimize cohesive workflows between teams.
- **Clinical Knowledge and Skill Application** enables education and coordination that best serve patients and their support systems.
- **Community Outreach** removes or reduces barriers that can affect care delivery and promotes health equity.
- **Electronic Health Record and Financial Acumen** ensures that data management and privacy are maintained through the use of relevant information systems.
- **Professional and Organizational Development** addresses the essential commitment to sustaining professional growth and the need to stay current in a changing environment.
- **Patient Advocacy** supports and promotes patients' rights and current and future needs.
- **Patient Education** addresses the unique role ONNs play in personalizing the education delivered to individuals with cancer and their caregivers.
- **Patient Care Management** addresses the development and implementation of care plans.
- **Care Coordination** ensures seamless transitions across the care continuum.
- **Evidence-Based Oncology Practice** includes integrating evidence-based resources and professional standards to drive care delivery.
- **Communication and Interpersonal Skills** addresses fostering trust and collaboration with patients, team members, and other support systems.

At the core of these competencies, ONNs must possess a strong clinical background in oncology, ideally holding specialty certification, to provide comprehensive, knowledgeable care to the patient population being served. They also must promote the oncology nursing and navigation professions by adhering to evidence-based practice, participating in quality improvement initiatives, and advocating for patients' needs at every phase along the cancer continuum—from survivorship to end of life (PONT, 2022).

Application of Competencies to Practice

Using standardized and validated competencies as the foundation for an ONN role ensures that the individual in the role and the role itself are based on evidence and aid in standardization across organizations. The *ONN Core Competencies* were developed and revised to reflect the diverse practice settings, team compositions, and disease types that ONNs experience in their practice. These competencies can be applied in the practice area in many ways (see Figure 4-1). Once implemented into practice, validation of competencies to ensure that ONNs are meeting these expectations is necessary. The measurement of competencies, or validation, may differ between organizations or institutions. For example, ONS provides checklists, handouts of the Navigation Standards, and clinical ladders that can be integrated into practice settings or used for self-assessment.

ONNs draw on clinical expertise and specialized knowledge to help assess and mitigate barriers to care that stem from social determinants of health, such as financial toxicities, food insecurity, transportation and housing needs, and access to quality care by providing resources directly to patients and caregivers. ONNs can also make referrals to other modalities, such as social services and case management, for additional assistance (Kline et al., 2019; World Health Organization, 2024). Screening for practical, social, spiritual, or physical issues can be performed by using a validated tool for assessing distress, such as the National Comprehensive Cancer Network Distress Thermometer, at the time of initial assessment and as needed throughout the treatment journey (National Comprehensive Cancer Network, 2025). A tool to measure distress enables ONNs to determine if patients have concerns regarding their physical symptoms, ability to care for themselves or others, work situation, or any other aspect of their care. If a need is identified, ONNs can assist patients with appropriate resources.

FIGURE 4-1 **Uses for Competencies in Practice**

- Creating of orientation and training plans
- Developing of competency validation checklists
- Writing job descriptions
- Assisting leaders in screening applications
- Developing education programs or curricula
- Evaluating performance
- Benchmarking and setting programmatic goals
- Marketing and promotion of the oncology nurse navigator role

Note. Based on information from Oncology Nursing Society & Oncology Nursing Certification Corporation, 2024.

Summary

Through several iterations and evolutions, the realm of patient navigation has expanded to include patients at every point on the cancer continuum—from screening and early diagnosis to survivorship or end of life. With navigation services reimbursable by the Centers for Medicare and Medicaid Services as of January 1, 2024, the role will likely undergo many more changes in the years to come to ensure that these services are accessible to all (Centers for Medicare and Medicaid Services, 2023). After more than three decades, it is clear that no matter how different cancer care may look in the future, competent ONNs will be there every step of the way to provide guidance, advocacy, and support.

The author would like to acknowledge Barbara G. Lubejko, MS, RN, for her contribution to this chapter that remains unchanged from the previous edition of this book.

References

Anderson, S., Kirton, C., Kolambel, R., & Ruiz, S. (2021). Patient lay navigator program: An approach to enhancing patients' access to psychosocial support and reducing non-clinical barriers associated with care [Abstract]. *Journal of Oncology Navigation and Survivorship, 12*(11). https://www.jons-online.com/issues/2021/november-2021-vol-12-no-11/4143:patient-lay-navigator-program-an-approach-to-enhancing-patients-access-to-psychosocial-support-and-reducing-nonclinical-barriers-associated-with-care#:~:text=Lay%20patient%20navigators%20are%20trained%20volunteer%20community%20members,and%20emotional%20support%20to%20patients%20diagnosed%20with%20cancer

Association of Oncology Social Work. (2024). *Scope and standards of practice: Scope of practice in oncology social work*. https://aosw.org/resources/scope-and-standards-of-practice

Board of Oncology Social Work Certification. (2022). Become a certified oncology social worker: OSW-C™. https://oswcert.org/getcertified

Case Management Society of America. (n.d.). *What is a case manager?* https://cmsa.org/who-we-are/what-is-a-case-manager

Centers for Medicare and Medicaid Services. (2023, November 2). *CMS finalizes physician payment rule that advances health equity* [Press release]. https://www.cms.gov/newsroom/press-releases/cms-finalizes-physician-payment-rule-advances-health-equity

Garnett, D., Hardy, L., Fitzgerald, E., Fisher, T., Graham, L., & Overcash, J. (2020). Nurse case manager: Measurement of care coordination activities and quality and resource use outcomes when caring for the complex patient with hematologic cancer. *Clinical Journal of Oncology Nursing, 24*(1), 65–74. https://doi.org/10.1188/20.CJON.65-74

Kline, R.M., Rocque, G.B., Rohan, E.A., Blackley, K.A., Cantril, C.A., Pratt-Chapman, M.L., ... Shulman, L.N. (2019). Patient navigation in cancer: The business case to support clinical needs. *Journal of Oncology Practice, 15*(11), 585–590. https://doi.org/10.1200/JOP.19.00230

Lubejko, B.G., Bellfield, S., Kahn, E., Lee, C., Peterson, N., Rose, T., ... McCorkle, M. (2017). Oncology nurse navigation: Results of the 2016 role delineation study. *Clinical Journal of Oncology Nursing, 21*(1), 43–50. https://doi.org/10.1188/17.CJON.43-50

National Comprehensive Cancer Network. (2025). *NCCN Clinical Practice Guidelines in Oncology (NCCN Guidelines®): Distress management* [v. 1.2025]. https://www.nccn.org

National Heart, Lung, and Blood Institute. (2014). *Role of community health workers*. https://www.nhlbi.nih.gov/health/educational/healthdisp/role-of-community-health-workers.htm

Oncology Nursing Society. (2017). *2017 oncology nurse navigator core competencies*. https://www.ons.org/oncology-nurse-navigator-competencies

Oncology Nursing Society & Oncology Nursing Certification Corporation. (2024). *Oncology nurse navigator competencies*. https://www.ons.org/oncology-nurse-navigator-competencies

Professional Oncology Navigation Task Force. (2022). Oncology navigation standards of professional practice. *Clinical Journal of Oncology Nursing, 26*(3), E14–E25. https://doi.org/10.1188/22.CJON.E14-E25

Robbins, L.M., & DeMeyer, E.S. (2022, June 17). *FAQs about oncology case manager roles.* https://cancernursingtoday.com/post/faqs-about-oncology-case-manager-roles

Sherman, D.E., & Fessele, K.L. (2019). Financial support models: A case for use of financial navigators in the oncology setting. *Clinical Journal of Oncology Nursing, 23*(5, Suppl. 2), 14–18. https://doi.org/10.1188/19.CJON.S2.14-18

Smith, G.L., Banegas, M.P., Acquati, C., Chang, S., Chino, F., Conti, R.M., ... Yabroff, K.R. (2022). Navigating financial toxicity in patients with cancer: A multidisciplinary management approach. *CA: A Cancer Journal for Clinicians 72*(5), 437–453. https://doi.org/10.3322/caac.21730

Wang, T., Huilgol, Y.S., Black, J., D'Andrea, C., James, J., Northrop, A., ... Esserman, L.J. (2021). Pre-appointment nurse navigation: Patient-centered findings from a survey of patients with breast cancer. *Clinical Journal of Oncology Nursing, 25*(5), E57–E62. https://doi.org/10.1188/21.CJON.E57-E62

Watabayashi, K., Steelquist, J., Overstreet, K.A., Leahy, A., Bradshaw, E., Gallagher, K.D., ... Shankaran, V. (2020). A pilot study of a comprehensive financial navigation program in patients with cancer and caregivers. *Journal of the National Comprehensive Cancer Network, 18*(10), 1366–1373. https://doi.org/10.6004/jnccn.2020.7581

World Health Organization. (2024). *Social determinants of health.* https://www.who.int/health-topics/social-determinants-of-health#tab=tab_1

CHAPTER 5

Models of Oncology Navigation

Amanda Bruffy, MBAHM, BSN, RN, CNRN, OCN®, and
Deborah M. Christensen, MSN, APRN, AOCNS®

> **KEY TOPICS**
> navigation models, patient navigation, oncology nurse navigation

Overview

Over the past three decades, navigation has evolved from community-based models focused on prevention and screening to models operating across the entire cancer care continuum with clinical and non-clinical personnel in the navigator role. This evolution reflects the growing complexity of cancer care and emphasizes the value of navigation in bridging gaps and improving outcomes across diverse patient populations.

Professionally licensed nurses and social workers primarily fill the navigator role in the clinical setting (e.g., hospitals, clinics, screening centers), where assistive personnel function outside of the healthcare setting. Hybrid navigation models also exist, with patients with cancer and their loved ones benefiting from a blend of oncology nurse navigators (ONNs) and non-clinically trained navigators. Oncology navigation can be described as assisting patients in navigating the complexities of the healthcare system. This team effort may include community health workers, promotores/promotoras de salud, and financial navigators (Franklin et al., 2022). Distinctive role definitions are displayed in Table 5-1.

This chapter will describe ONN interventions, with a focus on the various navigation models and settings that use ONNs and non-clinical navigators as resources.

Oncology Navigation Roles

Oncology navigation is a team effort. Navigators collaborate closely with other healthcare professionals, including physicians, social workers, care coordinators, and support staff, to guide patients and their loved ones through the medically complex and emotionally challenging journey of a cancer diagnosis. This support can range

TABLE 5-1. Oncology Navigation Role Definitions

Role	Definition
Oncology navigation	Individualized assistance offered to patients, families, and caregivers to help overcome healthcare system barriers and facilitate timely access to quality health and psychosocial care from prediagnosis through all phases of the cancer experience
Professional navigator	A trained individual employed and paid by a healthcare-, advocacy-, or community-based organization to fill the role of oncology navigator
Oncology patient navigator	A professional who provides individualized assistance to patients and families affected by cancer to improve access to healthcare services; does not have or use clinical training
Clinical	
Oncology nurse navigator	A professional registered nurse with oncology-specific clinical knowledge who offers individual assistance to patients, families, and caregivers to help overcome healthcare system barriers
Oncology social worker	A professional social worker with a master's degree in social work and a clinical license (or equivalent as defined by state laws) with oncology-specific and clinical psychosocial knowledge who offers individual assistance to patients, families, and caregivers to help overcome healthcare system barriers
Non-Clinical	
Community health worker	A person living within a community and chosen by community members or organizations to provide basic health and medical care to their community
Promotores/promotoras de salud	A frontline public health worker and trusted member of a community who usually has an especially close understanding of the community served
Financial navigator	A professional who helps patients manage the financial aspects of their cancer care, including understanding insurance coverage, finding financial assistance, and addressing out-of-pocket costs

Note. Based on information from Association of Community Cancer Centers, 2019; Bell-Brown et al., 2023; Franklin et al., 2022; Smithwick et al., 2023.

from explaining complex medical information to connecting patients with external resources. ONNs also provide emotional support and refer patients to psychosocial services. The complexity inherent to cancer care can be overwhelming. Addressing healthcare fragmentation by supporting care transitions between departments (e.g., surgery, medical and radiation oncology, radiology) is a primary ONN intervention.

Oncology navigation staff selection and delivery models will continue to evolve to meet the needs of patients, providers, institutions, and communities (Gentry, 2021). Although there may not be uniformity, navigation programs should incorporate the

Oncology Nursing Society's *Oncology Nurse Navigator Competencies* and the *Oncology Navigation Standards of Professional Practice*. These documents provide expert guidance yet may be applied differently depending on the navigator staff mix, setting, and model used to form a navigation program. The competencies are specific to the ONN role and outline the knowledge, skills, and proficiencies needed to effectively support patients and families at a single point in the cancer care continuum or across the entire care continuum (Oncology Nursing Society & Oncology Nursing Certification Corporation, 2024). The oncology nursing standards outline the knowledge and skills ONNs should have to provide high-quality, competent, and ethical services to patients with cancer. The standards can also be used as benchmarks for employers to inform policymakers and aid the public in understanding the navigator role (Franklin et al., 2022).

Staff Selection Strategies

Healthcare institutions may employ blended navigation teams in which clinical and non-clinical navigators support patients and caregivers. In Winget et al. (2019), one cancer center used a blended staffing model based on the complexity of a patient's situation. Non-clinical navigators resourced a broad range of patients, whereas ONNs navigated patients receiving at least two treatment modalities. Patients reported positive experiences, including getting help with complex scheduling, alleviating anxiety through access to information and educational resources, and receiving assistance with activities outside traditional health care (Winget et al., 2019).

Institutions mixing these professional navigators reported clinical navigators providing significantly more treatment-related support and non-clinical navigators engaging in more logistical coordination and resources (Ciccarelli et al., 2020; Wells et al., 2022). Clinical navigators are more likely to work in healthcare organizations and be funded by operational budgets. Community-based and nonprofit organizations primarily use grant funding to employ non-clinical navigators (often community members) or function with volunteers acting as peer navigators (Wells et al., 2022). Organizations should evaluate internal and external resources, different staffing mixes, and a variety of navigation models to determine the best fit for their patient population.

Customary Navigation Models

Institutions and clinics can implement a navigation program using one of several defined navigation models. The navigation staff mix, available funding, institutional resources, and community needs affect the choice of the model (Corbett et al., 2020).

General Oncology Navigation

General ONNs support patients regardless of cancer type. They must understand the nuances of the various types of cancer and the corresponding support services.

This model may work well for small organizations or centers specializing in a subset of disease types, such as gynecologic or gastrointestinal oncology. General navigators may function within a cancer continuum–specific or longitudinal navigation model.

The value of general navigation services exists across the scope of health care. Still, it remains rooted in oncology, where it has been shown to promote timely access to care, support improved communication, and maintain continuity of care (Baileys et al., 2018).

Disease-Specific Navigation

In the disease-specific navigation model, navigators specialize in a specific disease (e.g., breast, lung, pancreas) or body system (e.g., genitourinary, gynecologic, central nervous system) affected by cancer. Academic centers and other institutions have successfully used this model to provide comprehensive, patient-centered navigation. At St. Elizabeth Healthcare in Kentucky, ONNs were associated with general oncology providers and reported spending more time on clerical duties than direct patient care. Because of St. Elizabeth's successful lung cancer screening program, a thoracic navigation program was implemented, followed by gastrointestinal, genitourinary, and head and neck patient navigation. Metrics demonstrated improved time from diagnosis to treatment and notably reduced patient time and travel expenses resulting from expert care coordination (Bonfilio, 2023).

Care Continuum–Specific Navigation

Similar to disease-specific navigators serving a specific group of patients based on diagnosis, care continuum–specific navigators provide services within an identified phase of the patient journey: prevention and screening (early detection), diagnosis, treatment, survivorship, palliative care (people living with advanced, chronic, or terminal cancer), and end of life (Chan et al., 2023). In this model, interventions may be provided by clinical, non-clinical, generalist, or disease-specific navigators with the defining point of working within a specific phase. For example, non-clinical navigators primarily provide services within the early-detection space. In contrast, clinically trained personnel or hybrid teams navigate during the diagnosis, treatment, palliative care, and end-of-life phases of the cancer care continuum (Chan et al., 2023). Table 5-2 details levels of evidence related to navigation interventions on patient outcomes during the early detection, diagnostic, treatment, and survivorship phases of patient care.

Longitudinal Oncology Navigation

The distinct phases of the cancer care continuum are represented in longitudinal navigation models, which may involve clinical and non-clinical personnel at the community, health system, and clinic levels. The primary focus of navigation efforts in these settings and phases is to ensure consistent barrier assessments and ongoing support as patients move from one setting and phase to another. Longitudinal documentation allows care teams to identify and address ongoing healthcare- and

TABLE 5-2. Interventions During Early Detection, Diagnosis, Treatment, and Survivorship

Phase	Outcome Measure	Rating (1–3)[a]
Early detection	Improved cancer screening rates	3
Diagnosis	Reduced time to diagnosis	3
Treatment	Reduced time from diagnosis to treatment	2
	Reduced hospital readmissions	3
	Improved clinical trial enrollment and adherence	1
Survivorship	Adherence to surveillance appointments	3
	Improved decision-making and treatment knowledge	3
	Improved communication	1
	Reduced cancer-related fatigue	1
	Improved patient satisfaction with care	3
	Improved cancer survivor quality of life	3

[a] Ratings include limited evidence (1), some evidence (2), and strong evidence (3).

Note. Based on information from Chan et al., 2023.

patient-related barriers and coordinate care from the community setting throughout the patient journey (Corbett et al., 2020). Oncology navigation across the cancer care continuum establishes trusting relationships and a consistent point of contact.

Specialized Navigation Models

Cancer survivorship begins at diagnosis. Many patients describe unmet medical, physical, social, and emotional needs throughout the cancer care continuum (Hsu et al., 2024). People are living longer with advanced and metastatic cancer, often with profound losses in quality of life (Mollica et al., 2022). Furthermore, financial challenges resulting from cancer treatment costs, lost time at work, or insufficient insurance can significantly affect adherence to treatment and survivorship plans and access to medical care, further exacerbating inequities in cancer care (Abrams et al., 2021; Hsu et al., 2024). Survivorship and financial navigation are specialized navigation models evolving from these identified gaps in cancer care.

Survivorship Navigation

Survivorship is an extended phase of care that extends through palliative care for patients with advanced or metastatic cancer to the end of life. Survivorship can be complicated by lingering side effects, multiple referrals to specialists (e.g., rehabilitation, sexual health, counseling), cumulative toxicities, and feelings of abandonment (Chan et al., 2023). Navigation roles in survivorship may include a singular classification or a blend of clinical and non-clinical navigators. Advanced care providers, such as nurse practitioners, physician assistants, and clinical nurse specialists, often staff survivorship clinics where post-treatment patients receive follow-up medical care. Survivorship ONNs provide clinical education, coordinate palliative care, and support the emotional needs of patients and caregivers through referrals to support groups or professional services as needed. Non-clinical navigators can assist with surveillance scheduling, provide survivorship resources, and give emotional support during this transitional time (Oppong et al., 2024).

The role of the survivorship navigator can aid programs in their quest for accreditation. To meet accreditation standards, healthcare systems that are certified by the American College of Surgeons Commission on Cancer and National Accreditation Program for Breast Cancers must focus on addressing survivorship needs. To this end, survivorship navigators can provide screening and educational recommendations for life after cancer, facilitate timely follow-up care, ensure that referrals to specialists are completed, and address the psychosocial fallout from cancer and its treatments (American College of Surgeons Commission on Cancer, 2020, 2023).

Financial Navigation

Financial navigation focuses on the burdens associated with preventing, diagnosing, and treating illnesses to diminish the financial toxicities related to each phase of care. Financial burden and financial toxicity can affect patients and their families, influencing their decision-making when considering treatment options (Offodile et al., 2022).

Cancer centers may lack the resources for financial assistance or navigation because of the level of training and education this role requires to be proficient and offer individualized attention to patients (Bell-Brown et al., 2023). Financial toxicity is not a physical ailment that can be seen, which could cause it to be viewed as less important than navigation services for more tangible ailments. However, proactively addressing financial concerns and guiding patients through institution-offered financial assistance, co-pay assistance programs, and grant applications can reduce anxiety and address inequity in treatment access and outcomes (Offodile et al., 2022). Chapter 8 discusses the impact of financial toxicity and navigator interventions.

Setting-Specific Navigation

Community-Engaged Navigation

Community-based advocacy groups and cancer centers use a community-engaged navigation model to ensure timely healthcare delivery. Non-clinical navigators play critical roles in the community setting, educating community members, providing services remotely, and facilitating screening for early detection. Community-engaged navigation involves improving outreach to individuals to overcome barriers to care, including practical, cultural, financial, and physical barriers. The goal of this intervention is to ensure that those who are in most need, including ethnic and cultural minorities, people with disabilities, and underinsured and uninsured people, have appropriate resources, education, and access to care. Many cancer centers are partnering with community-based outreach programs for mobile care in conjunction with clinical navigators. Table 5-3 outlines the duties of navigators in different community care settings (Ver Hoeve et al., 2022). The use of navigation across the cancer care

TABLE 5-3. Patient Navigation Efforts Throughout the Cancer Care Continuum

Cancer Care Continuum	Patient Navigation and Tasks
Outreach	Navigators use knowledge of the communities in their catchment area to increase awareness of cancer prevention and early detection. Tasks may include: • Attend meetings with community health partners. • Prepare educational materials for distribution.
Screening	Navigators work to increase the uptake of cancer screening. Tasks may include: • Focus on targeted populations and risk areas within the communities. • Go to the populations; use innovative methods to reach people.
Diagnosis	Navigators follow up on suspicious screening results and improve timeliness to diagnostic resolution. Tasks may include: • Use a variety of patient contact methods. • Use medical training to facilitate explanations with patients and providers.
Treatment	Navigators assist patients as they initiate and adhere to treatment. Tasks may include: • Reduce barriers to attending cancer treatment appointments. • Provide resources to assist with barriers associated with treatment.
Survivorship	Navigators help individuals adjust to post-treatment cancer survivorship. Tasks may include: • Connect patients with survivorship community resources. • Facilitate re-connection with primary care provider.
Palliative	Navigators assist individuals who are transitioning to palliative/hospice care. Tasks may include: • Provide family with community resources. • Ensure end-of-life tasks (e.g., living will) have been set up.

Note. From "Implementing Patient Navigation Programs: Considerations and Lessons Learned From the Alliance to Advance Patient-Centered Cancer Care," by E.S. Ver Hoeve, M.A. Simon, S.M., Danner, A.J. Washington, S.D. Coples, S. Percac-Lima, ... H.A. Hamann, 2022, *Cancer, 128*(14), p. 2807 (https://doi.org/10.1002/cncr.34251). Copyright 2022 by American Cancer Society. Reprinted with permission.

continuum targets the expertise of nurses and other healthcare professionals to overcome barriers.

Rural Navigation

Rural locations are typically defined as areas outside cities and large towns characterized by low population density, open spaces, and limited infrastructure. People living in rural areas face limited access to specialized oncology care, financial challenges caused by time away from home and work to travel for treatment, and low recruitment in clinical trials—all of which affect overall health outcomes and quality care (Levit et al., 2020). Innovative approaches can address rural cancer care barriers, such as opening satellite clinics, expanding oncology telehealth options, and virtual navigation.

For example, patients in rural Ohio and Appalachia lack adequate access to diagnostic, treatment, and support services in addition to high rates of poverty, poor health status, low health literacy, lack of insurance, and distrust of the healthcare system. The James Cancer Hospital at Ohio State University has been working with this population to improve outcomes. Clinical and non-clinical navigators, including community health workers, provide cancer prevention and screening education. The James also partners with community-based programs, such as mobile mammography, to bring resources to the people. Navigators can assist patients with cancer with appointment scheduling and resources for travel and lodging (Levit et al., 2020).

Academic and urban cancer centers often institute satellite clinics in rural areas. This hub-and-spoke model can reduce travel time and expenses and address other rural barriers. For example, some clinics employ navigators within the rural location or provide navigation services from the anchor location, termed *virtual navigation*. This type of navigation can be challenging for ONNs, as they must learn to assess patients accurately and provide services using audio and video technologies, which can cause further complications if patients lack access to and understanding of technologic assets. Navigators address rural barriers through collaborative care with professionals at the hub locations (e.g., genetic counselors, financial navigators, social workers), with the overall goal of increasing patient access to quality cancer care (Levit et al., 2020; Rowett & Christensen, 2020).

Summary

Clinical and non-clinical navigators address the needs of patients and caregivers in community settings, oncology clinics, and academic centers. Oncology navigation programs are shaped based on patient and community needs and resources. Additionally, organizations must consider available funding sources, institutional resources, and navigation staffing. American College of Surgeons Commission on Cancer and National Accreditation Program for Breast Centers certification requirements mandate institutions to offer navigation services; however, the individual organization determines the staffing mix and model.

Customary navigation models include generalist (all cancer types), disease-specific (physical location or body system), continuum-specific (single point of care on the cancer care continuum), and longitudinal (across the cancer care continuum). Survivorship and financial navigation models have evolved to address gaps in cancer care and offer specialized support during particularly vulnerable situations.

The *Oncology Navigation Standards of Professional Practice* outline the skills and knowledge needed to effectively navigate patients and their loved ones through the complexity of cancer care. The standards can be used as benchmarks, inform policy, and educate the public on the navigator's purpose and role. Specific to the ONN, the *Oncology Nurse Navigator Competencies* describe the knowledge and skills required to guide patients through oncology care expertly—be it at a single point in the cancer care continuum or longitudinally.

Regardless of the navigator's role definition, setting, or model, the ultimate goal remains the same: to "advocate with and on behalf of people at risk for cancer, cancer patients, survivors, families, and caregivers to protect and promote the needs and interests of people impacted by cancer" (Franklin et al., 2022, p. E15).

The authors would like to acknowledge Jean Sellers, RN, MSN, and Steven Patierno, PhD, for their contribution to this chapter that remains unchanged from the previous edition of this book.

References

Abrams, H.R., Durbin, S., Huang, C.X., Johnson, S.F., Nayak, R.K., Zahner, G.J., & Peppercorn, J. (2021). Financial toxicity in cancer care: Origins, impact, and solutions. *Translational Behavioral Medicine, 11*(11), 2043–2054. https://doi.org/10.1093/tbm/ibab091

American College of Surgeons Commission on Cancer. (2020). *Optimal resources for cancer care: 2020 standards*. https://www.facs.org/quality-programs/cancer/coc/2020-standards

American College of Surgeons Commission on Cancer. (2023). *Optimal resources for breast care: 2024 standards*. https://accreditation.facs.org/accreditationdocuments/NAPBC/Standards/Optimal_Resources_for_Breast_Care_2024.pdf

Association of Community Cancer Centers. (2019). *Elevating survivorship: Results from two national surveys*. https://www.accc-cancer.org/docs/documents/oncology-issues/articles/2019/mj19/mj19-elevating-survivorship.pdf?sfvrsn=e2b4783_13

Baileys, K.A., McMullen, L., Lubejko, B., Christensen, D., Haylock, P.J., Rose, T., ... Srdanovic, D. (2018). Nurse navigator core competencies: An update to reflect the evolution of the role. *Clinical Journal of Oncology Nursing, 22*(3), 272–281. https://doi.org/10.1188/18.CJON.272-281

Bell-Brown, A., Watabayashi, K., Delaney, D., Carlos, R.C., Langer, S.L., Unger, J.M., ... Shankaran, V. (2023). Assessment of financial screening and navigation capabilities at National Cancer Institute community oncology clinics. *JNCI Cancer Spectrum, 7*(5), pkad055. https://doi.org/10.1093/jncics/pkad055

Bonfilio, S. (2023). Developing a disease-site specific oncology patient navigation program. *Oncology Issues, 38*(5), 7–17. https://doi.org/10.3928/25731777-20230920-03

Chan, R.J., Milch, V.E., Crawford-Williams, F., Agbejule, O.A., Joseph, R., Johal, J., ... Hart, N.H. (2023). Patient navigation across the cancer care continuum: An overview of systematic reviews and emerging literature. *CA: A Cancer Journal for Clinicians, 73*(6), 565–589. https://doi.org/10.3322/caac.21788

Ciccarelli, H., Csik, V.P., Rogers, A., Scheid, K., & Vadseth, C. (2020). Delineating roles in a hybrid nurse and patient navigation model can reduce care variation. *Journal of Oncology Navigation and Survivorship, 11*(1). https://www.jons-online.com/issues/2020/january-2020-vol-11-no-1/2761-delineating-roles-in-a-hybrid-nurse-and-patient-navigation-model-can-reduce-care-variation

Corbett, C.M., Somers, T.J., Nuñez, C.M., Majestic, C.M., Shelby, R.A., Worthy, V.C., ... Patierno, S.R. (2020). Evolution of a longitudinal, multidisciplinary, and scalable patient navigation matrix model. *Cancer Medicine, 9*(9), 3202–3210. https://doi.org/10.1002/cam4.2950

Franklin, E., Burke, S., Dean, M., Johnston, D., Nevidjon, B., & Booth, L.S. (2022). Oncology navigation standards of professional practice. *Clinical Journal of Oncology Nursing, 26*(3), E14–E25. https://doi.org/10.1188/22.CJON.E14-E25

Gentry, S. (2021, December 13). The journey of oncology navigation. *American Nurse.* https://www.myamericannurse.com/the-journey-of-oncology-navigation

Hsu, M., Boulanger, M.C., Olson, S., Eaton, C., Prichett, L., Guo, M., ... Feliciano, J.L. (2024). Unmet needs, quality of life, and financial toxicity among survivors of lung cancer. *JAMA Network Open, 7*(4), e246872. https://doi.org/10.1001/jamanetworkopen.2024.6872

Levit, L.A., Byatt, L., Lyss, A.P., Paskett, E.D., Levit, K., Kirkwood, K., ... Schilsky, R.L. (2020). Closing the rural cancer care gap: Three institutional approaches. *JCO Oncology Practice, 16*(7), 422–430. https://doi.org/10.1200/OP.20.00174

Mollica, M.A., Smith, A.W., Tonorezos, E., Castro, K., Filipski, K.K., Guida, J., ... Gallicchio, L. (2022). Survivorship for individuals living with advanced and metastatic cancers: National Cancer Institute meeting report. *Journal of the National Cancer Institute, 114*(4), 489–495. https://doi.org/10.1093/jnci/djab223

Offodile, A.C., II, Gallagher, K., Angove, R., Tucker-Seeley, R.D., Balch, A., & Shankaran, V. (2022). Financial navigation in cancer care delivery: State of the evidence, opportunities for research, and future directions. *Journal of Clinical Oncology, 40*(21), 2291–2294. https://doi.org/10.1200/JCO.21

Oncology Nursing Society & Oncology Nursing Certification Corporation. (2024). *Oncology nurse navigator competencies.* https://www.ons.org/sites/default/files/2024-10/onn-competencies-final.pdf

Oppong, B.A., Rumano, R.P., & Paskett, E.D. (2024). Expanding the use of patient navigation: Health coaching–based navigation as a novel approach to addressing deficits in breast cancer survivorship support. *Breast Cancer Research and Treatment, 205*(1), 1–3. https://doi.org/10.1007/s10549-023-07213-6

Rowett, K.E., & Christensen, D. (2020). Oncology nurse navigation expansion of the navigator role through telehealth. *Clinical Journal of Oncology Nursing, 24*(3), 24–31. https://doi.org/10.1188/20.CJON.S1.24-31

Smithwick, J., Nance, J., Covington-Kolb, S., Rodriguez, A., & Young, M. (2023). "Community health workers bring value and deserve to be valued too:" Key considerations in improving CHW career advancement opportunities. *Frontiers in Public Health, 11,* 1036481. https://doi.org/10.3389/fpubh.2023.1036481

Ver Hoeve, E.S., Simon, M.A., Danner, S.M., Washington, A.J., Coples, S.D., Percac-Lima, S., ... Hamann, H.A. (2022). Implementing patient navigation programs: Considerations and lessons learned from the Alliance to Advance Patient-Centered Cancer Care. *Cancer, 128*(14), 2806–2816. https://doi.org/10.1002/cncr.34251

Wells, K.J., Wightman, P., Cobian Aguilar, R., Dwyer, A.J., Garcia-Alcaraz, C., Saavedra Ferrer, E.L., ... Calhoun, E. (2022). Comparing clinical and non-clinical cancer patient navigators: A national study in the United States. *Cancer, 128*(Suppl. 13), 2601–2609. https://doi.org/10.1002/cncr.33880

Winget, M., Holdsworth, L., Wang, S., Veruttipong, D., Zionts, D., Rosenthal, E.L., & Asch, S.M. (2019). Effectiveness of a lay navigation program in an academic cancer center. *JCO Oncology Practice, 16*(1), e75–e83. https://doi.org/https://doi.org/10.1200/JOP.19.00337

CHAPTER 6

Determining Community and Program Needs

Kristin Ferguson, DNP, MBA, RN, OCN®

> **KEY TOPICS**
> community needs assessment, internal community, external community, barriers to care

Overview

Over the past 25 years, oncology navigation has evolved to assist individuals in overcoming personal, provider, and system barriers to care across the trajectory of the cancer experience. Outcomes from government-funded demonstration projects have been largely positive, resulting in increased participation in cancer screening activities; decreased time from abnormal cancer-related findings to cancer diagnosis for breast, cervical, colorectal, and prostate cancers; and improved health outcomes (Chan et al., 2023; Nelson et al., 2020). The benefits of navigation are mainly observed in groups historically marginalized or lacking resources due to social determinants of health (Carethers et al., 2020; Soto-Perez-de-Celis et al., 2021).

Although navigation is offered to patients across the United States, tremendous variation exists in how it is defined and delivered. In 2023, the National Comprehensive Cancer Network, American Cancer Society (ACS) Cancer Action Network, and National Minority Quality Forum announced three areas of policy focus to decrease the cancer care gap and reduce disparities in cancer treatments and outcomes. One policy focus is for organizations to provide more oncology navigation services to decrease barriers to care (Schatz et al., 2023). Determining community needs is essential to meeting this goal.

Various agencies offer cancer center accreditation, designation, and certification for the purpose of setting high-quality and evidence-based standards, key performance indicators, research initiatives, and patient care practices (Joseph, 2024; Misra et al., 2019; Russell & Ko, 2023). Cancer program accreditation validates compliance with standards reflecting program infrastructure and management, clinical services across the continuum of care, quality outcomes, and data collection (Joseph, 2024).

For many oncology physician practices and cancer centers, the initial impetus for implementing oncology navigation may have been because of requirements of the American College of Surgeons Commission on Cancer (ACoS CoC), the National Accreditation Program for Breast Centers (NAPBC), and the Enhancing Oncology Model (EOM), a Centers for Medicare and Medicaid Services (CMS) program.

This chapter will introduce accreditation agencies in cancer care, with the acknowledgment that not all cancer programs are aligned in the pursuit of accreditation. It will also explore and delineate the process of identifying community, patient, and institutional needs and service gaps from the introduction and implementation of formal or informal community needs assessments.

Cancer Program Accreditations and Requirements

American College of Surgeons Commission on Cancer

In 2012, the ACoS CoC *Standard 3.1: Patient Navigation Process* was introduced and defined as "individualized assistance offered to patients, families, and caregivers to help overcome health care system barriers and facilitate timely access to quality medical and psychosocial care and can occur from prior to a cancer diagnosis through all phases of the cancer experience" (ACoS CoC, 2012, p. 75). In 2020, patient navigation was removed, and *Standard 8.1: Addressing Barriers to Care* was added. This standard requires each facility within a network to address barriers to care in its demographic and geographic area (ACoS CoC, 2024). This change may have been caused by hospitals mistakenly defining the navigation process as synonymous with a navigator position, equating the implementation of a position with that of a process or a program.

National Accreditation Program for Breast Centers

Patient navigation is a criterion for NAPBC accreditation. These programs require navigation services to begin when a patient presents to an accredited facility (ACoS, 2023). Examples of this may include assessing patients' physical, psychological, and social needs, facilitating timely transitions between medical and surgical teams, or addressing surveillance issues during survivorship (ACoS, 2023).

Enhancing Oncology Model

EOM, which replaced the Oncology Care Model, requires participating practices to identify and address health-related social needs using screening tools, such as the National Comprehensive Cancer Network Distress Thermometer and the

Accountable Health Communities Health-Related Social Needs Screening Tool. Additional requirements include collecting electronic patient-reported outcomes and providing core functions of oncology navigation (CMS, 2022). The *EOM 2024 Health Equity Plan Guide* outlines how participating organizations can create quality improvement plans to identify health disparities and target priority populations (Centers for Medicare and Medicaid Innovation, 2024).

Although the ACoS CoC, NAPBC, and EOM accreditations and requirements do not mandate a formal community needs assessment, this oncology-focused community health process continues to be a valuable strategy for determining and addressing the disparities, barriers, and needs of communities served by cancer programs (ACoS CoC, 2024).

Determining Program Needs

Assessing patients' needs and barriers to care before identifying appropriate interventions is a fundamental part of the nursing process. Similarly, identifying the gaps in services within a community or population is an essential step in addressing community needs. A community needs assessment is a general needs assessment. In contrast, a community health needs assessment is focused on a population's health-related needs and is a government requirement for tax-exempt hospitals (U.S. House of Representatives, 2010). Either assessment can be used to inform navigation and cancer programs.

The first step in determining program needs is to define the community. Traditionally, a community is viewed as the patient population served by a local or regional healthcare system. An external community assessment explores the needs of external community residents, considering disparities, barriers to care, and available resources. External resources include community-based organizations, oncology providers, and other specialists to whom a navigator can refer patients for care (Patlak et al., 2018).

An internal community assessment includes patients receiving care from a cancer program, internal providers, and health system resources. Funding, space, professional development and training, supervision, and technologic infrastructure are internal sources that can also influence navigation program needs.

External Community Assessment

Gather External Data

Patient populations are frequently defined in terms of the community the facility or practice serves, commonly termed the *patient service area*. Hospital admission, discharge, or insurance data can describe the service area, which is defined by zip codes or counties. Information coming from the hospital or cancer program is referred to as *primary data.* Sources of publicly available demographic information are considered *secondary data.* Sources of community assessment data are displayed in Figure 6-1.

Local, city, and state agencies, such as city or state health departments, and national governmental agencies, such as the Centers for Disease Control and Prevention and the U.S. Census Bureau, offer web-based demographic information via reports. City and state agencies also publish information about community environments impacting health and access to health services, such as geographic variables, industrial exposure to carcinogens, weather, or transportation issues. Another option is collaboration with local community organizations that maintain demographic or community needs information to facilitate grant applications or program development.

Cancer-specific secondary data are available from several sources, such as ACS; the National Cancer Institute's Surveillance, Epidemiology, and End Results

---

FIGURE 6-1   Sources of Community Assessment Data

- Cancer registries: facility and state
  - Internal facility departments: marketing and business development; billing and claims
  - Oncology administrators who have developed return-on-investment reports to obtain approval for large equipment purchases or program development
- National Cancer Database: www.facs.org/quality-programs/cancer/ncdb
  - Jointly sponsored by the American College of Surgeons and the American Cancer Society
  - Contains Commission on Cancer–accredited hospital cancer registry data
  - Limited public access: https://oliver.facs.org/BMPub
  - Detailed access to accredited cancer programs (password protected)
- Local, regional, and state public health department websites: state bureaus of health statistics and research—discoverable by internet searches by state
- Local or regional chambers of commerce—discoverable by internet search by location
- National Cancer Institute Surveillance, Epidemiology, and End Results Program: https://seer.cancer.gov
- American Cancer Society cancer facts and statistics publications: www.cancer.org/research/cancer-facts-statistics.html
- U.S. Census Bureau
  - People and Households: www.census.gov/topics/population.html
  - Income and Poverty: www.census.gov/topics/income-poverty.html
- Cancer and other community organizations that support public health issues
  - Leukemia and Lymphoma Society, Pennsylvania Breast Cancer Coalition, Livestrong, etc.—all gather extensive community needs data to identify their funding strategic direction; local and regional offices are the best options.
- Local, regional, and state organizations supporting various diverse or underserved populations
- The Community Toolbox: https://ctb.ku.edu/en, a service of the Work Group for Community Health and Development at the University of Kansas—provides free information and resources

Program and its State Cancer Profiles; the National Cancer Database; and state cancer registries. The National Cancer Database, a joint initiative of ACoS CoC and ACS, is a robust national clinical oncology database with more than 40 million records. The data are submitted from the cancer registries of more than 1,500 ACoS CoC–accredited facilities, representing approximately 72% of all newly diagnosed cancer cases in the United States. National Cancer Database data are used to analyze and track patients with cancer, their demographic information, treatments, and outcomes. Trends in cancer care are used to create regional and state benchmarks for participating hospitals and inform quality improvement initiatives (ACoS, n.d.).

To address barriers to care, CMS and accreditation organizations recognize that patients may be referred to other healthcare facilities or the community for services such as mental health counseling, support groups, cancer rehabilitation, assistance with homecare needs, financial support resources, and transportation. The availability of services will vary from one community to another. Access to subspecialty physicians and services may be limited in rural areas. In these settings, it will be helpful to gather information about tertiary or quaternary referral centers and providers, referral processes, and options for transportation if needed.

Most city and state governments and community organizations provide web-based information about support services or links to resources for additional information. Navigators need to verify information about community resources obtained from web-based sources. Maintaining up-to-date, web-based information is timely and expensive; it is common for these sources to include outdated information, especially when many programs have limited financial resources.

Stakeholders or key informants who participate in a needs assessment are a valuable link and source of information about programs and services. Key informants also may be a source of information about informal resources, specifically involving disparity populations such as LGBTQ+ (lesbian, gay, bisexual, transgender, queer, or questioning, or other identities) individuals, racial and ethnic minorities, immigrants, and others. A good practice is to make contact with someone at each identified community resource to establish a relationship and develop an accurate understanding of services, any specific criteria or processes for referral, and the most appropriate contact person.

Navigation programs should also consider assessing the availability of nontraditional care approaches. Needs assessments should include the availability of telemedicine options, as these services can help to improve access to care, especially in remote locations (Kwok et al., 2022). Since the COVID-19 pandemic in 2020, telehealth has been increasingly used to conduct appointments and assess patients and their environments (Paterson et al., 2020). Some access barriers to care can be addressed by providing patients with internet-based resources. Patients have identified internet cancer support groups as desirable because of time commitments, the absence of the need to travel, the ability to communicate with others regardless of living in an isolated area, and anonymity; however, it is important to realize that not all patients will have equal access to the internet or have enough digital literacy to use internet support groups effectively enough to gain benefit (Lepore et al., 2018).

Identify External Barriers

Exploring the demographic characteristics of the external patient population can help identify disparities and potential barriers to care. Although preventable illness, injury, disability, and death affect all segments of society, life expectancy and other key health outcomes vary greatly by race, age, sexual and gender minorities, socioeconomic status, and geographic location (Agency for Healthcare Research and Quality, 2023; Kamen et al., 2023). For example, it has been well documented that individuals with low socioeconomic status are more likely to be diagnosed with cancer at a later stage and have lower survival rates than individuals with high socioeconomic status. Barriers or factors contributing to poor health outcomes include low income, inadequate insurance, inability to take time off from work for doctor appointments, and poor health practices, such as adherence to recommendations for screening, diet, and exercise (National Cancer Institute, 2024).

Internal Community Assessment

Gather Internal Data

The internal community consists of the analytic and nonanalytic patients included in the hospital cancer registry or community residents receiving care from physician practices. Analytic patients are those who are first diagnosed or receive their first course of treatment at a facility's cancer program. Although several classifications of nonanalytic patients exist, in general, they are patients who have received their diagnosis and all of their first course of treatment elsewhere and have subsequently presented to the facility cancer program with disease recurrence or persistence (ACoS, 2023). Healthcare providers, system structures, processes, and available resources represent the internal community.

The internal community has key informants who are valuable sources of primary data. The internal assessment process includes interviews, surveys, or focus groups involving physicians, nurses, social workers, radiation therapists, physical therapists, office personnel, and other staff who play a role in the patient's cancer journey.

Determine Internal Barriers

When assessing the internal community patient population, primary data from the cancer registry, hospital admissions, discharge, and insurance or physician practice billing records can provide information identifying disparaged populations and potential barriers to care. The same primary data sources can be used to define *community* in terms of high-risk populations or those with complex needs who may encounter barriers or challenges related to their care needs. For example, although the risk of being diagnosed with cancer increases with age and the people most likely to be diagnosed are adults aged 65 years or older, people aged 50–64 years with a cancer diagnosis are increasing (Siegel et al., 2024).

Colon cancer diagnoses among people aged 50 years or younger have risen and remain unexplained, creating the need for regulatory agencies to recommend changes in screening patterns (Collins, 2024). Black men have the highest overall mortality rate, 19% higher than White men, and Black women with endometrial cancer have a mortality rate two times higher than White women due to barriers that include a later diagnosis (Collins, 2024). Monitoring current trends in cancer data registries can help provide information about populations that may be disproportionately affected by cancer and need more support services to decrease barriers to screening, treatment, and healthy outcomes.

Patients with head and neck cancer are another subset of the internal patient community that may face disparities and barriers to care. Low socioeconomic status, low income, heavy alcohol and tobacco misuse, poor nutrition, lack of education, and an inactive lifestyle have all been associated with increased risk for the development of head and neck cancers. In addition, many of these lifestyle risk factors are modifiable, such as visits to the dentist and oral cancer screenings (Akinkugbe et al., 2020). Depending on the histology and stage of disease, patients with head and neck cancer may require multimodal therapy associated with numerous adverse effects, some of which may persist beyond initial treatment. The disparities and barriers to care in this population could likely be the focus of a navigation process.

Barriers to care can also be assessed through provider and hospital systems data. Provider-related factors that serve as barriers include biases, attitudes, and time constraints. System-related factors that can impose barriers to care include the scheduling process, communication patterns, and the availability of supportive resources. Figure 6-2 provides examples of internal and external barriers.

Consider Process Mapping

Process mapping is another method of gathering information about system-related barriers. The benefit of this quality improvement tool is that it allows participants to focus on a complex healthcare process that involves many individuals across numerous office functions or departments (Antonacci et al., 2018). Through this exercise, the participants, who are key informants, produce a visual representation of a process as it currently exists. For example, process mapping might be used to assess barriers to access to care when a new patient undergoing a screening mammogram has an abnormal result highly suspicious for malignancy. The participants create a visual representation of every step in the process, from the point of the initial abnormal imaging result to the first course of definitive treatment. Other individuals and departments involved in the mapping process may include scheduling personnel from diagnostic imaging (e.g., mammography, ultrasound, magnetic resonance imaging), physician offices (e.g., surgery, medical and radiation oncology), the preadmission department,

FIGURE 6-2. Potential Internal and External Barriers to Care

Internal Community		External Community
Provider Barriers • Age • Race, ethnicity, and gender • Communication skills • Attitudes, perceptions, and biases • Cultural sensitivity • Practice patterns • Language • Lack of familiarity, trust • Time constraints • Conflicting obligations • Organizational efficiency skills • Office personnel and processes • Views about patient support resources	**Health System Barriers** • System fragmentation • Hours of operation • Options for subspecialty provider access • Internal and external communication • Scheduling processes • Geographic environment, safety • Lack of resources for translation • Personnel staffing levels • Personnel knowledge and attitudes • Availability of public transportation, parking • Availability of support programs and resources • Organizational efficiency • Patterns of documentation	**Patient Barriers** • Age • Race, ethnicity, gender, and cultural influences • Education level • Employment, income, assets, and insurance status • Literacy and health literacy • Mental status, cognition • Language • Environmental issues (e.g., weather, roads) • Comorbidities, disability • Housing • Availability of social supports • Family care responsibilities • Transportation availability

the laboratory, the operating room, and hospital or short procedure registration. Financial counselors, breast care coordinators, clinical trial personnel, preadmission education (e.g., lymphedema therapy), and others may also be involved. Every point of contact and the processes of moving along the path are outlined. Although process mapping is often used to generate quality improvement strategies, it can significantly contribute to the identification of barriers that are then at least partly addressed by the development of a navigation process.

Use Surveys and Focus Groups

Surveys and focus groups are additional strategies to obtain primary data from community residents. These strategies can be used alone or in combination so that the data gathered are complementary. Surveys—available in English or languages predominantly used in the targeted community—should be conducted at community-based health centers, organizations, events, and hospital clinics. This activity can assist navigators and other individuals in gathering input from community members, especially vulnerable populations (Katchur et al., 2018). The same settings can be used to recruit focus group participants.

The advantage of using focus groups is that they provide data about barriers to health care and community member insights about how to address barriers (Aflague et al., 2023). This approach allows for a more detailed exploration of community member views because they involve small group settings, and the questions are most often open-ended with opportunities for continued dialogue. Focus groups can be structured to gather input from subsets of the community population. For example, a focus group of older adults would likely reveal needs that are very different from a focus group involving another population. Specific population interventions can be identified through focus groups targeting specific issues, such as exploring rural cancer screening challenges leading to disparities in breast and cervical cancer diagnoses (Carnahan et al., 2021) or developing culturally informed lifestyle interventions for Native Hawaiian, Chamoru, and Filipino breast cancer survivors (Aflague et al., 2023). It has also been suggested that by offering community members an opportunity to participate and express their views, interventions to promote health equity will be more sustainable than if they are not included in designing interventions (Subica & Brown, 2020).

Other strategies for contacting community residents for surveys or focus groups include social media, web-based advertising, mailed postcards, and fliers distributed or posted throughout the community in businesses, churches, and community centers. Collaboration with local partnerships, volunteers, community outreach workers, visiting nurses, student nurses, community organization staff members, and others can assist with the dissemination of surveys and focus group information (Katchur et al., 2018).

Needs Assessment Data and Program Monitoring

Information gathered through a community needs assessment or community health needs assessment can be used to determine the goals for a navigation process. Goal-setting questions include what should be achieved through the navigation program, what barriers and gaps in care it will address, and what personnel (clinical or non-clinical) can best meet the identified needs. Examples of navigator program goals are provided in Figure 6-3.

Implementing and sustaining an oncology navigation program or process requires resource space, supplies, equipment, information technology support, personnel (wages and benefits), orientation, training, continuing education, and administrative oversight (Pratt-Chapman & Willis, 2013). A needs assessment explores the availability of these facilities or practice resources.

The program also needs infrastructure components to support the delivery of navigation services, including financial support, personnel effort and time, job descriptions, delineation of activities between potentially overlapping disciplines (e.g., social work and nursing), sources of supervision and oversight, informatics, supplies, space, policies and procedures, determination of the capacity or number of patients that can be navigated, documentation processes, communication strategies, a quality

FIGURE 6-3	Examples of Patient Navigator Program Goals

- Optimize access to lung cancer care services for military veterans receiving health care through the XYZ Veterans Health System.
- Establish a patient-centered, value-based approach to care for patients receiving oral anticancer therapies.
- Improve community-based clinical trial participation for providers and underserved patients from the XYZ portion of ABC County, Pennsylvania.
- Develop an interprofessional clinic to improve care access, minimize treatment interruptions, promote symptom management, and decrease costs for patients with head and neck cancer.
- Promote early detection and timeliness of care for community residents with colorectal cancer.
- Implement a gero-oncology program to improve the quality of care access and address the needs of individuals aged ≥ 65 years.
- Reduce barriers to treatment through value-based approaches to care for individuals receiving multimodal therapies for rectal, gynecologic, and lung cancers.

monitoring and improvement plan, and marketing strategies for providers, staff, and patients. Ideally, to support navigation processes, a program infrastructure must be in place. Table 6-1 shows an example of a needs assessment template.

Few healthcare organizations would continue to support programs and services without evaluation based on predetermined metrics and outcome measures. Given the tremendous diversity among healthcare facilities, communities, and available resources, cancer programs have looked to metrics and outcomes based on their program goals, populations, navigation processes, and ability to collect and analyze data. However, as navigation continues, standardization of metrics and outcomes is vital so that much-needed research can be conducted to assess the contribution of navigation to quality care processes and health outcomes. The Academy of Oncology Nurse and Patient Navigators has developed 35 baseline metrics that focus on three areas: business performance/return on investment, clinical outcomes, and patient experience (Strusowski et al., 2017). It has suggested that all navigation programs, regardless of their structure, should be evaluating and monitoring these metrics. Programs may follow additional metrics based on their communities and goals.

Examples of Best Practices in Navigation Processes

The focus of navigation processes that target barriers to care may be limited to one phase of the cancer continuum, such as prevention and screening or diagnostic evaluation, or may include the entire journey through survivorship and end-of-life care. In some situations, navigation processes focus on the needs of patients with a specific cancer diagnosis. The following are examples of best practices that address barriers to care access.

TABLE 6-1 Community Needs Assessment Template Components and Examples of Data Entries

Assessment Components		Examples
Description of the community	External community patient population	Patient service area by zip codes or communities surrounding the facility Specific population within external community (e.g., refugees, people who are unhoused or unsheltered, residents of low-income housing)
	External community resources	Local, city, and state government support services (e.g., health clinics, screening programs) Patient advocacy or health-related organization support services (e.g., American Cancer Society) Public transportation system
	Internal facility patient population	Disease site–specific focus (e.g., breast or colorectal cancer) High-risk populations (e.g., recipients of multimodal therapy, individuals with no social support)
	Internal system resources	Onsite support services (e.g., social work, financial counseling, cancer rehabilitation) Disease site–specific programs and interprofessional case conferences Academic health system affiliation and telemedicine health services
Identification of disparities	Categories as identified by the American College of Surgeons Commission on Cancer	Socioeconomic status Disability Gender Immigrant or refugee status Age Geography Sexuality of gender identity Pregnant women Veterans
Identified barriers or gaps in service	Patient related	Language, health literacy, physical disability, comorbidities, rural geography, competing family or work responsibilities, poor health practices, age > 65 years
	Provider related	Older age, language, time constraints, competing priorities, location, limitations in support staff, patient hours, options for communication with providers
	System related	Location; limitations in patient hours, subspecialty physician services, communication access, staffing patterns, and support resources

(Continued on next page)

TABLE 6-1. Community Needs Assessment Template Components and Examples of Data Entries *(Continued)*

Assessment Components		Examples
Community needs assessment and process	May involve one or multiple approaches	Community health needs assessment conducted as part of the Patient Protection and Affordable Care Act (section 501(c)(3)) for hospitals to maintain tax-exempt status Subcommittee of the facility's cancer committee Working groups with community partners and facility representatives Focus groups
Community needs assessment data sources	May involve one or multiple approaches	Hospital business and cancer registry; data from the Centers for Disease Control and Prevention, the National Cancer Institute's Surveillance, Epidemiology, and End Results Program, and the American Cancer Society; and local public health data Primary data from key informants

Timeliness of Care

One of the most significant barriers to care is the amount of time it takes for people diagnosed with cancer to establish appointments in a timely manner. These individuals are often overwhelmed and unaware of how difficult it can be to schedule appointments with multiple providers and clinics (i.e., medical oncology, surgical oncology, radiation oncology, infusion center, radiology, financial counselor). This delay can often negatively impact treatment outcomes (Graboyes et al., 2023; LeClair et al., 2022). Many studies have compared oncology navigation to no navigation services for patients with different cancer diagnoses. A retrospective study revealed that implementing a patient navigator program improved the timeliness of care for patients with esophageal cancer, especially in patients undergoing complex, multimodal curative therapy. Navigation services in this study consisted of coordination of appointments, expedited and streamlined referrals, patient education, and psychosocial support (Arora et al., 2023).

Dessources et al. (2020) prospectively enrolled patients with cervical cancer stage IB1 to IVA from 2012–2016 into a navigation program with financial, medical, and psychosocial aspects of care after noticing many patients were not completing all components of primary chemoradiotherapy, resulting in worse survival. When compared to a similar cohort of patients from 1998–2008, the percentage of patients receiving five or more cycles of weekly cisplatin increased from 74% to 93%, and the median treatment time was reduced from 67 days in the non-navigated patients to 55 days in the cohort with navigation support. Approximately 95% of patients with navigator support completed primary chemoradiotherapy within 63 days, compared to

52% of non-navigated patients (Dessources et al., 2020). Navigation care can significantly improve the timeliness of recommended treatment in various settings and cancer types.

Supporting Patients With Cancer Who Are Unhoused

Individuals who are unhoused or unsheltered experience a significant lack of resources, often including healthcare coverage, basic housing, and access to food. A retrospective analysis of one academic county hospital in Seattle, Washington, showed that 17% of patients diagnosed with non-small cell lung cancer from 2012–2018 were unhoused at the time of their treatment. Those with advanced disease had a median survival of 0.58 years when compared to 1.30 years in those patients who were housed. This significant inequity in outcomes is likely caused by delays in biopsies, missed appointments, and other factors (Concannon et al., 2020).

Despite the rise in interest in health equity initiatives, people who are unhoused are rarely included in clinical trials or abstracts (Mayo et al., 2023), and studies are limited as to the impact that oncology navigation can have in improving their access to care and decreasing their barriers to treatment. Only four studies were identified as evaluating the number of unhoused individuals diagnosed with cancer and how oncology navigation models affected their care from 2000–2021 (Carmichael et al., 2023).

At Rhode Island Hospital, oncology navigators meet with patients in person and then flag high-risk patients. Navigators keep track of when patients are admitted so they can meet with them in person and identify any barriers to attending their next appointment. Using patient navigators for those with complex cancers, such as pancreatic cancer in patients who are unhoused and recommended to have surgery, can help them keep appointments and attain clearance for surgery (Louie et al., 2021).

In addition to improving access and adherence to cancer treatments, it is likely that oncology navigation services will positively impact access to cancer screenings. Mortality from lung cancer in unhoused individuals is double that of the general population. In Boston, Massachusetts, patients are being randomized to standard of care versus standard of care plus navigation services to include assistance in making and attending appointments, lung cancer education, and smoking cessation support (Baggett et al., 2022). Services such as these are the cornerstone of oncology navigation and can significantly impact patient outcomes.

Boosting Black Population Clinical Trial Participation

The University of Southern California Norris Comprehensive Cancer Center, a National Cancer Institute–designated cancer center and part of an integrated health system, provides tertiary and quaternary services to several Los Angeles communities. However, in the South Central Los Angeles community, where 64% of the patients diagnosed with cancer are Black, relatively few sought treatment from the cancer center—a contributing factor to existing concerns about minority participation in oncology clinical trials (Holmes et al., 2012). Across the country, several well-documented barriers limit Black participation in oncology clinical trials, including fears about research, mistrust of healthcare providers, socioeconomic factors, competing family and work priorities, transportation issues, and communication challenges. In addition, provider and system barriers that impede clinical trial participation include limited awareness of available trials, lack of appropriate trials or access to trials, restrictive eligibility criteria, inadequate resources to support clinical trial conduct, and competing priorities for providers and health systems (ACS Cancer Action Network, 2018).

The Norris Comprehensive Cancer Center developed a program to address disparities and barriers to Black women's participation in breast cancer trials. The cancer center formed a partnership with a nonprofit professional organization with more than 250 Black physician members. Collaborative relationships were established with South Central Los Angeles community-based practices, including breast and surgical oncology, medical oncology, and a Los Angeles Department of Public Health Administration ambulatory center. The cornerstone of this program was the implementation of an oncology nurse navigator (ONN) role that combined processes used by oncology research nurses and processes for outreach to community physicians and patients (Holmes et al., 2012). ONNs made weekly visits to the community physician practices to share information about available trials, receive and coordinate referrals, and provide culturally sensitive patient education about breast cancer and treatment approaches, including clinical trial options. ONNs also worked with physicians to confirm patient eligibility and obtain informed consent. Assistance was provided to coordinate and schedule appointments and procedures, including accompanying patients, if needed, who were unfamiliar with their surroundings or especially anxious. ONNs assessed and addressed specific patient barriers, such as transportation, insurance, and medication co-pays. Emphasis was placed on establishing relationships with patients and providers, serving as a patient advocate, and promoting clinical trials. ONNs were also responsible for trial conduct activities, such as toxicity assessment, symptom management, specimen procurement, and data collection (Holmes et al., 2012).

Over two years, 59 of the 132 screened Black women were found to be eligible for breast cancer trial participation. Of the eligible patients, 51 (86%) were ultimately enrolled in one or more trials; eight declined to participate. Accrual for Black women rose from 3% at baseline to 7% at the time of evaluation. This outcome was viewed as a positive, considering that the American adult accrual rate for all demographic groups had remained at approximately 3% for many years (Nass et al., 2010). Patient navigators can assist in increasing clinical trial accruals by educating prospective patients and identifying eligible patients to study coordinators. When patients are approached and offered to enroll in a clinical trial, approximately 50% of the time, they accept. Yet, one survey showed that only 8.9% of patients were ever invited to participate in a clinical trial due to barriers including age, lower socioeconomic status, living in areas without clinical trials being offered, and complex eligibility criteria (National Cancer Institute, 2022).

Summary

The inclusion of navigation processes in oncology payment reform and accreditation requirements demonstrates recognition by government and national quality programs of the importance of assisting patients through a fragmented healthcare system. Conducting a community needs assessment is essential for identifying patients' barriers to accessing oncology care. A needs assessment should consider both external and internal factors to provide a comprehensive understanding of the needs, gaps, and available resources within the community.

From this analysis, navigation program goals and metrics can be established, with decisions on whether to use clinical, non-clinical, or a combination of personnel guided by the findings. Continuous monitoring and reassessment are necessary to maintain program sustainability, identify best practices, and ensure that patients receive timely access to quality care.

The author would like to acknowledge Cindy Stern, RN, MSN, CCRP, for her contribution to this chapter that remains unchanged from the previous edition of this book.

References

Aflague, T.F., Hammond, K., Delos Reyes, B., Rios, D., De Leon, E., Leon Guerrero, R.T., & Esquivel, M.K. (2023). Barriers, facilitators, and strategies for developing a culturally informed lifestyle intervention for Native Hawaiian, CHamoru, and Filipino breast cancer survivors: Mixed-methods findings from focus group participants. *International Journal of Environmental Research and Public Health*, 20(12), 6075. https://doi.org/10.3390/ijerph20126075

Agency for Healthcare Research and Quality. (2023). *2023 national healthcare quality and disparities report.* https://www.ahrq.gov/research/findings/nhqrdr/index.html

Akinkugbe, A.A., Garcia, D.T., Brickhouse, T.H., & Mosavel, M. (2020). Lifestyle risk factor related disparities in oral cancer examination in the U.S.: A population-based cross-sectional study. *BMC Public Health*, 20(1), 153. https://doi.org/10.1186/s12889-020-8247-2

American Cancer Society Cancer Action Network. (2018). *Barriers to patient enrollment in therapeutic clinical trials for cancer: A landscape report.* https://www.fightcancer.org/sites/default/files/National%20Documents/Clinical-Trials-Landscape-Report.pdf

American College of Surgeons. (n.d.). *About the National Cancer Database.* https://www.facs.org/quality-programs/cancer-programs/national-cancer-database/about

American College of Surgeons. (2023). *Optimal resources for breast care 2024 standards.* https://accreditation.facs.org/accreditationdocuments/NAPBC/Standards/Optimal_Resources_for_Breast_Care_2024.pdf

American College of Surgeons Commission on Cancer. (2012). *Cancer program standards 2012: Ensuring patient-centered care* (v.1.2.1). https://apos-society.org/wp-content/uploads/2016/06/CoCStandards.pdf

American College of Surgeons Commission on Cancer. (2024). *Optimal resources for cancer care 2020.* https://www.facs.org/quality-programs/cancer/coc/2020-standards

Antonacci, G., Reed, J.E., Lennox, L., & Barlow, J. (2018). The use of process mapping in healthcare quality improvement projects. *Health Service Management Research*, 31(2), 74–84. https://doi.org/10.1177/0951484818770411

Arora, N., Lo, M., Hanna, N.M., Pereira, J., Digby, G., Bechara, R., Merchant, S.J., ... Chung, W. (2023). Influence of a patient navigation program on timeliness of care in patients with esophageal cancer. *Cancer Medicine, 12*(10), 11907–11914. https://doi.org/10.1002/cam4.5882

Baggett, T.P., Teixeira, J.B., Rodriguez, E.C., Anandakugan, N., Sporn, N., Chang, Y., ... Rigotti, N.A. (2022). Patient navigation to promote lung cancer screening in a community health center for people experiencing homelessness: Protocol for a pragmatic randomized controlled trial. *Contemporary Clinical Trials, 113*, 106666. https://doi.org/10.1016/j.cct.2021.106666

Carethers, J.M., Sengupta, R., Blakey, R., Ribas, A., & D'Souza, G. (2020). Disparities in cancer prevention in the COVID-19 era. *Cancer Prevention Research, 13*(11), 893–896. https://doi.org/10.1158/1940-6207.CAPR-20-0447

Carmichael, C., Smith, L., Aldasoro, E., Gil Salmerón, A., Alhambra-Borrás, T., Doñate-Martínez, A., ... Grabovac, I. (2023). Exploring the application of the navigation model with people experiencing homelessness: A scoping review. *Journal of Social Distress and Homelessness, 32*(2), 352–366. https://doi.org/10.1080/10530789.2021.2021363

Carnahan, L.R., Abdelrahim, R., Ferrans, C.E., Rizzo, G.R., Molina, Y., & Handler, A. (2021). Rural cancer disparities: Understanding implications for breast and cervical cancer diagnoses. *Clinical Journal of Oncology Nursing, 25*(Suppl. 1), 10–16. https://doi.org/10.1188/21.CJON.S1.10-16

Centers for Medicare and Medicaid Innovation. (2024). *Enhancing oncology model (EOM): 2024 health equity plan guide* (V.2). https://www.cms.gov/priorities/innovation/media/document/eom-health-equity-plan

Centers for Medicare and Medicaid Services. (2022). *The enhancing oncology model (EOM): Request for applications*. https://www.cms.gov/priorities/innovation/media/document/eom-rfa

Chan, R.J., Milch, V.E., Crawford-Williams, F., Agbejule, O.A.R., Joseph, R., Johal, J., ... Hart, N.H. (2023). Patient navigation across the cancer care continuum: An overview of systematic reviews and emerging literature. *CA: A Cancer Journal for Clinicians, 73*(6), 565–589. https://doi.org/10.3322/caac.21788

Collins, S. (2024, January 17). *2024—First year the US expects more than 2M new cases of cancer*. https://www.cancer.org/research/acs-research-news/facts-and-figures-2024.html

Concannon, K.F., Thayer, J.H., Wu, Q.V., Jenkins, I.C., Baik, C.S., & Linden, H.M. (2020). Outcomes among homeless patients with non-small-cell lung cancer: A county hospital experience. *JCO Oncology Practice, 16*(9), e1004–e1014. https://doi.org/10.1200/jop.19.00694

Dessources, K., Hari, A., Pineda, E., Amneus, M.W., Sinno, A.K., & Holschneider, C.H. (2020). Socially determined cervical cancer care navigation: An effective step toward health care equity and care optimization. *Cancer, 126*(23), 5060–5068. https://doi.org/10.1002/cncr.33124

Graboyes, E.M., Chappell, M., Duckett, K.A., Sterba, K., Halbert, C.H., Hill, E.G., ... Calhoun, E. (2023). Patient navigation for timely, guideline-adherent adjuvant therapy for head and neck cancer: A national landscape analysis. *Journal of the National Comprehensive Cancer Network, 21*(12), 1251–1259. https://doi.org/10.6004/jnccn.2023.7061

Holmes, D.R., Major, J., Lyonga, D.E., Alleyne, R.S., & Clayton, S.M. (2012). Increasing minority patient participation in cancer clinical trials using oncology nurse navigation. *American Journal of Surgery, 203*(4), 415–422. https://doi.org/10.1016/j.amjsurg.2011.02.005

Joseph, K.-A. (2024). Does cancer accreditation designation mean better quality care and long-term oncological outcomes? *Annals of Surgical Oncology, 31*(5), 2804–2805. https://doi.org/10.1245/s10434-024-14962-1

Kamen, C.S., Dizon, D.S., Fung, C., Pratt-Chapman, M.L., Agulnik, M., Fashoyin-Aje, L.A., ... Maingi, S. (2023). State of cancer care in America: Achieving cancer health equity among sexual and gender minority communities. *JCO Oncology Practice, 19*(11), 959–966. https://doi.org/10.1200/op.23.00435

Katchur, K., Reed, R., & Coyle, B. (2018). Hitting the mark. *Oncology Issues, 33*(1), 36–41. https://doi.org/10.1080/10453356.2018.1400872

Kwok, C., Degen, C., Moradi, N., & Stacey, D. (2022). Nurse-led telehealth interventions for symptom management in patients with cancer receiving systemic or radiation therapy: A systematic review and meta-analysis. *Supportive Care in Cancer, 30*(9), 7119–7132. https://doi.org/10.1007/s00520-022-07052-z

LeClair, A.M., Battaglia, T.A., Casanova, N.L., Haas, J.S., Freund, K.M., Moy, B., ... Lemon, S.C. (2022). Assessment of patient navigation programs for breast cancer patients across the city of Boston. *Supportive Care in Cancer, 30*(3), 2435–2443. https://doi.org/10.1007/s00520-021-06675-y

Lepore, S.J., Rincon, M.A., Buzaglo, J., Golant, M., Lieberman, M.A., Bass, S.B., & Chambers, S. (2018). Digital literacy linked to engagement and psychological benefits among breast cancer survivors in Internet-based peer support groups. *European Journal of Cancer Care, 28*(4), e13134. https://doi.org/10.1111/ecc.13134

Louie, A.D., Nwaiwu, C.A., Rozenberg, J., Banerjee, D., Lee, G.J., Senthoor, D., & Miner, T.J. (2021). Providing appropriate pancreatic cancer care for people experiencing homelessness: A surgical perspective. *ASCO Educational Book, 41.* https://doi.org/10.1200/EDBK_100027

Mayo, Z.S., Campbell, S.R., Shah, C.S., Weleff, J., & Kilic, S.S. (2023). Improving treatment interventions and cancer outcomes in persons experiencing homelessness: A population underrepresented in equity initiatives. *International Journal of Radiation Oncology, Biology, Physics, 115*(2), 302–304. https://doi.org/10.1016/j.ijrobp.2022.09.059

Misra, S., Fan, J., Yanala, U., & Are, C. (2019). The value of Commission on Cancer accreditation: Improving survival outcomes by enhancing compliance with quality measures. *Annals of Surgical Oncology, 26*(6), 1585–1587. https://doi.org/10.1245/s10434-019-07335-6

Nass, S.J., Moses, H.L., & Mendelsohn, J. (Eds.). (2010). *A national cancer clinical trials system for the 21st century: Reinvigorating the NCI Cooperative Group Program.* https://doi.org/10.17226/12879

National Cancer Institute. (2022). Clinical trial participation among US adults. *Hints Brief, 48.* https://hints.cancer.gov/docs/Briefs/HINTS_Brief_48.pdf

National Cancer Institute. (2024, March 21). *Cancer disparities.* https://www.cancer.gov/about-cancer/understanding/disparities

Nelson, H.D., Cantor, A., Wagner, J., Jungbauer, R., Fu, R., Kondo, K., ... Quiñones, A. (2020). Effectiveness of patient navigation to increase cancer screening in populations adversely affected by health disparities: A meta-analysis. *Journal of General Internal Medicine, 35*(10), 3026–3035. https://doi.org/10.1007/s11606-020-06020-9

Paterson, C., Bacon, R., Dwyer, R., Morrison, K.S., Toohey, K., O'Dea, A., ... Hayes, S.C. (2020). The role of telehealth during the COVID-19 pandemic across the interdisciplinary cancer team: Implications for practice. *Seminars in Oncology Nursing, 36*(6), 151090. https://doi.org/10.1016/j.soncn.2020.151090

Patlak, M., Trang, C., & Nass, S.J. (2018). *Establishing effective patient navigation programs in oncology: Proceedings of a workshop.* National Academies Press. https://doi.org/10.17226/25073

Pratt-Chapman, M., & Willis, A. (2013). Community cancer center administration and support for navigation services. *Seminars in Oncology Nursing, 29*(2), 141–148. https://doi.org/10.1016/j.soncn.2013.02.009

Russell, T.A., & Ko, C. (2023). History and role of quality accreditation. *Clinics in Colon and Rectal Surgery, 36*(4), 279–284. https://doi.org/10.1055/s-0043-1761592

Schatz, A.A., Chambers, S., Wartman, G.C., Lacasse, L.A., Denlinger, C.S., Hobbs, K.M., ... Winn, R.A. (2023). Advancing more equitable care through the development of a Health Equity Report Card. *Journal of the National Comprehensive Cancer Network, 21*(2), 117–124.e3. https://doi.org/10.6004/jnccn.2023.7003

Siegel, R.L., Giaquinto, A.N., & Jemal, A. (2024). Cancer statistics, 2024. *CA: A Cancer Journal for Clinicians, 74*(1), 12–49. https://doi.org/10.3322/caac.21820

Soto-Perez-de-Celis, E., Chavarri-Guerra, Y., Ramos-Lopez, W.A., Alcalde-Castro, J., Covarrubias-Gomez, A., Navarro-Lara, Á., ... Goss, P.E. (2021). Patient navigation to improve early access to supportive care for patients with advanced cancer in resource-limited settings: A randomized controlled trial. *Oncologist, 26*(2), 157–164. https://doi.org/10.1002/onco.13599

Strusowski, T., Sein, E., Johnston, D., Gentry, S., Bellomo, C., Brown, E., ... Messier, N. (2017). Standardized evidence-based oncology navigation metrics for all models: A powerful tool in assessing the value and impact of navigation programs. *Journal of Oncology Navigation and Survivorship, 8*(5), 220–237.

https://www.researchgate.net/publication/326632056_Standardized_Evidence-Based_Oncology_Navigation_Metrics_for_All_Models_A_Powerful_Tool_in_Assessing_the_Value_and_Impact_of_Navigation_Programs/link/5b59d2540f7e9bc79a666de0/download?_tp=eyJjb250ZXh0Ijp7ImZpcnN0UGFnZSI6InB1YmxpY2F0aW9uIiwicGFnZSI6InB1YmxpY2F0aW9uIn19

Subica, A.M., & Brown, B.J. (2020). Addressing health disparities through deliberative methods: Citizens' panels for health equity. *American Journal Public Health, 110*(2), 116–173. https://doi.org/10.2105/AJPH.2019.305450

U.S. House of Representatives. (2010, May 1). *Compilation of Patient Protection and Affordable Care Act.* https://housedocs.house.gov/energycommerce/ppacacon.pdf

CHAPTER 7

Measuring Nurse-Led Patient Outcomes

Tricia Strusowski, MS, RN, Stephanie Bonfilio, MSN, RN, OCN®, ONN-CG, and Chris Gosselin, MBA, BSN, RN

> **KEY TOPICS**
> navigation metrics, return on investment, value-based models

Overview

Multisystem and single institutional research have consistently demonstrated the value of navigation interventions in patient and provider satisfaction, improving treatment adherence, securing patient loyalty, and reducing healthcare spending and penalties through decreased use of emergency departments and hospital readmissions. These interventions, the result of outcomes data developed for more than a century, have led to the creation of the standards, roles, and definitions that guide oncology nurse navigation in its present state.

The first record of a nurse using outcomes data to improve patient care can be traced back to Florence Nightingale's work in the late 1840s. However, it was not until the 1970s that the U.S. Department of Health and Human Services began to use metrics in earnest to improve patient access to care and lower healthcare costs (Gormley et al., 2024).

Another 20 years passed until, in 1994, the American Nurses Association launched the Nursing Safety and Quality Initiative to examine factors and outcomes related to the nursing process, known as *nursing-sensitive outcomes*. This idea of nursing-sensitive outcomes would be further refined over the next 30 years, leading to beneficial metrics that would help to develop standards for oncology navigation. For example, between 2001 and 2002, the Oncology Nursing Society (ONS) Advanced Practice Nurse Retreat Project Team generated the first list of nursing-sensitive outcomes, evaluating nursing interventions related to patients (e.g., symptom management, financial impact of care) and healthcare professionals (Visintini & Palese, 2023). In 2003, ONS defined nursing-sensitive outcomes directly related to independent nursing care or nursing interventions provided as part of the care team.

The challenges inherent in using standardized metrics comparatively are ongoing issues in nursing research, such as having data collection inconsistencies and determining which outcomes result from independent or collaborative nursing interventions (Visintini & Palese, 2023).

This chapter will review the development of oncology navigation standards and role definitions, competencies, and defined metrics. It will explain how national accreditation and value-based care models can be used when selecting metrics to measure navigation services, describe the Centers for Medicare and Medicaid Services (CMS) Principal Illness Navigation (PIN) reimbursement codes, and identify methods for using standardized metrics to measure patient experience, clinical outcomes, and return on investment (ROI).

Establishing Navigation Metrics

Although the foundational work of oncology navigation began in the 1990s, it was not until 2016 that the Academy of Oncology Nurse and Patient Navigators (AONN+) created a multidisciplinary task force to establish navigation metrics. Contributing publications and documentation leading to the establishment of the AONN+ metrics include the following:

- ONS's *Oncology Nurse Navigator Competencies*
- AONN+ Knowledge Domains
- American Cancer Society (ACS) National Navigation Roundtable patient navigation job roles
- George Washington Cancer Center Patient Navigation Core Competencies

The AONN+ metrics task force also reviews national oncology standards, such as the American College of Surgeons Commission on Cancer (ACoS CoC) and the National Accreditation Program for Breast Centers, value-based cancer care initiatives, and Quality Oncology Practice Initiatives (QOPI) certification. The extensive literature review supported the development of the navigation metrics. See Table 7-1 for information on core competencies, knowledge domains, and practice standards for oncology navigation.

American College of Surgeons Commission on Cancer Standards

ACoS CoC is a consortium of professional organizations dedicated to improving the survival and quality of life of patients with cancer through standard setting, prevention, research, education, and monitoring of comprehensive quality of care. Many ACoS CoC standards can be used to support the navigator's role and program enhancement through metrics. For example, navigators can partner with providers or support service staff on quality improvement initiatives described in the following (ACoS CoC, 2024):

- *Standard 7.1: Accountability and Quality Improvement Measures*
- *Standard 7.2: Monitoring Concordance with Evidence-Based Guidelines*
- *Standard 7.3: Quality Improvement Initiative*

TABLE 7-1	Core Competencies and Practice Standards
National Organization	**Associated Websites**
Academy of Oncology Nurse and Patient Navigators Knowledge Domains	www.jons-online.com/issues/2017/may-2017-vol-9-no-5/1623:value-impact-of-navigation-programs https://aonnonline.org/toolkits
American Cancer Society National Navigation Roundtable	https://navigationroundtable.org/wp-content/uploads/Workforce-Development-Job-Performance-Behaviors.pdf
Association of Oncology Social Work Scope of Practice in Oncology Social Work	https://aosw.org/resources/scope-and-standards-of-practice
George Washington Cancer Center Patient Navigation Core Competencies	www.jons-online.com/issues/2015/april-2015-vol-6-no-2/1320-core-competencies-for-oncology-patient-navigators https://link.springer.com/article/10.1007/s00520-019-04739-8/tables/1
National Association of Social Workers Practice Standards and Guidelines	www.socialworkers.org/Practice/Practice-Standards-Guidelines
Oncology Nursing Society Competencies	www.ons.org/career-development/competencies
Professional Oncology Navigation Taskforce *Oncology Navigation Standards of Professional Practice*	www.jons-online.com/issues/2022/march-2022-vol-13-no-3/4399-oncology-navigation-standards-of-professional-practice

National Accreditation Program for Breast Centers

The National Accreditation Program for Breast Centers provides the structure and resources needed to develop, evaluate, and facilitate interprofessional, integrated, and comprehensive breast cancer services. Accredited breast cancer programs are expected to meet or exceed national benchmarks. Even if an organization is not seeking accreditation, oncology navigators can use these national benchmarks to select metrics measuring the effect of navigation on patients with breast cancer. For example, *Standard 5.8: Patient Navigation* specifies the need for patients to have a professional navigator (clinical or non-clinical) from diagnosis and throughout the cancer journey. The navigation process must also accomplish the following (ACoS, 2024):

- Facilitate timely transitions between diagnosis, surgical intervention, and medical oncology.

- Address survivorship and surveillance throughout the treatment phase of care.
- Alert the radiology team if chemotherapy is not initiated or if it is completed early.

Alternative Payment Models

Alternative payment models (APMs) provide financial incentives to practices that demonstrate high-quality and cost-efficient care (Shaughnessy et al., 2022). These models can apply to a specific clinical condition, care episode, or population.

Value-Based Payment Model

The Centers for Medicare and Medicaid Innovation's Enhancing Oncology Model (EOM), which replaced the Oncology Care Model, is a five-year voluntary program designed to improve oncology care and reduce costs through payment incentives and required quality improvement activities. EOM aims to improve care coordination and patient health outcomes while holding oncology practices accountable for the total cost of care. Requirements related to oncology navigation include connecting patients to support services and community resources and evaluating and addressing health-related social needs, such as food insecurities, housing instability, financial concerns, and transportation issues (CMS & Centers for Medicare and Medicaid Innovation, 2024).

Merit-Based Payment Model

On January 1, 2017, Medicare's legacy quality reporting programs were consolidated and streamlined into the Merit-Based Incentive Payment System (MIPS). This consolidation reduced the aggregate financial penalties physicians faced and provided more significant potential for bonus payments. Physicians and practices can obtain financial benefits based on the quality of care they deliver (American Medical Association, 2023).

Although navigation is not a merit-based requirement, oncology navigators have demonstrated improvements in quality-of-care delivery, including reduced time to treatment, increased adherence to treatment, and a positive impact on quality metrics (e.g., hospital readmissions, emergency department visits) (Chan et al., 2023; Chen et al., 2024).

Patient-Centered Payment Model

Created in 2015 and updated in 2018, the American Society of Clinical Oncology's Patient-Centered Oncology Payment model details care delivery requirements related to navigation interventions. Specifically, "all patients are provided navigation for support services and community resources specific to the practice patient population, on-site psychosocial distress screening is performed, and referral for the provision of psychosocial care is provided as needed" (Ward et al., 2020, p. 266). Navigation-specific metrics, such as the number of patients referred to psychosocial support services, could inform documentation needed for practices to meet requirements.

Each of these examples demonstrates how oncology navigation can be leveraged to support oncology practices and potentially be used to indicate ROI.

Centers for Medicare and Medicaid Principal Illness Navigation Billing Codes

In January 2024, CMS released new billing codes for reimbursement of navigation interventions. The G-codes (CMS codes used in billing for non-physician services and quality reporting) represent the culmination of years of research showing the benefits of oncology navigation. PIN G-codes can be used for navigation services performed by clinical and non-clinical personnel. CMS provision of services for PIN includes the following (American Society of Clinical Oncology, 2024; Pratt-Chapman et al., 2024):
- Providing a person-centered assessment
- Identifying or referring patient (and caregiver or family) to appropriate supportive services
- Coordinating with practitioner, home, and community-based care
- Providing health education
- Building patient self-advocacy skills
- Navigating healthcare access and the health system
- Facilitating behavioral change as necessary for meeting diagnosis and treatment goals
- Facilitating and providing social and emotional support
- Leveraging knowledge of the condition or lived experience when applicable to provide support, mentorship, or inspiration to meet treatment goals

CMS describes PIN services as navigation performed by certified or trained personnel as part of the treatment plan for one serious, high-risk disease that is expected to last at least three months and places the patient at significant risk of hospitalization or nursing home placement, acute exacerbation/decompensation, functional decline, or death. The condition should require the development, monitoring, or revision of a disease-specific care plan. It also may require frequent adjustments in the medication or treatment regimen or substantial assistance from a caregiver (American Society of Clinical Oncology, 2024).

Continued Development and Application of Navigation Metrics

In 2017, AONN+ announced the 35 evidence-based navigation metrics, applying to navigation programs regardless of the setting or navigation model used. Metrics are based on the eight certification domains and are divided into three main categories: patient experience, clinical outcomes, and business performance (Johnston & Strusowski, 2018).

The release of standardized metrics changed the landscape of navigation, with institutions looking to structure their programs around these core metrics but questioning how to standardize data collection to optimize program growth and outcomes. Knowing this, a team of navigation experts from AONN+, ACS, and Chartis, a national consulting company, launched a multisite exploratory study with the primary objective of structuring metrics implementation, validating navigation metrics, identifying barriers to measurement, and determining how to overcome these barriers (AONN+, 2020). A secondary objective was to develop and release a tool kit reporting best practices and lessons learned during this study. The institutional review board–approved research was completed in 2018, and in August 2020, AONN+ and ACS released the *Navigation Metrics Toolkit* (AONN+, 2020; see Chapter 18).

The *Navigation Metrics Toolkit* guides navigation programs through metric implementation, focusing on the 10 navigation metrics evaluated in the study (AONN+, 2020):
- Barriers to care
- Time from diagnosis to initial treatment
- Navigation caseload
- Number of navigated patients readmitted to the hospital at 30, 60, and 90 days
- Psychosocial distress screening
- Social support referrals
- Palliative care referrals
- Identifying patient learning style preference
- Navigation knowledge at the time of orientation
- Patient experience and satisfaction with care

National Navigation Roundtable Survey

In the late 2010s, as significant progress was made nationally to establish measurable outcomes and assess the value of oncology navigators, organizations still faced challenges in collecting metrics to sustain navigation programs. The ACS's National Navigation Roundtable supports the growth of oncology navigation by using work conducted across multiple organizations to move the field forward. In 2019, the National Navigation Roundtable Evidence-Based Promising Practices Task Group conducted a survey of 38 items, including program characteristics, respondent characteristics, program data collection, and navigation metric questions that incorporated perceived difficulty in measuring specific items. Approximately 750 navigators and administrators responded, with 72% indicating that they tracked some metrics for their program. However, only 22% of respondents admitted to any metrics tracking that proved financially beneficial or offered any data regarding ROI (Battaglia et al., 2022).

Additionally, the survey revealed several barriers to collecting and reporting navigation metrics, including time constraints, technology challenges, a lack of navigator knowledge of technology solutions and software, and minimal to no technology support (see Figure 7-1).

Electronic health records (EHRs) may not offer easy navigation metrics tracking, requiring navigators and administrators to use additional software or Excel spread-

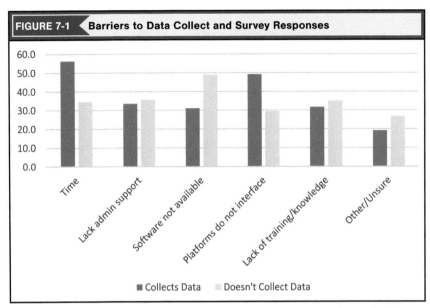

Note. From "Barriers and Opportunities to Measuring Oncology Patient Navigation Impact: Results From the National Navigation Roundtable Survey," by T.A. Battaglia, L. Fleisher, A.J. Dwyer, D.E. Wiatrek, K.J. Wells, P. Wightman, ... E. Calhoun, 2022, *Cancer, 128*(Suppl. 13), p. 2573. Copyright 2022 by the authors. Reprinted with permission from T.A. Battaglia.

sheets. Approximately 60% of survey respondents noted they used at least two or more databases to collect and manage data; however, only half reported using the collected data to create reports. Organizations participating in oncology accreditation programs were more likely to collect and report on outcomes data across the care continuum (Battaglia et al., 2022).

Navigation Metrics Implementation

Small steps, added together, can lead to sizeable programmatic growth and accomplishments. An essential first step in applying navigation metrics is determining what to track. A new navigation program will likely face different implementation challenges than an established one. Regardless of the stage of development, program size, navigation structure, or institution type, the following questions can help navigation program organizers select realistic, attainable, and valuable metrics for their program and healthcare facilities.

What Is Essential to the Key Stakeholders?

Showing evident value contributing to overall program goals is key to securing buy-in for a navigation program. For example, if an oncology program seeks to decrease hospital admissions for patients with cancer or increase patient experience scores, it is helpful to demonstrate how navigators can significantly impact these efforts. These goals are directly linked to standardized navigation metrics that can be implemented to help with navigation program sustainability.

What Initial Metrics Seem to Be the Most Achievable?

A small win is important for building ongoing success. Is there a simple metric to track that will allow the team to report navigation-specific data to senior leaders to work on program buy-in? For example, a navigation program may choose to measure referrals to its navigators or measure referrals from its navigators to support services and resources.

The AONN+ Navigation Metrics Toolkit Institutional Review Board study identified five core metrics that directly correlate to the role of oncology navigators: barriers to care, navigator interventions, navigation caseloads, navigator knowledge at the time of orientation, and psychosocial distress screening (AONN+, 2020; see Table 7-2). Understanding these metrics can assist the navigation team and key stakeholders

TABLE 7-2. Core Navigation Metrics

Metric	Measurement and Definition
Barriers to care	The number and list of specific barriers to care identified by the navigator per month Barriers to care definition: obstacles that prevent a patient with cancer from accessing care, services, resources, and support
Navigator interventions	The number of specific referrals or interventions offered to navigated patients per month Intervention definition: the act of intervening, interfering, or interceding with the intent of modifying the outcome
Navigation caseloads	The number of new cases, open cases, and closed cases navigated per month New cases definition: new patient cases referred to the navigation program per month Open cases definition: patient cases that remain open per month Closed cases definition: the number of patient cases closed per month; formal closing of a patient case from the navigation program
Navigator knowledge at the time of orientation	Percentage of new hires that have completed institutionally developed navigator core competencies
Psychosocial distress screening	The number of navigated patients per month who received psychosocial distress screening with a validated tool at a pivotal medical visit Pivotal medical visit definition: period of high distress for the patient when psychosocial assessment should be completed Validated tool examples: Functional Assessment of Cancer Therapy–General National Comprehensive Cancer Network Distress Thermometer

Note. Based on information from Academy of Oncology Nurse and Patient Navigators, 2020.

in improving care delivery. It is important to start tracking one or two measures and increase tracking sequentially. The five core metrics support value-based cancer care and national oncology standards, and are essential tools to guide navigation programs regardless of size, model, or setting (AONN+, 2020).

Tracking navigator caseloads is key to measuring the navigation program's growth and development. These data can be used to establish a standard for determining when to close a patient case and how long cases remain open for different disease sites.

Examining the number of barriers per patient and the most commonly assessed barriers based on disease site or facility can help identify resource needs and areas of focus for navigator interventions. Quantifying barriers to care can contribute to a level of individual patient acuity, adding value to the caseload metric. Nurses and navigation personnel are precious resources, so determining if there are ways to offload or automate processes to support patients through some of the more common barriers is important, and to do that, barriers must be assessed. Evaluating the number of navigator interventions and how these are associated with the barriers assessed can help teams determine program and staffing needs as well as productivity measurements. Psychosocial distress screening can be a high priority for organizations. Caring for the patient as a whole, understanding their goals and barriers, and providing resources to help them manage are central to patient-centered care (Johnston et al., 2017).

Establishing and maintaining a standard for navigator competency ensures structure and standardization among the internal navigator team. Using evidence-based and nationally recognized navigator standards and competencies allows programs to measure their standards against others nationwide. It also creates a foundation for growth for individual navigators and overall programs (AONN+, 2020).

How Will the Data Be Collected?

Data collection should be tailored to an organization's available resources. The simplest way to capture the data is through documentation already being performed within discrete fields in the EHR, as this helps ensure the data move with less chance of intentional or unintentional manipulation. Intentional manipulation involves making specific changes to data to change outcomes, whereas unintentional manipulation happens when pieces of data get deleted or misaligned. Many healthcare systems have moved to this type of documentation system; however, the exact type varies. Even still, most EHRs can capture discrete data fields that can later be used for creating reports. This data-capturing technique allows navigators to minimize or eliminate duplicate documentation to capture and report the identified metrics. This frequently requires help and support from information system teams; however, even with minimal support and less-than-optimal EHRs, navigators can find ways to document and track their data. Although Excel files are not ideal, and significant effort must go into verifying Health Insurance Portability and Accountability Act (more commonly known as HIPAA) adherence, this is an option to capture the information needed for metrics tracking.

Metrics must be validated and have clear definitions regardless of the method used. This clarity helps team members understand why they are documenting distinctive items in a specific way and helps ensure that documentation is uniform and accurate. Although this can be time consuming, it will create building blocks for additional metrics. For collecting and reporting metrics outcomes, navigators can use the resources available and discussed in this chapter, as well as different internal teams and departments that may have performed similar methodologies, outside hospitals, and navigation programs. It is integral to work with billing and coding departments, information systems teams, quality departments, tumor registries, and others within an organization to optimize metric collection without duplication of effort.

Once these core metrics are captured, it is important to expand the metric collection to support additional growth, such as allocating additional staffing resources, improving patient outcomes, minimizing readmission rates, and detailing any additional information the organization needs for accreditation or designation status.

How Will the Information Be Reported, and Who Will It Be Shared With?

The answer to this question depends on how the data are collected. If navigators use an EHR for documentation and data collection, reports can be created within these systems with the help of information systems. If using a program such as Excel, reports can also be generated to develop graphs and visuals related to navigation metrics.

It is integral to share metrics and outcomes with the navigation team to identify performance improvement opportunities that may become evident. Having transparent conversations and including the team in the metrics collecting and reporting processes allows for additional insight from those on the front lines of the navigation program. Furthermore, metrics must be reported to administrative partners, senior leadership, and key stakeholders. Significant is the need to show metrics related to ROI (e.g., readmission rates, number of no-shows, charge captures) and patient experiences (e.g., palliative care referrals, diagnosis to treatment, patient satisfaction and experience scores). Sharing these data supports ongoing growth and program improvement and, more importantly, builds and fosters overall buy-in to the navigation program.

What Stakeholders Can Help Inform Navigation Programs?

The most important stakeholders in any organization are the patients. Programs can glean significant insights by engaging with patient advisory boards, community leaders, and staff members. Building reports and data to support patients and staff will help program leaders understand when, where, and what patients will get the most benefit of support through navigation. Additional stakeholders, such as cancer center directors, the operations team, and healthcare providers, can inform a navigation program.

How Can Return on Investment Metrics Be Collected and Used?

Measuring ROI can be challenging, but it is achievable. A simple way to obtain ROI is by determining cost versus revenue. However, navigation historically has not been a billable service. Using the number of patients as a measurement, examples of

ROI metrics identified in the *Navigation Metrics Toolkit* include the following (Johnston et al., 2017):
- Referred for diagnostic workup after abnormal screening
- Completed diagnostic workup
- Adhered to institutional treatment pathways
- Received patient education
- Referred to revenue-generating support services
- Sought care outside the diagnosing institution (outmigration)
- Visited the emergency department
- Readmitted to hospital

The average rate of hospital readmission for patients with cancer can be as high as 30% (Stabellini et al., 2023). Navigators and administrators can analyze how a navigation program can decrease this rate, leading to healthcare savings.

Adherence is also another beneficial way to evaluate ROI. The following questions can help identify metrics applicable to barriers within an organization:
- Are patients more or less likely to attend treatment with or without a navigator?
- How likely are patients to transition to another organization because they do not feel they have someone who cares and connects with them?
- How likely will patients tell the provider in their 20-minute appointment slot that they cannot afford gas to come to their appointments?

Kline et al. (2019) examined five institutions that found unique ways to evaluate navigator interventions, demonstrating tangible results for patients and the institutions (see Table 7-3). Commonalities across institutions showed increased satisfaction in patients and members of the healthcare team. Metrics demonstrating decreased hospitalizations and acute care visits were equated with revenue by saving on penalties and healthcare spending (e.g., measuring the number of patients treated at the diagnosing facility, decreases in no-show rates, and patient outcomes). One institute noted improved patient survival, leading researchers to conclude that oncology navigation can increase revenue in a fee-for-service payment system and decrease costs for organizations using a bundled payment structure (Kline et al., 2019).

What Are Effective Methods for Selecting and Displaying Navigation Metrics?

Clinical dashboards can effectively showcase multiple reports, giving administrators and the interprofessional team a concise view of data. They are used to track key activities and display performance goals (benchmarks). For example, visually showing navigation case volumes increasing and touch points per patient decreasing can send a powerful message.

Steps in setting up a dashboard will vary based on the method. Spreadsheets can formulate charts and graphs for display on a dashboard. EHRs often have built-in reporting systems that update as the data are entered. Best practices in healthcare data visualization include the following (State Health and Value Strategies, 2022):
- Consider the purpose of the dashboard and the intended end user (e.g., navigators, physicians, administrators, focus groups).
- Prioritize and validate the data for display.

TABLE 7-3. Examples of Research Results From Navigation Programs

	The Patient Care Connect Program	Levine Cancer Center	University of Pennsylvania Health System	Sarah Cannon Cancer Institute	Northern California Healthcare System
Location	University of Alabama, Birmingham, Alabama	Charlotte, North Carolina	3 hospitals in Pennsylvania	65 hospitals across 7 states	Northern California
Staffing model	Non-clinical navigators	Clinical and non-clinical navigators	Clinical navigators (RNs)	Clinical navigators (RNs)	Clinical navigators (RNs)
Interventions	Administered distress screening to identify and address barriers	Interacted with each patient an average of 1.7 times in 30 days	Identified and addressed barriers to care	Coordinated care across institutions	Interacted with patients with breast cancer at suspicious diagnosis
Findings compared with a control group	Decreased emergency department, hospital, and intensive care visits	Reduced use of health care in the acute care setting and decreased readmission rates	Decreased outmigration and increased use of infusion and radiology services	Increased patient retention (> 90%) for all cancers; breast cancer retention nearly doubled from the previous 50% retention rate.	Increased patient retention (35%)
Return on investment	Inpatient and outpatient costs per patient declined by $781.29 in navigated patients.	Savings occurred associated with reduced acute care costs and 30-day readmission penalties.	Revenue increased, associated with a 27% increase in infusion services and 17% increase in radiation oncology services.	Revenue increased, associated with an increase in patient retention.	Revenue increased, associated with the retention of 2 patients equated to the cost for 1 nurse navigator.

Note. Based on information from Kline et al., 2019.

- Create the chart or figure and provide a descriptive title.
- Include data labels and sources.
- Seek help from information technology staff as needed.
- Avoid cluttering the dashboard with more information than needed.

Summary

Milestones in oncology navigation include the development of national standards and role definitions, competencies for clinical and non-clinical navigators, uniform metrics for measuring the impact of navigation interventions, and CMS-established billing codes for services provided by professional navigators. These achievements resulted from the combined efforts of AONN+, ONS, ACS, George Washington University, and oncology accreditation agencies, to name a few.

To enhance the value of navigation interventions and provide patient and provider satisfaction, navigation leaders must select and collect data that supports program success and sustainability. ROI data have been promising, as demonstrated in multiple studies. Navigation leaders must select and collect data that supports program success and sustainability. The fundamental steps when implementing navigation metrics are discussing the metrics with key stakeholders, involving navigators in collecting data, and participating in quality improvement initiatives. Once solid metrics are in place and consistently monitored, the data tell the navigation program's story.

The authors would like to acknowledge Kris Blackley, MSN, RN, BBA, OCN®, for her contribution to this chapter that remains unchanged from the previous edition of this book.

References

Academy of Oncology Nurse and Patient Navigators. (2020). *Navigation metrics toolkit*. https://www.aonnonline.org/images/resources/navigation_tools/2020-AONN-Navigation-Metrics-Toolkit.pdf

American College of Surgeons. (2024). *Optimal resources for breast care: 2024 standards*. https://accreditation.facs.org/accreditationdocuments/NAPBC/Standards/Optimal_Resources_for_Breast_Care_2024.pdf

American College of Surgeons Commission on Cancer. (2024). *Optimal resources for cancer care: 2020 standards*. https://www.facs.org/quality-programs/cancer/coc/2020-standards

American Medical Association. (2023, September 18). *Understanding Medicare's Merit-Based Incentive Payment System (MIPS)*. https://www.ama-assn.org/practice-management/payment-delivery-models/understanding-medicare-s-merit-based-incentive-payment

American Society of Clinical Oncology. (2024). *Care management services and proposed social determinants of health codes: A comparison*. https://society.asco.org/sites/new-www.asco.org/files/content-files/practice-patients/documents/2024-01-Care-Management-SDOH-CHI-PIN-Comparison.pdf

Battaglia, T.A., Fleisher, L., Dwyer, A.J., Wiatrek, D.E., Wells, K.J., Wightman, P., ... Calhoun, E. (2022). Barriers and opportunities to measuring oncology patient navigation impact: Results from the National

Navigation Roundtable survey. *Cancer, 128*(Suppl. 13), 2568–2577. https://doi.org/10.1002/cncr.33805

Centers for Medicare and Medicaid Services & Centers for Medicare and Medicaid Innovation. (2024). *Oncology Model: EOM 2024 health equity plan guide* [version 2.0]. https://www.cms.gov/priorities/innovation/media/document/eom-health-equity-plan

Chan, R.J., Milch, V.E., Crawford-Williams, F., Agbejule, O.A., Joseph, R., Johal, J., ... Hart, N.H. (2023). Patient navigation across the cancer care continuum: An overview of systematic reviews and emerging literature. *CA: A Cancer Journal for Clinicians, 73*(6), 565–589. https://doi.org/10.3322/caac.21788

Chen, M., Wu, V.S., Falk, D., Cheatham, C., Cullen, J., & Hoehn, R. (2024). Patient navigation in cancer treatment: A systematic review. *Current Oncology Reports, 26*(5), 504–537. https://doi.org/10.1007/s11912-024-01514-9

Gormley, E., Connolly, M., & Ryder, M. (2024). The development of nursing-sensitive indicators: A critical discussion. *International Journal of Nursing Studies Advances, 7*, 100227. https://doi.org/10.1016/j.ijnsa.2024.100227

Johnston, D., Sein, E., & Strusowski, T. (2017). Academy of Oncology Nurse and Patient Navigators announces standardized metrics. *Journal of Oncology Navigation and Survivorship, 8*(2). https://www.accc-cancer.org/docs/Documents/acccbuzz/0217-jons-whitepaper

Johnston, D., & Strusowski, T. (2018). AONN+ evidence-based oncology navigation metrics crosswalk with national oncology standards and indicators. *Journal of Oncology Navigation and Survivorship, 9*(6). https://www.jons-online.com/issues/2018/june-2018-vol-9-no-6/1852-aonn-evidence-based-oncology-navigation-metrics-crosswalk-with-national-jons-oncology-standards-and-indicators

Kline, R.M., Rocque, G.B., Rohan, E.A., Blackley, K.A., Cantril, C.A., Pratt-Chapman, M.L., ... Shulman, L.N. (2019). Patient navigation in cancer: The business case to support clinical needs. *JCO Oncology Practice, 15*(11), 585–590. https://doi.org/10.1200/JOP.19.00230

Pratt-Chapman, M.L., McMahon, J., Pena, N., Gallardo, E., Angell, K., Quiring, J., ... Kushalnagar, P. (2024). CMS payment for principal illness navigation: How do I credential my navigators? *Journal of Oncology Navigation and Survivorship, 15*(3). https://www.jons-online.com/issues/2024/march-2024-vol-15-no-3/5030-cms-payment-for-principal-illness-navigation-how-do-i-credential-my-navigators

Shaughnessy, E., Johnson, D.C., Lyss, A.J., Parikh, R.B., Peskin, S.R., Polite, B.N., ... Goh, L. (2022). Oncology alternative payment models: Lessons from commercial insurance. *American Journal of Managed Care, 28*(3), 98–100. doi.org/10.37765/ajmc.2022.88835

Stabellini, N., Nazha, A., Agrawal, N., Huhn, M., Shanahan, J., Hamerschlak, N., ... Montero, A.J. (2023). Thirty-day unplanned hospital readmissions in patients with cancer and the impact of social determinants of health: A machine learning approach. *JCO Clinical Cancer Informatics, 7*. https://doi.org/10.1200/cci.22.00143

State Health and Value Strategies. (2022). *Tracking Medicaid coverage post the continuous coverage requirement: Using data dashboards to monitor trends*. https://www.shvs.org/wp-content/uploads/2022/01/Tracking-Medicaid-Coverage-Post-the-Continuous-Coverage-Requirement_Using-Data-Dashboards-to-Monitor-Trends.pdf

Visintini, C., & Palese, A. (2023). What nursing-sensitive outcomes have been investigated to date among patients with solid and hematological malignancies? A scoping review. *Nursing Reports, 13*(3), 1101–1125. https://doi.org/10.3390/nursrep13030096

Ward, J.C., Bourbeau, B., Chin, A.L., Page, R.D., Grubbs, S.S., Kamin, D.Y., ... Rappaport, M. (2020). Updates to the ASCO Patient-Centered Oncology Payment Model. *JCO Oncology Practice, 16*(5), 263–269. https://doi.org/10.1200/JOP.19.00776

CHAPTER 8

Interventions Addressing Financial Toxicity

Dan Sherman, MA, LPC

> **KEY TOPICS**
> financial toxicity, financial navigation, insurance optimization

Overview

The devastating consequences of financial toxicity (FT) affect a sizable portion of patients with cancer. FT negatively impacts overall patient well-being, treatment adherence, quality of care, and quality of life, resulting in an increased mortality risk (Chan et al., 2019; Longo, 2022; National Cancer Institute [NCI], 2024). Solving this problem is not necessarily easy, as multiple, complex, systemwide variables foster the experience of FT. Examples include the high cost of pharmaceutical products, income inequalities, the complexities of the U.S. health insurance system, the lack of focus on the issue within health institutions, and the lack of formal educational programs preparing healthcare staff (Hussaini et al., 2022; Wheeler et al., 2022).

Because of its complexity, a dedicated role within a medical institution is favored to mitigate the adverse effects of FT. If adequately trained, navigators can take steps to prevent FT and intervene in the early stages of diagnosis and treatment initiation. Financial navigation includes oncology nurse navigators, oncology social workers, and financial navigators collaborating to address FT in oncology. Financial navigation describes oncology professions addressing any part of the cascade of factors leading to FT.

This chapter will review factors contributing to FT and present critical solutions and proactive interventions to consider when developing or improving a financial navigation program.

Impact of Financial Toxicity

Variables such as age, pre-illness debt load, high cost of cancer treatment, employment status, type and staging of cancer, race, and income inequality all contribute to FT in patients with cancer (NCI, 2024). However, the two most common variables are that the majority of Americans lack a basic understanding of their health insurance policy and the coverage options to select from, and a high percentage are underinsured with their elected policy (NCI, 2024). Deductibles and out-of-pocket responsibilities continue to rise yearly, as evidenced by the $9,200 out-of-pocket responsibilities in the health insurance Marketplace and $9,350 maximum out-of-pocket (MOOP) responsibilities in Medicare Advantage plans in 2025 (Freed et al., 2024b).

On average, there are 100 Marketplace policies and 43 Medicare Advantage plans to choose from in communities across the United States (Pollitz et al., 2023). Navigating patients through the maze of these insurance plans is complicated and overwhelming for even the most seasoned oncology navigator. Furthermore, these coverage instruments have premium and cost-sharing subsidies for lower-income beneficiaries, and understanding how to access these programs is daunting, evidenced by the low enrollment numbers into the Medicare Savings Program (MSP) and Extra Help (formerly Low-Income Subsidy) for Medicare beneficiaries. More than a third of Medicare beneficiaries are not enrolled in these government safety net programs simply because the beneficiary and the health system are unaware of their availability (Popham et al., 2020).

However, the decision-making process in selecting Marketplace policies and Medicare plans has never been more critical, as the average cost of treating cancer has exceeded more than $100,000 (NCI, 2024). Financial navigators can assess patients for economic challenges, connect them with programs and resources to prevent or mitigate FT, and refer them to proactive help (Bell-Brown et al., 2023).

Financial consequences can affect any patient with cancer; however, in patients with healthcare disparities, the margin widens. For example, non-White and Hispanic patients with breast cancer have worse cancer outcomes, including being diagnosed at a later stage, receiving less treatment as per standard of care, and having higher mortality (Yedjou et al., 2019). Moreover, Hispanic and Black cancer survivors are more likely to forgo prescription medications because of cost (Panzone et al., 2021). These patients also are more likely to lose their housing because of FT (Jagsi et al., 2018). Younger patients are at a higher risk for lasting FT because they face higher economic burdens, have fewer savings, and are at higher risk for compromised long-term outcomes due to a lack of appropriate follow-up care and preventive medicine (Corrigan et al., 2022).

Even considering the increased attention to FT within health institutions, there is little to no evidence that the burden is diminishing for patients with cancer (NCI, 2024). The increased risk of death from economic distress is driven by factors such as overall poorer well-being, impaired health-related quality of life, lower treatment adherence, decreased income and asset depletion, and subpar quality of care (Ma et al., 2021). Developing proactive and systematic methods to mitigate FT is therefore urgently needed. Figure 8-1 depicts the association between financial distress and mortality.

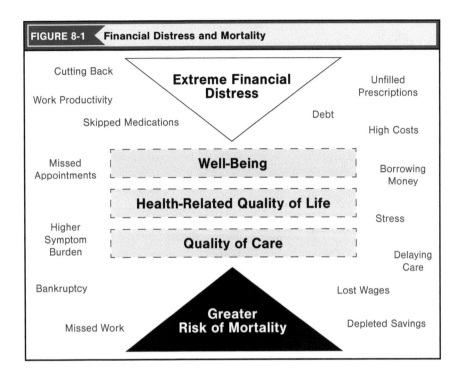

FIGURE 8-1. Financial Distress and Mortality

Financial Navigation Considerations

As the options for obtaining health insurance through an employer, the Marketplace, Medicaid, or Medicare continue to get more complex, there is a growing need for an increased level of expertise within health institutions to educate patients on how insurance plans could shield them from FT (Levitt & Altman, 2023). Oncology programs developing or desiring to improve their financial advocacy programs should consider the importance of defining the financial navigator model, creating a systematic process to treat FT, and fostering a culture of ongoing education for their navigation team.

Financial Navigation Models

The Traditional Financial Counseling model, Financial Advocacy model, and Financial Navigation model are three common approaches found in oncology programs in the United States (Sherman & Fessele, 2019). Unfortunately, the titles are used interchangeably in most health settings, further complicating the development of a robust financial navigation program. Understanding how these models are defined and how they can build upon each other can assist administrators and navigators in developing interventions to address FT.

Traditional Financial Counseling Model

The Traditional Financial Counseling model has been in the hospital setting for decades. This model primarily focuses on assisting patients with applying for Medicaid, seeking hospital charity programs, determining cost estimates, and exploring payment options that may include loans through credit agencies. It is limited in its ability to effectively address the experience of FT, as the tools used to reduce patient responsibility are effective only for a small portion of patients with cancer. Medicaid and hospital-based charity programs are reserved for patients and families who have low incomes. A second concern with this model is the financial counselors' need for access to clinical information. The staff members in this role are often not part of the treatment team and thus not knowledgeable of the patient's clinical journey, resulting in counselors reacting to rather than proactively treating FT (Sherman & Fessele, 2019).

Financial Advocacy Model

The Financial Advocacy model has emerged as a response to the limitations of the Traditional Financial Counseling model. Pharmacy staff, oncology social workers, oncology nurse navigators, and other advocates within the oncology service line are adapting their roles to deal with the massive influx of patients expressing financial distress. This model uses specific community-based programs designed to lessen the financial burden on patients, such as co-pay assistance, premium assistance, and patient assistance programs (PAPs). In addition, attention to patients' basic needs, such as housing costs, transportation, and utility expenses, is often a central part of the Financial Advocacy model. Staff functioning as financial advocates typically have self-educated to find programs to help decrease financial burden (Mangir et al., 2020; Michigan Cancer Consortium, 2018).

At times, the Financial Advocacy model can be proactive. However, it is often reactive and based on a referral process. Although this model has made some progress in decreasing FT, it cannot effectively mitigate it for those receiving radiation treatments, surgical intervention, and all the other nonpharmaceutical medical care (Sherman & Fessele, 2019).

Financial Navigation Model

The Financial Navigation model absorbs the two previous models but also adds proactive insurance optimization to decrease FT. In this model, the navigator is embedded within the oncology program and works closely with the treatment team to seek optimal care with the least financial responsibility being transferred to patients. The Financial Navigation model has been piloted and showed promise with patients with cancer as a strategy to ease FT (Phillips, 2023; Yezefski et al., 2018).

Financial navigators can address FT by proactively educating patients about the complexities of the numerous health insurance options available. This navigation can contribute to the decision-making of treatment options and treatment timing. Ultimately, this model helps maximize patients' healthcare coverage and minimize out-of-pocket costs.

Healthcare providers should seek to understand the distinct differences between these models and how they differ in their ability to alleviate FT for patients with cancer. Furthermore, qualifications, experiences, and educational backgrounds will vary significantly for each model (Sherman & Fessele, 2019).

Systematic Process Development

FT is often not addressed at diagnosis. However, the reality is that patients with a new cancer diagnosis will experience anxiety about the potential financial consequences (NCI, 2024). It is an error to believe that these patients are too overwhelmed to deal with or discuss the financial ramifications of their diagnosis. Avoiding this challenging conversation will only exacerbate the situation. Early intervention to treat pending FT is usually the best approach, especially if mitigation techniques include insurance optimization. Therefore, developing a systematic process to proactively identify and meet with patients who are at the most significant risk of developing FT is essential (NCI, 2024; Sherman & Fessele, 2019).

Educational Trainings

The Association of Cancer Care Centers has created a Financial Advocacy Bootcamp program that provides a foundation for financial advocacy navigators. The free-for-members program is based on self-learning modules and includes education on most financial advocacy topics that navigators should understand (www.accc-cancer.org/home/learn/financial-advocacy/boot-camp).

Triage Cancer provides live seminars addressing some of the financial aspects of cancer care. Education focuses on the legal aspects of the economic barriers that patients with cancer experience. The organization also has a webpage with links to worksheets and guides for helping navigators with educational resources to assist patients in navigating finances (https://triagecancer.org/free-cancer-resources-by-topic).

The NaVectis Group offers consulting and training services to healthcare institutions desiring to implement or improve a financial navigation program (https://navectis.com/services). One-on-one financial navigation training is followed by a minimum of 12 months of mentorship that helps foster the continued growth necessary to become a seasoned financial navigator. Additional training programs should be developed that oncology navigators can use, as staff members in these roles should not be learning on the job as their primary source of education.

Digital Solutions

The path to capturing solutions to address FT can be operationally complex and time consuming. Given the outsized patient needs compared to the capacity of most programs to manage them, it is increasingly more challenging to run a successful financial navigation program without the aid of technology (Sheehan et al., 2023). Examples of digital solutions include TailorMed, AssistPoint, RxLightning, and Atlas. An organization's investment in digital financial navigation solutions has three primary benefits:

- Centralization: It is common for facilities within the same health system to take separate approaches to financial navigation. These financial assistance silos drive

inefficiency, underutilization of resources, and poor patient experiences. Deploying technology across the organization allows data to be centralized, giving all teams broader access to resources and better visibility into program performance.
- Proactive identification of at-risk patients: Identifying at-risk patients is typically inconsistent and reactive. Predictive analytics technology can evaluate entire patient populations to identify high-risk patients proactively. Such insights allow navigators to initiate hardship discussions much sooner to ensure that patients can afford treatment and the health system can avoid uncompensated care.
- Process modernization: Technology can automate many financial navigation processes, including matching and enrolling eligible patients in funding sources such as co-pay cards and free drug programs. Software solutions also simplify the cumbersome task of filling out enrollment forms and enhance communication among staff.

Assessment Tools

As FT is highly prevalent in the oncology setting, a need exists for the early identification of at-risk patients. However, despite the pervasiveness and adverse impacts of FT in cancer care, no definitive screening measures have been widely integrated into clinical practice (Samaha et al., 2024). Multiple screening tools have been developed or are being developed that can aid in this process, such as the FACIT-COST and the National Comprehensive Cancer Network Distress Thermometer (Prasad et al., 2021; Samaha et al., 2024).

Patients with a new cancer diagnosis should have a minimum of one touchpoint with a navigator who assesses for financial distress. Specific patient populations include, but are not limited to, the following:
- Self-pay patients, Medicare A/B only, aged 64–65 years, enrolling in or newly enrolled in Medicare
- Marketplace enrollees with a predicted decrease in income as the result of treatment needs
- Patients whose treatment regimen includes pharmaceutical interventions and have a co-pay assistance program available
- Patients with advanced-stage disease with an employer-based coverage benefit for being assessed in the early stages of diagnosis

These patients need assistance with obtaining health coverage through the Marketplace, navigating Medicare options, potentially enrolling in a Consolidated Omnibus Budget Reconciliation Act (COBRA) program, becoming educated regarding short-and long-term disability benefits, and securing Social Security Disability Insurance.

Patients and providers benefit when a financial assessment occurs as early as possible to treat anticipatory financial distress proactively—seeing patients proactively will give the navigator additional tools to treat FT compared to seeing them after FT has occurred (Longo, 2022). Follow-up assessments are also recommended and can occur within a few months after treatment initiation. By then, there is likely a clearer understanding of the effects of the diagnosis and treatments on financial well-being. Assessing patients at the beginning of the calendar year is also recommended, as deductibles and out-of-pocket responsibilities will likely be renewed. Figure 8-2 lists items to consider when assessing patients for FT.

Financial Resources

Internal and Local Programs

Hospital-based oncology providers have programs to help reduce the financial burden for patients in lower income brackets. Some providers have transportation and food resources readily available. Most hospital-based providers also offer financial aid that removes or decreases the out-of-pocket responsibilities for patients.

FIGURE 8-2	Financial Navigation Checklist
☐	Proactively screen for patients needing assistance (rather than working with only uninsured patients or those who approach navigators for help).
☐	Educate patients on their insurance status, benefit coverage, and expected costs of planned treatment.
☐	Educate patients on the best insurance plans for their needs and provide guidance on applying for primary or secondary insurance as necessary.
☐	Be knowledgeable of the treatment plan to anticipate the expected cost of treatment.
☐	Continuously review and verify patients' insurance status throughout their treatment (as plans or employment may change).
☐	Monitor for patients undergoing treatment with missed payments or unpaid balances.
☐	Use tools such as the FACIT-COST survey or the National Comprehensive Cancer Network Distress Thermometer to assess patients' financial stress.
☐	Routinely assess symptom burden and the medication list; directly ask patients if they are taking their medications if there is a disconnect.
☐	Identify and help patients apply for financial assistance programs, including co-pay assistance, foundation support, drug replacement programs, hospital charity programs, and basic needs financial assistance options.
☐	Connect patients to other healthcare team members, such as financial advocates, navigators, and social workers, to help them find additional support for living expenses and transportation assistance.
☐	Educate other healthcare team members about financial navigation so that they can refer patients whom they identify as needing financial support.

Federal regulations require that nonprofit hospitals provide charity care and other community benefits for patients who meet specific financial criteria (U.S. Government Accountability Office, 2023). Some patients may not qualify for assistance because of income status at the time of diagnosis. However, they may become eligible a few months into treatment, as a significant portion of patients with cancer experience a decrease in household income after treatment initiation (Alzehr et al., 2022).

Multiple local resources, such as transportation services, food banks, charities, and religious organizations, can assist with the basic needs of the people in their community. Programs such as Meals on Wheels, the National Association of Area Agencies on Aging, the United Way, and community health centers can assist patients experiencing FT.

External Assistance Programs

A variety of external assistance programs are available to those diagnosed with cancer or other chronic medical conditions. These programs can be subcategorized into basic needs programs, PAPs, co-pay assistance programs, and premium assistance programs.

Basic Needs Programs

Basic needs programs are national charities (beyond the local resources) that can assist with non-medical bills, such as car payments, mortgages, rent, food, transportation, and gas cards. Examples of national charities that help in this way are the Patient Advocate Foundation, Pink Fund, Cancer Care, Family Reach, Pink Aid, Leukemia and Lymphoma Society, American Cancer Society, and Share a Smile.

The Cancer Financial Assistance Coalition (www.cancerfac.org) is a well-crafted online tool for identifying financial assistance programs for patients with cancer.

Patient Assistance Programs

PAPs are typically available for patients who lack insurance coverage or whose insurance policy does not cover a specific medication, usually because of off-label use. In these circumstances, it is in the financial interest of patients and providers to secure free drugs directly from the pharmaceutical company. Most pharmaceutical companies have simplified the application process for obtaining free medication, often resulting in the approval process taking less than three days from the date of application.

Once approved, navigators need to work directly with the program to determine if the drug delivery will be upfront, meaning that they will ship the drug before treating the patient or replace the drug after treatment has occurred. Some pharmaceutical companies provide retroactive approvals up to 12 months from the date of application. As providers receive the drug for free from the manufacturer, patients cannot be billed for the cost of the medication.

An online tool, NeedyMeds (https://needymeds.org), assists users in finding these free drug programs. Pharmacy programs that can lower patients' oral prescription costs, such as GoodRx, Cost Plus, or SingleCare, are also available. These online tools find low prices and discounts on oral prescriptions by searching surrounding retail pharmacies for deals or coupons for needed medications.

Co-Pay Assistance Programs

Co-pay assistance programs are available for patients with co-pay responsibilities for oral or infused pharmaceutical products. These programs are provided directly by pharmaceutical companies or through independent co-pay assistance foundations. Pharmaceutical co-pay cards are available for patients with commercial coverage who are receiving a brand name drug or a biosimilar. An increasing number of manufacturer co-pay card programs do not have financial requirements to qualify, guaranteeing enrollment for most commercially insured patients. These programs will, at times, also cover administration charges for an infused product. As each pharmaceutical company has a unique process for assisting patients with their co-pay responsibilities, navigators must learn the specific rules of each assistance program to optimize these opportunities.

Co-pay assistance programs are generally reserved for Medicare beneficiaries, as patients with public coverage cannot use the pharmaceutical co-pay card programs. However, unlike pharmaceutical co-pay programs, which are continuously available for commercially insured patients, independent co-pay assistance foundation availability will depend on the funding level of the grant. Examples of independent co-pay assistance foundations available for patients who meet enrollment criteria are shown in Table 8-1.

Commonly, navigators will have less than 90 minutes to secure a grant once it becomes available, as these programs work on a first-come, first-serve basis. However,

TABLE 8-1. Examples of Independent Co-Pay Assistance Foundations

Foundation	Website
Accessia Health	www.accessiahealth.org
CancerCare	www.cancercare.org
Good Day's Chronic Disease Fund	www.mygooddays.org
HealthWell Foundation	www.healthwellfoundation.org
Leukemia and Lymphoma Society	www.lls.org/support-resources
Musella Brain Tumor Foundation	www.braintumorcopays.org
National Organization for Rare Disorders	www.rarediseases.org
The Assistance Fund	www.tafcares.org

the Patient Access Network Foundation and The Assistance Fund have waiting lists that patients or navigators can use to increase their chances of approved enrollment once funding is available. Independent co-pay assistance foundations have income requirements to qualify for assistance, typically below 400%–500% of the federal poverty level (FPL). Health organizations that do not use paid software programs can use an online tool called Fund Finder, available through the Patient Access Network Foundation website (https://fundfinder.panfoundation.org). This free, easy-to-use tool assists in identifying foundation support for patients and only requires an email address to enroll.

Premium Assistance Programs

Premium assistance programs are commonly available through independent co-pay assistance foundations and some basic needs programs. These programs can be highly effective in helping reduce the cost of health insurance premiums. Patients diagnosed with cancer often have a decrease in income, making costly health insurance premium payments unattainable. Securing premium assistance in these circumstances can often prevent the loss of health insurance coverage.

Insurance Optimization

Insurance optimization seeks to improve health insurance coverage by reducing the out-of-pocket responsibilities that patients have for care (Sherman & Fessele, 2019). These opportunities are available for Medicare patients, making it essential to understand how Medicare Parts D, A, and B, and the two safety net programs from the U.S. Social Security Administration and the Centers for Medicare and Medicaid Services (CMS) work to help low-income beneficiaries.

Medicare Part D

Medicare Part D is the prescription drug coverage within the Medicare system. Starting in 2025, Part D has three coverage levels: deductible, initial coverage, and catastrophic coverage. The coverage gap, also known as the donut hole, was eliminated at the end of 2024. During the annual deductible phase, beneficiaries pay 100% of the prescription drug costs until the deductible of $590 for calendar year 2025 has been met. During the initial coverage phase, beneficiaries pay up to 25% coinsurance for covered Part D drugs. This phase ends when beneficiaries have reached the annual out-of-pocket threshold of $2,000 (including the deductible) for 2025. During the catastrophic coverage phase, beneficiaries pay no cost sharing for covered Part D drugs (CMS, 2024b).

The Extra Help safety net program (also named Low Income Subsidy), administered through the U.S. Social Security Administration, significantly reduces the co-pay responsibilities for all oral medications filled through the Part D system. Three distinct levels of assistance are available (Medicare Rights Center, 2025):

- Level 1 enrollees are Medicare beneficiaries with both Medicare and Medicaid (dual eligible) and live in a nursing home. They have zero co-pays for all their Part D–covered oral medications.
- Level 2 enrollees are dual eligible but do not live in a nursing home. In calendar year 2025, these enrollees will have a $1.60 co-pay for generic medications and a $4.80 co-pay for brand-name medications.
- Level 3 enrollees are all other Medicare beneficiaries who fall below 150% FPL and meet the asset qualifier, set at $17,600 for single individuals and $35,130 for couples in 2025. These enrollees have a $4.90 co-pay responsibility for generic medications and a $12.15 responsibility for brand-name medications. The co-pay responsibilities and asset qualifiers change yearly, so navigators must stay current with these changes to ensure that patients who qualify get enrolled.

Medicare beneficiaries can apply for the Extra Help program at a Social Security Administration office or online (www.ssa.gov; U.S. Social Security Administration, 2024). An estimated 30% of Medicare beneficiaries who qualify for this program are not currently enrolled (CMS, 2024b). Therefore, oncology navigators should educate patients about potentially enrolling if they meet the requirements.

An additional change to Medicare Part D in 2025 is the Medicare Prescription Payment Plan, also known as the "smoothing" program. It will allow Part D beneficiaries to "smooth" out their cost-sharing responsibilities throughout the year. In other words, the $2,000 MOOP will be spread out through the year rather than beneficiaries needing to cover the entire expense in one month. Anyone with a Medicare Part D prescription drug plan can enroll in the monthly payment plan, either before the beginning of or in any month during the plan year (CMS, 2024b). Key features of this program include the following (CMS, 2024c):

- The Medicare Prescription Payment Plan is a voluntary program. Part D beneficiaries must opt in and can do so at any time of the year; they can also disenroll at any time.
- Once beneficiaries have out-of-pocket prescription costs, they will be billed monthly directly from the Part D sponsor. They are not billed at the point of sale and will, therefore, have zero co-pay at the retail pharmacy. This will continue if they remain part of the Medicare Prescription Payment Plan. Furthermore, beneficiaries will not need to spend a certain out-of-pocket amount before joining the program.
- All Medicare Part D beneficiaries are eligible to enroll in the smoothing program regardless of income status.

Potential concerns about the program include the following (Dusetzina et al., 2024):

- There may be confusion at the point of sale. Part D beneficiaries will have a zero co-pay at the retail pharmacy and will be billed monthly by the Part D sponsor.
- Beneficiaries may also need clarification regarding paying the Part D sponsor directly rather than at the retail pharmacy for responsible co-pays.
- Although protections have been put in place to prevent the Part D sponsors from disenrolling members from the Part D plan when the beneficiaries do not pay the

sponsor, questions remain regarding how aggressive the Part D sponsor will be in collecting the co-pays from the beneficiaries.
• From an insurance optimization standpoint, it would benefit beneficiaries to meet the $2,000 Part D MOOP at the beginning of the year by using a co-pay assistance foundation. In scenarios where co-pay assistance programs have been secured, a smoothing program may not be in beneficiaries' best interests.

Navigators must be prepared to help patients understand smoothing program benefits and potential concerns. Patients will likely need help understanding how the program may or may not help their specific financial situation (Dusetzina et al., 2024).

Medicare Parts A and B

MSP addresses Medicare's medical components (Parts A and B). It is administered through states' U.S. Health and Human Services Departments or Medicaid offices and is available for Medicare beneficiaries who fall below 135% FPL and meet the state asset qualifier (if applicable). For most states, the 2025 asset qualifier is $9,660 for single individuals and $14,470 for married couples. Some states have higher income thresholds and asset qualifiers (or no asset qualifiers). Furthermore, some income disregards are available within the MSP program, such as the first $20 of all income, the first $65 of earned income, and 50% of the remaining earned income. The National Council on Aging (2025) lists each state's income threshold and asset qualifier for the MSP program.

Four distinct programs exist within MSP (National Council on Aging, 2025):
• Qualified Medicare Beneficiary (QMB) is available for Medicare beneficiaries who fall below 100% FPL (in most states) and meet the state asset qualifier. It covers all cost-sharing responsibilities and pays the Part A premium (if there is one) and the Part B premium for beneficiaries. In other words, a beneficiary will have zero financial responsibility for all Medicare-covered services.
• The Specified Low-Income Medicare Beneficiary (SLMB) qualification is for individuals below 120% FPL (in most states) and who meet the state asset qualifier. It covers beneficiaries' Part B premiums.
• Qualified Individual (QI) beneficiaries must fall below 135% FPL (in most states) and meet the state asset qualifier. If funding remains available in the state budget, this program will cover the beneficiaries' Part B premiums.
• Qualified Disabled Working Individual (QDWI) beneficiaries need to be working, younger than age 65 years, have Medicare due to disability, be below 400% FPL, meet the state asset qualifier, and have a monthly premium for Part A. This program covers Part A premiums for beneficiaries who do not have enough work credits to qualify for premium-free Part A coverage.

Medicare Advantage Versus Medicare Supplement Plans

Navigators can start looking for insurance optimization opportunities for Medicare beneficiaries after understanding the two safety net programs, Extra Help and

MSP. Because of the complexity of Medicare, beneficiaries are often lost in a maze of coverage options available within this system. If Medicare beneficiaries do not have a group secondary policy or qualify for Medicaid, they have only one of two other options to avoid the unlimited 20% responsibility for Part B–covered services: Medicare Advantage (also known as Part C) or Medicare Supplement policy. Currently, 47% of Medicare beneficiaries are enrolled in Medicare Advantage plans, and less than 20% are enrolled in a supplemental policy (Ochieng et al., 2024; Xu et al., 2023).

Medicare Advantage Plans

Medicare Advantage plans are sold through private insurance companies and replace original Medicare. Insurance companies that sell these plans will often entice beneficiaries to enroll by offering extra benefits, such as dental, vision, and hearing benefits, health club memberships, a flexible spending card to cover some over-the-counter products, and, at times, reimbursement to cover all or a portion of the Part B premium. Medicare Advantage plans are prevalent because of these benefits and low monthly premiums; however, they can leave beneficiaries with high out-of-pocket responsibilities (up to $9,350 in 2025). The average out-of-pocket responsibility for Medicare Advantage plans in 2023 was $4,850 for health maintenance organization (HMO) plans and $5,628 for in-network preferred provider organization (PPO) plans (Freed et al., 2024a).

Enrollment into Medicare Advantage plans occurs without underwriting, guaranteeing the policy to any Medicare beneficiary regardless of medical condition. Medicare beneficiaries can enroll when they first become eligible for Medicare or during the national Open Enrollment Period (OEP) between October 15 and December 7 every year. These plans also have several Special Enrollment Periods (SEPs) that Medicare beneficiaries can use to optimize their coverage. The most common SEPs for these plans are (a) January 1 through March 31, when beneficiaries can change their advantage plan to a different one or revert to their original Medicare coverage, (b) within 60 days of Low Income Subsidy approval, and (c) January 1 through November 30 and December 8–31 every year, if beneficiaries have access to a five-star Medicare Advantage plan. Navigators can search for these five-star plans using the Medicare Plan Finder Tool at the Medicare website (www.medicare.gov/plan-compare). The effective date of all new Medicare Advantage plans is the first of the following month of enrollment. The latter two SEPs apply mainly to Medicare Parts A and B–only beneficiaries, as this population may struggle with unlimited 20% financial responsibility for outpatient medical care.

Medicare Supplement Plans

Medicare Supplement plans are secondary coverage instruments to original Medicare. These plans cover most or all of the deductibles, co-pays, and coinsurance responsibilities of original Medicare. Most importantly, Medicare Supplement plans A, B, C, D, F, G, M, and N cover the 20% responsibility that comes with Part B coverage (see Table 8-2). Medicare Supplement plans do not offer the extra benefits often available with Medicare Advantage plans but leave beneficiaries with significantly lower out-of-pocket responsibilities. For example, if beneficiaries have original Medicare and supplemental Plan G, they will only owe the Part B deductible for all Medicare-covered services, which is $257 in the calendar year 2025. However, unlike Medicare Advantage plans, where beneficiaries are not subjected to underwriting and have a yearly OEP, insurance companies that sell Medicare Supplement plans will require underwriting if beneficiaries are past six months of being new to Medicare Part B. As access for enrolling into Medicare Supplement policies is governed mainly by individual state laws, navigators should check with their specific state to determine if beneficiaries live in a state that provides a level of guaranteed issue for supplemental plans. Connecticut, Maine, Massachusetts, and New York mandate that insurance companies sell specific Medicare Supplement policies as a guaranteed issue policy regardless of when beneficiaries become eligible for Medicare.

Patient Protection and Affordable Care Act

With the passing of the Patient Protection and Affordable Care Act (ACA) in 2010, obtaining health insurance coverage improved for approximately 50% of Americans younger than age 65 years who lacked access to health insurance because of preexisting conditions (U.S. Department of Health and Human Services, 2022). Starting in 2014, individuals or families below 138% FPL have access to Medicaid through the Medicaid Expansion portion of the law. Those above 138% FPL can enroll in commercial coverage through the Marketplace and receive subsidies on premiums if their income is below 400% FPL (CMS, 2024a).

Medicaid Expansion

ACA changed the income criteria for access to Medicaid from 100% to 138% FPL and removed any consideration of assets status for Medicaid eligibility. It also removed the disability requirement to qualify for Medicaid, leaving Medicare eligibility, legal status, and income as the only requirements for eligibility. Some states have removed legal immigration status as a qualifier. This portion of ACA is called Medicaid Expansion.

However, because of a U.S. Supreme Court ruling in 2012, individual states were left to decide whether to expand Medicaid (Jones, 2013). At the time of publication, Alabama, Florida, Georgia, Kansas, Mississippi, South Carolina, Tennessee, Texas, Wisconsin, and Wyoming have not expanded Medicaid. In these states, the income criteria for enrolling in the Marketplace was lowered from 138% to 100% FPL, granting access to the Marketplace to a larger share of the residents of these states. However, these residents do not have access to premium and cost-sharing subsidies within the Marketplace if their income falls below 100% FPL. There are exceptions to this rule for individuals with less than five years of legal documentation to be in the United States. These individuals can access the subsidies available within the Marketplace, even if their income falls below 100% FPL because of their lack of access to Medicaid.

TABLE 8-2 Medicare Supplement Insurance Plans

Benefits	A	B	C	D	F*	G*	K**	L**	M	N
Part A coinsurance and hospital costs (up to an additional 365 days after Medicare benefits are used)	✓	✓	✓	✓	✓	✓	✓	✓	✓	✓
Part B coinsurance or copayment	✓	✓	✓	✓	✓	✓	50%	75%	✓	✓***
Blood benefit (first 3 pints)	✓	✓	✓	✓	✓	✓	50%	75%	✓	✓
Part A hospice care coinsurance or copayment	✓	✓	✓	✓	✓	✓	50%	75%	✓	✓
Skilled nursing facility care coinsurance	✗	✗	✓	✓	✓	✓	50%	75%	✓	✓
Part A deductible	✗	✓	✓	✓	✓	✓	50%	75%	50%	✓
Part B deductible	✗	✗	✓	✗	✓	✗	✗	✗	✗	✗
Part B excess charge	✗	✗	✗	✗	✓	✓	✗	✗	✗	✗
Foreign travel emergency (up to plan limits)	✗	✗	80%	80%	80%	80%	✗	✗	80%	80%
							Out-of-pocket limit in 2025**			
							$7,220	$3,610		

*Plans F and G also offer a high-deductible plan in some states. You must pay for Medicare-covered costs (coinsurance, copayments, and deductibles) up to the deductible amount of $2,870 in 2025 before your policy pays anything. (You can't buy Plans C and F if you were new to Medicare on or after January 1, 2020.)

**For Plans K and L after you meet your out-of-pocket yearly limit and your yearly Part B deductible ($250 in 2025), the Medigap plan pays 100% of covered services for the rest of the calendar year.

***Plan N pays 100% of the Part B coinsurance. You must pay a copayment of up to $20 for some office visits and up to a $50 copayment for emergency room visits that don't result in an inpatient admission.

Note. From *2025 Choosing a Medigap Policy*, by Centers for Medicare and Medicaid Services, 2025 (https://www.medicare.gov/publications/02110-choosing-a-medigap-policy-a-guide-to-health-insurance-for-people-with-medicare.pdf). In the public domain.

The Healthcare Marketplace in 2025

Individuals or families above the 100% FPL threshold in states that have not expanded Medicaid or the 138% FPL threshold in states that have expanded can access the Marketplace if they cannot obtain health insurance through other means. The Marketplace is a service that helps people shop for and enroll in health insurance through websites, call centers, and in-person assistance. The federal government operates the Health Insurance Marketplace at HealthCare.gov for 32 states. Currently, 18 states run their own state-based Marketplace service centers. ACA standardized health insurance policies by creating metal levels for individual/family and small group policies (see Table 8-3). Premium tax credits are applied to Marketplace plans in any of the four metal levels of coverage (Bronze, Silver, Gold, Platinum). Bronze plans tend to have the lowest premiums but the highest deductibles and cost-sharing responsibilities, leaving beneficiaries to pay more out-of-pocket when they receive covered healthcare services. Platinum plans have the highest premiums but lowest out-of-pocket costs (Ortaliza & Cox, 2024).

The premium tax credit subsidies are provided on a sliding scale based on projected household income for the year. Marketplace enrollees pay a percentage of their income toward the benchmark Silver plan. They also pay the premium difference if they elect a Marketplace plan that is not the benchmark Silver plan. The American Rescue Plan of 2021 and the Inflation Reduction Act of 2022 temporarily expanded the premium tax credit subsidies to all Marketplace enrollees through a sliding scale until the end of 2025 (see Table 8-4).

With the passing of these enhanced subsidies, premiums for Marketplace policies have never been lower. However, these enhanced subsidies will expire at the end of 2025 unless Congress acts (Kaiser Family Foundation, 2024). Furthermore, cost-sharing subsidies, also known as cost-sharing reduction, are available through a provision of ACA that allows those with modest incomes (up to 250% FPL) to enroll in Silver-level plans that have more robust benefits than a standard Silver plan (see Table 8-5). In 2025, MOOP in Marketplace policies can be as high as $9,200. Navigators can help educate patients whose projected income falls below 250% FPL with these cost-sharing subsidies (Kaiser Family Foundation, 2024). As a significant portion of patients with cancer experience a decrease in income after a diagnosis, ongoing

TABLE 8-3. Affordable Care Act Plan Comparisons 2025

Plan Category	Insurance Company Pays	Enrollee Pays
Bronze	60%	40%
Silver	70%	30%
Gold	80%	20%
Platinum	90%	10%

Note. Based on information from Healthcare.gov, n.d.-a.

TABLE 8-4	Affordable Care Act Compared to American Rescue Plan	
Income (% of Poverty)	Affordable Care Act (Base Law) % of Income Toward the Benchmark Silver Plan	American Rescue Plan/Inflation Reduction Act Through the End of 2025 % of Income Toward the Benchmark Silver Plan
Under 100%	Not eligible for subsidies	Not eligible for subsidies
100%–138%	2.07%	0%
138%–150%	3.10%–4.14%	0%
150%–200%	4.14%–6.52%	0%–2%
200%–250%	6.52%–8.33%	2%–4%
250%–300%	8.33%–9.83%	4%–6%
300%–400%	9.83%	6%–8.5%
Over 400%	Not eligible for subsidies	8.5%

Note. From *Explaining Health Care Reform: Questions About Health Insurance Subsidies*, by Kaiser Family Foundation, 2024 (https://www.kff.org/affordable-care-act/issue-brief/explaining-health-care-reform-questions-about-health-insurance-subsidies). Copyright 2024 by Kaiser Family Foundation. Licensed under CC BY-NC-ND 4.0 (https://creativecommons.org/licenses/by-nc-nd/4.0/).

income status assessment is needed throughout their cancer journeys (Alzehr et al., 2022). Patients currently enrolled in a Marketplace policy and experiencing a reduced household income should contact Marketplace customer assistance and provide notification of their income change.

Open Enrollment

OEP and SEP are two types of open enrollment opportunities for those who need access to health insurance through the Marketplace. The OEP runs from November 1 through January 15 each year. Individuals or families can enroll during this time frame in a Marketplace policy without regard to preexisting conditions. The effective date of the Marketplace policy will be January 1 if enrollment is completed in November or December. If enrollment occurs in January, then the effective date will be February 1 (Ortaliza & Cox, 2024). Navigators should assess if patients needing access to the Marketplace outside of the national OEP qualify for a SEP. Various SEP opportunities are available, and understanding these is essential for patients with cancer who find themselves without any health insurance coverage after a cancer diagnosis. The three most common SEP opportunities include the following (HealthCare.gov, n.d.-b):
• Recent loss of credible coverage: Patients have up to 60 days from the date of loss of credible coverage to enroll in the Marketplace. As most patients are terminated from employment once their Family and Medical Leave of Absence or short-term

TABLE 8-5 Maximum Annual Limitation on Cost-Sharing

Taxable Income (% Federal Poverty Level)	Actuarial Value of a Silver Plan	MOOP for Individual/Family 2024	MOOP for Individual/Family 2025
Under 100%	70%	$9,450/$18,900	$9,200/$18,400
100%–150%	94%	$3,150/$6,300	$3,050/$6,100
150%–200%	87%	$3,150/$6,300	$3,050/$6,100
200%–250%	73%	$7,550/$15,100	$7,350/$14,700
Over 250%	70%	$9,450/$18,900	$9,200/$18,400

MOOP—maximum out-of-pocket cost

Note. From *Explaining Health Care Reform: Questions About Health Insurance Subsidies*, by Kaiser Family Foundation, 2024 (https://www.kff.org/affordable-care-act/issue-brief/explaining-health-care-reform-questions-about-health-insurance-subsidies/). Copyright 2024 by Kaiser Family Foundation. Licensed under CC BY-NC-ND 4.0 (https://creativecommons.org/licenses/by-nc-nd/4.0/).

disability policy expires, which most often results in loss of coverage, ongoing assessment of the patient is necessary to help patients take advantage of this SEP opportunity.
- Decrease in household income: Current Marketplace enrollees who experience a significant decrease in household income, from above 250% to below 250% FPL, should notify the Marketplace of this change. This income change can generate a SEP, allowing enrollees to take advantage of the cost-sharing subsidies available in Silver plans (Kaiser Family Foundation, 2024).
- Projected income falls below 150% FPL: In September 2021, the U.S. Department of Health and Human Services finalized a new SEP in states that use Health Care.gov (optional for other states), granting year-round enrollment in the Marketplace if an applicant's projected household income does not exceed 150% FPL and if they are eligible for subsidies that cover the cost of the benchmark Silver plan. This SEP opportunity is vital to understand, especially for patients with cancer, who often experience decreased income during their cancer journey. Therefore, ongoing income assessment of the self-pay population is critical so that these patients do not miss SEP opportunities (Kaiser Family Foundation, 2024).

Summary

As the U.S. healthcare system continues to become more complex, measures should be put in place to mitigate further marginalization of patient populations who are affected by the devastating impact of FT. A wide range of assistance programs are available to patients with cancer, and navigators play an essential role in using these programs for this population. Navigators also play an indispensable role in guiding patients by educating them about the many insurance optimization opportunities available to Marketplace and Medicare beneficiaries. Making decisions after receiving a complex medical diagnosis such as cancer is challenging for anyone, but especially for patient populations that have been historically marginalized. Navigation programs can offer individualized services to patients to help them overcome healthcare system barriers, facilitate timely access to quality care, and help lessen financial burdens during and after treatment. Navigating the economic aspect of the cancer journey should, therefore, be included in any oncology navigation program.

The author would like to acknowledge Kanan Shah, BS, Yousuf Zafar, MD, MHS, and Fumiko Chino, MD, for their contribution to this chapter that remains unchanged from the previous edition of this book.

References

Alzehr, A., Hulme, C., Spencer, A., & Morgan-Trimmer, S. (2022). The economic impact of cancer diagnosis to individuals and their families: A systematic review. *Supportive Care in Cancer, 30*(8), 6385–6404. https://doi.org/10.1007/s00520-022-06913-x

Bell-Brown, A., Watabayashi, K., Delaney, D., Carlos, R.C., Langer, S.L., Unger, J.M., ... Shankaran, V. (2023). Assessment of financial screening and navigation capabilities at National Cancer Institute community oncology clinics. *JNCI Cancer Spectrum, 7*(5), pkad055. https://doi.org/10.1093/jncics/pkad055

Centers for Medicare and Medicaid Services. (2024a). *At risk: Pre-existing conditions could affect 1 in 2 Americans.* https://www.cms.gov/CCIIO/Resources/Forms-Reports-and-Other-Resources/preexisting

Centers for Medicare and Medicaid Services. (2024b). *Medicare and you 2025: The official U.S. government Medicare handbook.* https://www.medicare.gov/publications/10050-medicare-and-you.pdf

Centers for Medicare and Medicaid Services. (2024c). *What's the Medicare Payment Prescription Plan?* https://www.medicare.gov/publications/12211-whats-the-medicare-prescription-payment-plan.pdf

Chan, R.J., Gordon, L.G., Tan, C.J., Chan, A., Bradford, N.K., Yates, P., ... Miaskowski, C. (2019). Relationships between financial toxicity and symptom burden in cancer survivors: A systematic review. *Journal of Pain and Symptom Management, 57*(3), 646–660.e1. https://doi.org/10.1016/j.jpainsymman.2018.12.003

Corrigan, K.L., Fu, S., Chen, Y.-S., Kaiser, K., Roth, M., Peterson, S.K., ... Smith, G.L. (2022). Financial toxicity impact on younger versus older adults with cancer in the setting of care delivery. *Cancer, 128*(13), 2455–2462. https://doi.org/10.1002/cncr.34220

Dusetzina, S., Zuckerman, A.D., Keating, N., & Huskamp, H.A. (2024, February 8). Medicare Part D's new prescription payment plan may not reduce costs for all. *Health Affairs Forefront.* https://doi.org/10.1377/forefront.20240206.784421

Freed, M., Biniek, J.F., Damico, A., & Neuman, T. (2024a). *Medicare Advantage in 2024: Enrollment update and key trends.* Kaiser Family Foundation. https://www.kff.org/medicare/issue-brief/medicare-advantage-in-2024-enrollment-update-and-key-trends

Freed, M., Biniek, J.F., Damico, A., & Neuman, T. (2024b). *Medicare Advantage in 2024: Premiums, out-of-pocket limits, supplemental benefits, and prior authorization.* Kaiser Family Foundation. https://www.kff.org/medicare/issue-brief/medicare-advantage-in-2024-premiums-out-of-pocket-limits-supplemental-benefits-and-prior-authorization

HealthCare.gov. (n.d.-a). *How to pick a health insurance plan.* https://www.healthcare.gov/choose-a-plan/plans-categories

HealthCare.gov. (n.d.-b). *Keep or change your insurance plan.* https://www.healthcare.gov/keep-or-change-plan

Hussain, S.M.Q., Gupta, A., & Dusetzina, S.B. (2022). Financial toxicity of cancer treatment. *JAMA Oncology, 8*(5), 788. https://doi.org/10.1001/jamaoncol.2021.7987

Jagsi, R., Ward, K.C., Abrahamse, P.H., Wallner, L.P., Kurian, A.W., Hamilton, A.S., ... Hawley, S.T. (2018). Unmet need for clinician engagement regarding financial toxicity after diagnosis of breast cancer. *Cancer, 124*(18), 3668–3676. https://doi.org/10.1002/cncr.31532

Jones, E.C. (2013). Supreme Court decision on the Affordable Care Act: What does it mean for neurology? *Neurology Clinical Practice, 3*(1), 61–66. https://doi.org/10.1212/CPJ.0b013e318283ffb9

Kaiser Family Foundation. (2024). *Explaining health care reform: Questions about health insurance subsidies.* https://www.kff.org/affordable-care-act/issue-brief/explaining-health-care-reform-questions-about-health-insurance-subsidies

Levitt, L., & Altman, D. (2023). Complexity in the US health care system is the enemy of access and affordability. *JAMA Health Forum, 4*(10), e234430. https://doi.org/10.1001/jamahealthforum.2023.4430

Longo, C.J. (2022). Linking intermediate to final "real-world" outcomes: Is financial toxicity a reliable predictor of poorer outcomes in cancer? *Current Oncology, 29*(4), 2483–2489. https://doi.org/10.3390/curroncol29040202

Ma, S.J., Iovoli, A.J., Attwood, K., Wooten, K.E., Arshad, H., Gupta, V., ... Singh, A.K. (2021). Association of significant financial burden with survival for head and neck cancer patients treated with radiation therapy. *Oral Oncology, 115*, 105196. https://doi.org/10.1016/j.oraloncology.2021.105196

Mangir, C., Schneider, L., Santiago, A., Kajdic, R., Hudson-DiSalle, S., Dallara, E., ... Lucas, L. (2020). Current state and future needs of the financial advocacy workforce: Workload, responsibilities, and education. *Journal of Oncology Navigation and Survivorship, 11*(11), 3207. https://www.jons-online.com/issues/2020/november-2020-vol-11-no-11/3207

Medicare Rights Center. (2025). *Extra Help: Income and asset limits 2025.* https://www.medicarerights.org/fliers/Help-With-Drug-Costs/Extra-Help-Chart.pdf?nrd=1

Michigan Cancer Consortium. (2018). *Financial navigation for people undergoing cancer treatment.* https://navectis.com/wp-content/uploads/2020/02/FinancialNavigationReport_FinalAccessible20183.pdf

National Cancer Institute. (2024, May 29). *Financial toxicity and cancer treatment (PDQ®)–Health professional version.* https://www.cancer.gov/about-cancer/managing-care/track-care-costs/financial-toxicity-hp-pdq

National Council on Aging. (2025, March 24). *Medicare savings programs eligibility and coverage.* https://www.ncoa.org/article/medicare-savings-programs-eligibility-coverage

Ochieng, N., Cubanski, J., & Neuman, T. (2024, September 23). *A snapshot of sources of coverage among Medicare beneficiaries.* Kaiser Family Foundation. https://www.kff.org/medicare/issue-brief/a-snapshot-of-sources-of-coverage-among-medicare-beneficiaries

Ortaliza, J., & Cox, C. (2024). *The Affordable Care Act 101.* Kaiser Family Foundation. https://www.kff.org/health-policy-101-the-affordable-care-act/?entry=table-of-contents-what-is-the-affordable-care-act

Panzone, J., Welch, C., Morgans, A., Bhanvadia, S.K., Mossanen, M., Shenhav-Goldberg, R., ... Goldberg, H. (2021). Association of race with cancer-related financial toxicity. *JCO Oncology Practice, 18*(2), e271–e283. https://doi.org/10.1200/OP.21.00440

Phillips, C. (2023, April 21). *Financial navigation can reduce the financial toxicity of cancer care.* National Cancer Institute. https://www.cancer.gov/news-events/cancer-currents-blog/2023/cancer-care-financial-navigation-saves-money

Pollitz, K., Lo, J., & Wallace, R. (2023). *Standardized plans in the health care marketplace: Changing requirements.* Kaiser Family Foundation. https://www.kff.org/private-insurance/issue-brief/standardized-plans-in-the-health-care-marketplace-changing-requirements

Popham, L., Bedlin, H., Fried, L. & Hoadley, J. (2020). *Take-up rates in Medicare savings programs and the Part D low-income subsidy among community-dwelling Medicare beneficiaries age 65 and older.* https://www.advancingstates.org/sites/default/files/2020-CBA-DG02_-LIS-MSP-Issue-Brief_6-19b.pdf

Prasad, R.N., Patel, T.T., Keith, S.W., Eldredge-Hindy, H., Fisher, S.A., & Palmer, J.D. (2021). Development of a financial toxicity screening tool for radiation oncology: A secondary analysis of a pilot prospective patient-reported outcomes study. *Advances in Radiation Oncology, 6*(6), 100782. https://doi.org/10.1016/j.adro.2021.100782

Samaha, N.L., Mady, L.J., Armache, M., Hearn, M., Stemme, R., Jagsi, R., & Gharzai, L.A. (2024). Screening for financial toxicity among patients with cancer: A systematic review. *Journal of the American College of Radiology, 21*(9), 1380–1397. https://doi.org/10.1016/j.jacr.2024.04.024

Sheehan, S.M., Patel, S., Leach, C.R., Goldsack, J.C., & Robinson, E.J. (2023). Advancing digital innovation to improve equity and reduce financial toxicity in cancer treatment. *Journal of Clinical Oncology, 41*(16, Suppl.), e18644. https://doi.org/10.1200/JCO.2023.41.16_suppl.e18644

Sherman, D.E., & Fessele, K.L. (2019). Financial support models: A case for use of financial navigators in the oncology setting. *Clinical Journal of Oncology Nursing, 23*(5), 14–18. https://doi.org/10.1188/19.CJON.S2.14-18

U.S. Department of Health and Human Services. (2022). *Fact sheet: Celebrating the Affordable Care Act.* https://www.hhs.gov/about/news/2022/03/18/fact-sheet-celebrating-affordable-care-act.html

U.S. Government Accountability Office. (2023, April 26). *Testimony before the Subcommittee on Oversight, Committee on Ways and Means, House of Representatives: Tax administration: IRS oversight of hospitals' tax-exempt status.* https://www.gao.gov/assets/gao-23-106777.pdf

U.S. Social Security Administration. (2024, February). *Understanding the Extra Help with your Medicare prescription drug plan.* https://www.ssa.gov/pubs/EN-05-10508.pdf

Wheeler, S.B., Birken, S.A., Wagi, C.R., Manning, M.L., Gellin, M., Padilla, N., ... Rosenstein, D.L. (2022). Core functions of a financial navigation intervention: An in-depth assessment of the Lessening the Impact of Financial Toxicity (LIFT) intervention to inform adaptation and scale-up in diverse oncology care settings. *Frontiers in Health Services, 2*, 958831. https://doi.org/10.3389/frhs.2022.958831

Xu, L., Welch, P., Ruhter, J., Nguyen, N.X., Sheingold, S., DeLew, N., & Sommers, B.D. (2023, May 25). *Medicare Advantage overview: A primer on enrollment and spending.* Assistant Secretary for Planning and Evaluation: Office of Health Policy. https://aspe.hhs.gov/sites/default/files/documents/9b42ffbf2341726d5b63a9647b0aad15/medicare-advantage-overview.pdf

Yedjou, C.G., Sims, J.N., Miele, L., Noubissi, F., Lowe, L., Fonseca, D.D., ... Tchounwou, P.B. (2019). Health and racial disparity in breast cancer. *Advances in Experimental Medicine and Biology, 1152*, 31–49. https://doi.org/10.1007/978-3-030-20301-6_3

Yezefski, T., Steelquist, J., Watabayashi, K., Sherman, D., & Shankaran, V. (2018). Impact of trained oncology financial navigators on patient out-of-pocket spending. *American Journal of Managed Care, 24*(5, Suppl.), S74–S79. https://www.ajmc.com/view/impact-of-trained-oncology-financial-navigators-on-patient-outofpocket-spending

SECTION III
Noteworthy Navigation Topics From the Experts

Chapter 9. Personalized Communication Across the Cancer Care Continuum
Chapter 10. Navigating Each Phase of the Patient Journey
Chapter 11. Unique Navigation Issues
Chapter 12. Personalized Medicine and Novel Therapies
Chapter 13. Spiritual Considerations

CHAPTER 9

Personalized Communication Across the Cancer Care Continuum

Deborah M. Christensen, MSN, APRN, AOCNS®

> **KEY TOPICS**
> communication, age-appropriate strategies

Overview

Effective communication lies at the heart of oncology care, connecting patients, families, and healthcare teams. For oncology nurse navigators (ONNs), communication is not just about relaying information; it is about establishing relationships, inspiring hope, and guiding patients and their families through the complex and emotionally charged path of cancer care. ONNs work with patients of all ages and stages across the cancer care continuum. They may be responsible for clarifying diagnoses, explaining treatment options, and providing comfort and support to those facing recurrence or end-of-life care. Difficult conversations frequently arise during the cancer journey—from the identification of suspicious findings to treatment and end-of-life care. To be prepared for these conversations, ONNs also need to understand that different age groups process information and emotions differently, leading to the need for tailored communication strategies.

Mastering essential communication skills is necessary for overcoming challenges within the healthcare system. Patient and provider encounters are often brief, and patients may not have all their needs addressed (Prip et al., 2018). They also may receive test results before anyone on the clinical team, leading to misinterpretation of findings and medical terminology (Arvisais-Anhalt et al., 2022). ONNs can help patients and their families cope with a cancer diagnosis by using age-appropriate, culturally centered communication and various teaching methods to ensure that information is understood (Oncology Nursing Society & Oncology Nursing Certification Corporation, 2024).

This chapter will showcase effective communication methods at each stage of the cancer care continuum, including prediagnosis, diagnosis, treatment, survivorship, recurrence, and hospice through the end of life. It will also cover some of the unique needs and preferences of parents of pediatric patients, adolescents and young adults (AYAs), adults, and older adults. Additionally, evidence-based strategies to overcome communication barriers will be addressed.

Prediagnosis to Diagnosis: Navigating Uncertainty

Waiting for a diagnosis can be exceptionally difficult for patients and their loved ones. This period often involves scheduling appointments with specialists, undergoing diagnostic tests, and waiting for the results to return. This uncertainty can be a central part of the overall experience for patients and presents an ideal opportunity for ONNs to establish a therapeutic and supportive relationship. ONNs can assist patients by reviewing the typical wait time for test results, discussing potential next steps, assessing how patients would like to hear test results, and, when possible, being present when a diagnosis is disclosed.

ONNs can face significant challenges when excluded from discussions regarding a patient's prognosis, leading to frustration and a sense of being peripheral to the care process (Saleh, 2022). Without access to diagnostic and prognostic information, ONNs may feel ill-equipped to fulfill their roles as educators, advocates, and support systems, fearing they might inadvertently provide information that contradicts physician statements. This risks confusing patients and their families and raises concerns about being perceived as incompetent or indifferent. Moreover, ONNs may worry that such a communication gap may erode the trust that patients and families have in them (Saleh, 2022).

In the past, a familiar physician typically disclosed a cancer diagnosis. However, with the fast-paced changes in health care, this tradition has been replaced by various healthcare providers, such as specialists, hospitalists, and other medical professionals (Cantril et al., 2019). These providers may not have any previous relationship with specific patients, yet they deliver news that will change the patients' and their families' lives forever.

An alternative to this practice was implemented at breast imaging centers in Marin and Sonoma Counties in Northern California. A breast health nurse navigator (BNN) met with patients who required biopsies. The BNN provided education, ensured the biopsies were scheduled, and arranged for an in-person follow-up within three to four days to discuss the results. The pre-biopsy meeting was essential for the BNN to gather social and demographic details and encourage patients to bring a support person to the follow-up. During the follow-up, the BNN reviewed the pathology, described future steps, and provided written and visual information. This approach focused on patients' needs and was revered by patients and healthcare providers. Patients expressed being better informed and less anxious when meeting with the surgeon or oncologist (Cantril et al., 2019).

Being part of delivering bad news can happen at any time during the cancer care continuum when the message has the potential to impact patients and their families' lives negatively. The SPIKES and PEWTER models are structured approaches healthcare professionals can use to deliver bad news and guide delicate conversations with empathy and clarity (see Figure 9-1). Essential communication strategies from both models suggest preparing a comfortable and private space for a sensitive conversation, giving patients and their families the time and privacy they need to process the news emotionally. ONNs should be well informed about the diagnosis, treatment strategies, and any information that has been previously communicated to ensure message consistency and anticipate potential reactions. It is also important to assess patients' current understanding of the topic to tailor communication to their level and needs (Baile et al., 2000; Kitz et al., 2023).

Treatment: Supporting Informed Decision-Making

Communication regarding prognosis in oncology is a complex challenge for nurses. It is important for ONNs to accurately gauge how much information patients want to know about their prognosis. This enables ONNs to collaborate with the interprofessional team in respecting patient preferences and ensuring that patients receive the necessary information to make well-informed decisions about their care (Kim et al., 2020). ONNs can be conduits between oncologists and patients to ensure clear and compassionate communication and support informed decision-making. Effective communication informs, supports, and guides patients, whereas ineffective communication can lead to confusion and distress, especially in the treatment phase of care (Leblanc et al., 2019).

It is essential to understand how patients are processing their diagnoses. An ideal communication strategy is simply asking what their biggest concern is at that moment. Open-ended questions can receive the following responses:
- Am I going to die?
- I do not want to lose my hair!
- I have to keep working; my family relies on me.

ONNs can compassionately address these types of questions and continue to build on the trusting relationship.

Cancer literacy presents specific barriers different from general health literacy, largely because decisions related to cancer are usually more complicated, such as choosing screenings, selecting treatments, and managing side effects. Additionally, quickly making these decisions is often more critical in the context of cancer care (Sørensen et al., 2020).

Samoil et al. (2021) evaluated 146 peer-reviewed articles related to the impact of patients' health literacy on their treatment choices. Out of the 12 studies examining decision-making for cancer care, one study indicated that men with lower health literacy and higher anxiety about their prostate-specific antigen levels were more likely to choose a type of prostate cancer therapy known for its unwanted side effects. In another study, patients with low health literacy were less likely to choose breast reconstruction after a mastectomy. However, low health literacy did not appear to impact the decision to undergo surgical treatments. Similarly, another study found

FIGURE 9-1	SPIKES and PEWTER Communication Models for Delivering Bad News
SPIKES Model	
Setting Up	When delivering news, it is crucial to prioritize privacy, involve loved ones, sit down, make a connection with the patient, and manage time constraints and interruptions.
Perception	When breaking news to a patient, healthcare professionals should first assess what the patient already knows or suspects about the situation to tailor the information accordingly. This helps ensure that the patient understands the news.
Information	Respect the patient's preference regarding the amount of information they want to receive.
Knowledge	When giving medical information, use simple language, go at the patient's pace, and prepare them emotionally if bad news is coming.
Emotions and empathy	Observe the patient's reaction and respond empathetically. Acknowledge their emotions, offer support, and allow them to express their feelings.
Summary	Summarize the news and outline a future strategy for the patient, offering hope that aligns with reality.
PEWTER Model	
Prepare	Gather relevant information about the patient and find a private setting for the discussion without interruptions.
Emotion	Be prepared to recognize and address a range of emotional responses from patients, including shock, sadness, anger, or denial.
Warning	A warning statement helps patients prepare for bad news, preventing sudden emotional shock.
Tell	Deliver clear and straightforward news, avoiding medical jargon. Be honest, direct, and compassionate.
Empathize	Show empathy after delivering the news. Listen, acknowledge, and offer support. It is crucial for the patient to feel heard and understood.
Review and summarize	Summarize the next steps to ensure patient understanding, clarify misunderstandings, and answer questions.

Note. Based on information from Baile et al., 2000; Kitz et al., 2023.

that health literacy levels did not significantly affect the decision to begin hormone therapy for breast cancer treatment (Samoil et al., 2021).

Operating under the assumption that health information can pose comprehension difficulties for all patients and caregivers, ONNs should communicate in straightforward, universally understood terms. This approach enhances patient care and demonstrates respect for the patients' experiences. Clear and actionable information is universally valued by patients, aiding in informed decision-making and fostering a collaborative care environment where patients feel supported and empowered (Hyatt et al., 2021). Studies have shown that communication interventions tailored to the specific needs of patients with cancer and their families can bring many benefits, such as increased acceptance of the intervention and improved completion rates (Li et al., 2020).

Cancer Survivorship: Fostering Resilience

Cancer survivors face unique challenges. Transitioning from treatment to post-treatment often requires a higher level of engagement and communication with the healthcare team (Dahlke et al., 2022). Effective communication between patients and their healthcare teams is essential for providing high-quality, patient-centered care, and it has been linked to improved adherence to post-treatment protocols, patient satisfaction, and self-management. A survey conducted on 147 breast cancer survivors revealed communication gaps with healthcare teams while transitioning from treatment to post-treatment care (Dahlke et al., 2022). Healthcare providers must fulfill fundamental functions to meet cancer survivors' diverse needs, including establishing healing relationships, facilitating information exchange, attuning to emotional needs, navigating uncertainties, assisting in decision-making, and supporting patient self-care (Austin et al., 2019).

Quality communication between healthcare providers and patients has improved patient involvement in their care, leading to better care and health outcomes (Jenstad et al., 2024). Patient-centered communication is essential for self-management and influences patient outcomes, including self-efficacy. However, research indicates that patient-centered communication often falls short, especially for cancer survivors managing multiple chronic conditions, even a decade post-diagnosis. This suggests a disconnect beyond the initial transition period, highlighting the need for continued effective communication in cancer care (Austin et al., 2019). Strategies that ONNs can use to enhance communication in survivorship are available in Table 9-1.

Cancer Recurrence: Renewing Dialogue

A cancer recurrence is an emotional time for most patients, as they must face new decisions and life-altering changes. Research indicates that up to half of patients with advanced or incurable cancers do not fully comprehend their prognosis and, therefore, choose aggressive therapies, potentially setting up immense disappointment when cancer returns (Leblanc et al., 2019). Empathic responses are necessary during this time. Even if expected, recurrence requires a renewed dialogue between the healthcare team, patient, and their family.

ONNs can use the communication strategies in Figure 9-1 and Table 9-1 to empathetically address patients' psychosocial and physical needs with recurrent disease. As

TABLE 9-1. Strategies to Enhance Post-Treatment Communication

Strategy	Description
Establish trust and rapport	Create a supportive environment through empathetic interactions, making patients feel valued.
Open and clear information exchange	Provide understandable information about post-treatment care, side effects, and signs of recurrence, explaining medical terms in simple language and ensuring comprehension.
Emotional support	Listen and respond to the emotional needs of patients and families, validating their feelings and addressing their concerns.
Managing uncertainty	Discuss long-term side effects and coping strategies. Help family members understand that recovery is a process.
Shared decision-making	Help patients make informed decisions about follow-up care by weighing options and discussing preferences.
Promote self-management	Empower patients with self-care practices and resources for symptom management and lifestyle modifications.
Long-term follow-up	Discuss the importance of regular follow-ups to help manage the physical and emotional effects of cancer and its treatment.
Interdisciplinary collaboration	Collaborate with the healthcare team to ensure consistent communication and meeting patient needs, including referrals to specialists.
Continuous education	Stay updated on the latest cancer survivorship research and guidelines to provide current information and advice to patients.
Tailored communication	Personalize communication strategies to match each survivor's unique needs, cultural backgrounds, and preferences.
Feedback and adaptation	Collect patient feedback on communication effectiveness and adjust as needed to improve clarity and helpfulness.

Note. Based on information from Austin et al., 2019, 2021.

patients may move in and out of different therapy stages and deal with various late and long-term side effects, ONNs can explain the roles of multiple providers (e.g., specialists, primary care physicians, non-oncology experts, palliative care teams, social workers, other support services) in providing quality care.

Hospice and End of Life: Ensuring Peace and Comfort

For patients approaching the end of life, ONNs may find themselves in situations where they need to have complex and often emotional conversations with patients and family members about treatment decisions and advance directives. ONNs need to have the necessary communication skills to handle such situations effectively. These abilities include providing clinical care to anxious patients, answering questions about prognosis, dealing with disagreements between nurses and physicians, and introducing the concept of palliative care and hospice to patients and caregivers (Spine et al., 2022).

Practical end-of-life communication skills are fundamental for optimal patient and family care. The strategies discussed throughout this chapter can be refined through ongoing practice, real-world experience, and dedicated patience. Table 9-2 displays additional communication resources and training programs.

By committing to continuously improving their communication abilities, ONNs can profoundly influence the quality of care they offer to patients at a critical time in their lives. This commitment helps address patients' complex emotional and physical needs and supports families during challenging transitions, ensuring that all involved receive compassionate, respectful, and comprehensive care.

Age-Related Communication Considerations

By developing actionable insights and strategies, ONNs can communicate in a compassionate, clear, and responsive manner, addressing the specific challenges faced by parents of pediatric patients, AYAs, adults, and older adults from diagnosis through survivorship or end of life. The age ranges of these categories vary depending on the characteristics being examined and the source (National Cancer Institute,

TABLE 9-2. Palliative Care, End-of-Life, and Communication Training Resources

Resource	Website
COMFORT Communication: application that lists a variety of communication tools and strategies for healthcare providers	www.communicatecomfort.com/comfort-communication-app
Conversation Project: provides downloadable conversation guides	www.theconversationproject.org
Conversation Ready: includes a tool kit for respectful end-of-life conversations that align with patients' goals, values, and preferences	www.ihi.org/resources/tools/how-talk-your-patients-about-end-life-care-conversation-ready-toolkit-clinicians
Plain Language: offers communication checklists, handouts, and posters	www.plainlanguage.gov/resources/checklists
Vital Talk: offers one-page guides on difficult conversations, respecting emotions, and more	www.vitaltalk.org/resources/quick-guides

n.d.). The ranges established for this chapter are pediatrics (1–12 years), adolescents (13–19 years), young adults (20–39 years), adults (40–64 years), and older adults (65 years or older).

Pediatric Patients

The diagnosis of cancer in a child can cause profound emotional turmoil for parents, affecting their capacity to understand medical information and make decisions about their child's care (Sisk et al., 2021). By offering empathy, acknowledging the parents' emotional struggles, striving to relate to their experiences, and catering to each family's specific circumstances, ONNs can make a meaningful difference. ONNs need to balance straightforward information with kindness and understanding and consider the weight of their words when delivering bad news (Sisk et al., 2021).

ONNs must provide comprehensive patient education in an age-related manner, including potential side effects and what to do if and when they occur. Effective communication can help build trust between healthcare providers, parents, and children. Studies have shown that when parents are provided with detailed explanations about their child's condition, they feel more comfortable and confident and less guilty. This can also lead to a deeper trust in the healthcare provider's ability to provide the best care for their child. Transparency about the child's condition can help instill hope, and following through on promises can build further trust and confidence in the healthcare provider (Srinivas et al., 2023).

Another communication strategy is offering support and affirming parents' optimism about their child's prognosis and future aspirations. Parents indicated they appreciated healthcare professionals recognizing and celebrating their child's treatment milestones. Although fostering a positive outlook is essential, ONNs should avoid giving parents unfounded or unrealistic expectations (Srinivas et al., 2023). This is where clear communication among healthcare team members is critical in maintaining a consistent narrative for parents and their children. Additional communication strategies include using simple language, moderating the flow of information, and patiently addressing questions without showing frustration (Sisk et al., 2019; Srinivas et al., 2023).

Adolescents and Young Adults

AYAs with cancer face singular complexities during an already transitional life phase. This diverse age group of patients is at a juncture between pediatric and adult oncology care, which can lead to feelings of displacement within the healthcare system (Smith et al., 2020). AYAs have distinct experiences and communication needs compared to younger children and older adults. Along with physical, cognitive, emotional, and behavioral shifts, AYAs often endure a unique biologic profile, extended treatment durations, poorer prognoses, and intense feelings of despair and isolation (Smith et al., 2020).

Srinivas et al. (2023) analyzed responses from two studies asking AYAs to provide communication advice to clinicians. Respondents indicated that AYAs:
- Appreciate when healthcare providers inquire about their emotional well-being and that of their families.
- Recommend assessing the emotional atmosphere—reading the room—before sharing bad news.
- Suggest tailoring the communication approach to meet the family's specific emotional requirements.
- Express the need to feel supported and have ongoing availability, even after treatment ends or if they have moved to a different clinical team.
- Want to be part of the decision-making process and expect to be asked to engage in communication.
- Request optimism and an upbeat demeanor, even in adverse situations.
- Acknowledge the need for honesty and transparency.
- Expect their healthcare team to remain calm and help patients and families feel their care is in good hands.

Similar to other patient groups, AYA patients preferred explanations in simple language followed by written material for later review and to share with family. They also wanted to control both the timing and amount of information they received (Sisk et al., 2022; Srinivas et al., 2023).

Adults

Adults with cancer also have distinctive communication needs that require personalization. They are typically the primary decision-makers regarding their care, so they need detailed information to make informed choices independently. Therefore, adults prefer conversations to be straightforward and autonomous, focusing on individual needs and life context (Vicente et al., 2023). Adults have unique life experiences to draw upon when processing their diagnosis and treatment options, influencing how information is perceived and how decisions are made. In general, adult patients desire comprehensive information about their condition but also wish to have some control over the extent, format, and timing of this information (Leblanc et al., 2019).

Comprehensive care and support for adult patients with cancer requires understanding their concerns, including the physical aspects of cancer, as well as the emotional, social, and practical barriers they face. Adults may be the primary wage earners or caregivers in their households and worry about how their family will be cared for financially. They may be on a fixed income and have financial concerns. Adults can also feel isolated or perceive they are a burden to their loved ones (Dhakal et al., 2022). ONNs can build a trusting relationship by addressing these concerns at the onset of and throughout the cancer care continuum.

Although oncologists typically provide the most information about a patient's prognosis and treatment options, ONNs may need to clarify misconceptions and reinforce what patients and families understand about the prognosis. This highlights the importance of ONNs understanding patient preferences and being skilled in delivering information in a way that balances honesty with optimism.

Older Adults

The older adult population faces age-related communication challenges. Cognitive and sensory decline, such as vision changes and hearing deficits, can lead to poor communication and unmet information needs. ONNs must maintain patience, ask for feedback on preferred communication methods, and be flexible in adapting to their needs. Building a rapport with older adults and understanding their unique challenges will help provide compassionate and effective oncology care.

It is a common misconception that older adult patients are a homogenous group. This age group is incredibly diverse, with unique information preferences and needs (Bol et al., 2020). Recognizing and responding to this diversity is essential to ensure that patients receive the care they deserve.

Bol et al. (2020) identified three distinct communication profiles among older adult patients: information seekers, listeners, and information avoiders. Information seekers actively search for details to manage their concerns, whereas listeners may not engage or express their questions. Information avoiders require clear and concise communication about the purpose of the consultation to avoid feeling overwhelmed.

Information seekers often struggle with the inherent uncertainty regarding their diagnosis. ONNs can assist this group by prioritizing information and managing uncertainty rather than overwhelming them with data. They can encourage listeners to engage more and express their needs. Encouraging listeners emotionally may also improve their recall and consultation outcomes. For information avoiders, ONNs can offer support by clearly communicating the aim of the consultation to help patients gain focus and encourage their participation in decision-making, even if they prefer less information. By adopting a tailored approach to each patient's profile, ONNs can foster effective communication and enhance patient engagement and satisfaction with care.

Communication Strategies in Action

Communication strategies can provide structure for patient and caregiver conversations. These case studies demonstrate how age-appropriate communication and elements from SPIKES and PEWTER models can guide conversations during diagnosis, recurrence, and end of life.

A New Cancer Diagnosis

Rachel was diagnosed with invasive ductal carcinoma, stage IIIc, after her first mammogram at age 53 years. Despite feeling a lump in her right breast for 18 months, she was initially reluctant to seek medical care.

Rachel meets with Cindy, an ONN, to learn more about additional testing and treatment options. In a private consultation room, Cindy explores Rachel's existing knowledge about her situation. Cindy understands that most adults want straightforward information. However, she asks Rachel how much detail she prefers to hear. Overwhelmed, Rachel asks for basic information for now. Cindy uses simple language, acknowledges Rachel's emotions of guilt for waiting so long to seek treatment, and summarizes the next steps. Rachel feels supported and more at ease, knowing what to expect.

The Cancer Is Back

James, a 67-year-old Black male, is scheduled to meet with Kevin, an ONN, after metastatic spread was found during a surveillance scan. Before entering the conference room, Kevin reviews case details, noting a prostatectomy and a two-year history of androgen deprivation therapy. He also verifies the new treatment plan with the medical oncologist. Kevin introduces himself, clarifies James's understanding of the proposed plan, and validates his disappointment in having a recurrence. Kevin uses strategies from the PEWTER model to carefully balance treatment details with optimism while honoring James's quality-of-life goals and request to know the facts.

Transitioning to Hospice

After 18 months, Emily and Mark have come to the heartbreaking realization that further treatment will not improve their daughter Lily's condition. Grace, their ONN, is now guiding them through the transition to hospice care.

Grace provides the family with comprehensive information about hospice care, emphasizing it is a compassionate choice focused on 4-year-old Lily's comfort rather than continuing treatments that could cause more harm. She validates their feelings of guilt and remorse, emphasizing that choosing hospice care is not about giving up but about prioritizing Lily's quality of life. She reassures them that hospice care can be provided at home, where Lily can be surrounded by her family and familiar surroundings. Grace listens attentively, giving them time to express their emotions. She outlines the next steps and calls to provide ongoing support and reassurance the next day.

Summary

Healthcare communication, especially in oncology, is a delicate task. ONNs can provide empathy and clarity by using elements from structured communication models such as SPIKES and PEWTER. Simple language is vital to patients' understanding of their diagnosis and treatment options. During the shift to survivorship, or when there is cancer recurrence, ONNs can provide clear guidance and emotional support to patients, aiding their comprehension of the situation and fostering informed decision-making. The continuity of ONN support across the cancer care continuum becomes even more meaningful when discussing advance care planning and end-of-life decisions. Through these profound transitions, ONNs can blend compassion with clear communication to support patients and families.

ONNs can also adapt their communication style according to patient age and individual needs, ranging from pediatric patients and their parents to older adults with varying degrees of information processing abilities. As educators, advocates, and compassionate supporters, ONNs can tailor their communication to support hope while providing realistic expectations and ensuring patient dignity and preferences are respected throughout each phase of the cancer care continuum.

The author would like to acknowledge Cynthia Cantril, MPH, RN, OCN®, CBCN®, for her contribution to this chapter that remains unchanged from the previous edition of this book.

References

Arvisais-Anhalt, S., Lau, M., Lehmann, C.U., Holmgren, A.J., Medford, R.J., Ramirez, C.M., & Chen, C.N. (2022). The 21st Century Cures Act and multiuser electronic health record access: Potential pitfalls of information release. *Journal of Medical Internet Research, 24*(2), e34085. https://doi.org/10.2196/34085

Austin, J.D., Allicock, M., Fernandez, M.E., Balasubramanian, B.A., & Lee, S.C. (2021). Understanding the delivery of patient-centered survivorship care planning: An exploratory interview study with complex cancer survivors. *Cancer Control, 28*, 1–8. https://doi.org/10.1177/10732748211011957

Austin, J.D., Robertson, M.C., Shay, L.A., & Balasubramanian, B.A. (2019). Implications for patient-provider communication and health self-efficacy among cancer survivors with multiple chronic conditions: Results from the Health Information National Trends Survey. *Journal of Cancer Survivorship, 13*(5), 663–672. https://doi.org/10.1007/s11764-019-00785-7

Baile, W.F., Buckman, R., Lenzi, R., Glober, G., Beale, E.A., & Kudelka, A.P. (2000). SPIKES—A six-step protocol for delivering bad news: Application to the patient with cancer. *Oncologist, 5*(4), 302–311. https://doi.org/10.1634/theoncologist.5-4-302

Bol, N., Linn, A.J., Smets, E.M.A., Verdam, M.G.E., & van Weert, J.C.M. (2020). Tailored communication for older patients with cancer: Using cluster analysis to identify patient profiles based on information needs. *Journal of Geriatric Oncology, 11*(6), 944–950. https://doi.org/10.1016/j.jgo.2020.01.004

Cantril, C., Moore, E., & Yan, X. (2019). Diagnosis disclosure: Patient preferences and the role of the breast nurse navigator. *Clinical Journal of Oncology Nursing, 23*(6), 619–626. https://doi.org/10.1188/19.CJON.619-626

Dahlke, D., Yoshikawa, A., McAdam, M., Malatok, S., & Gonzales, E.D. (2022). An analysis of health care team communication needs among younger vs older breast cancer survivors: Web-based survey. *JMIR Cancer, 8*(1), e31118. https://doi.org/10.2196/31118

Dhakal, P., Wichman, C., Pozehl, B., Weaver, M.S., Fisher, A.L., Vose, J.M., Bociek, G.R., & Bhatt, V.R. (2022). Understanding the treatment preferences of adults with cancer. *Blood, 140*(Suppl. 1), 5070–5072. https://doi.org/10.1182/blood-2022-164863

Hyatt, A., Drosdowsky, A., Koproski, T., Milne, D., Rametta, M., McDonald, G., McKenzie, T., & Blaschke, S.-M. (2021). Identification of low health and cancer literacy in oncology patients: A cross-sectional survey. *Supportive Care in Oncology, 29*(11), 6605–6612. https://doi.org/10.1007/s00520-021-06164-2

Jenstad, L.M., Howe, T., Breau, G., Abel, J., Colozzo, P., Halas, G., ... Strachan, S. (2024). Communication between healthcare providers and communicatively-vulnerable patients with associated health outcomes: A scoping review of knowledge syntheses. *Patient Education and Counseling 119*, 108040. https://doi.org/10.1016/j.pec.2023.108040

Kim, S.-H., Kim, J.-H., Shim, E.-J., Hahm, B.-J., & Yu, E.-S. (2020). Patients' communication preferences for receiving a cancer diagnosis: Differences depending on cancer stage. *Psycho-Oncology, 29*(10), 1540–1548. https://doi.org/10.1002/pon.5447

Kitz, C.C., Barclay, L.J., & Breitsohl, H. (2023). The delivery of bad news: An integrative review and path forward. *Human Resource Management Review, 33*(3), 100971. https://doi.org/10.1016/j.hrmr.2023.100971

Leblanc, T.W., Marron, J.M., Ganai, S., McGinnis, M.M., Spence, R.A., Tenner, L., ... Hlubocky, F.J. (2019). Prognostication and communication in oncology. *Journal of Oncology Practice, 15*(4), 208–215. https://doi.org/10.1200/JOP.18.00647

Li, J., Luo, X., Cao, Q., Lin, Y., Xu, Y., & Li, Q. (2020). Communication needs of cancer patients and/or caregivers: A critical literature review. *Journal of Oncology, 2020*, 7432849. https://doi.org/10.1155/2020/7432849

National Cancer Institute. (n.d.). *Cancer Statistics Explorer Network*. https://seer.cancer.gov/statistics-network/

Oncology Nursing Society & Oncology Nursing Certification Corporation. (2024). *Oncology nurse navigator competencies*. https://www.ons.org/sites/default/files/2024-10/onn-competencies-final.pdf

Prip, A., Møller, K.A., Nielsen, D.L., Jarden, M., Olsen, M.-H., & Danielsen, A.K. (2018). The patient–healthcare professional relationship and communication in the oncology outpatient setting: A systematic review. *Cancer Nursing, 41*(5), E11–E22. https://doi.org/10.1097/NCC.0000000000000533

Saleh, A.M. (2022). Nurses' perceptions of prognosis-related communication. *Asian Pacific Journal of Cancer Prevention, 23*(3), 775–780. https://doi.org/10.31557/APJCP.2022.23.3.775

Samoil, D., Kim, J., Fox, C., & Papadakos, J. (2021). The importance of health literacy on clinical cancer outcomes: A scoping review. *Annals of Cancer Epidemiology, 5*(3), 1–30. https://doi.org/10.21037/ace-20-30

Sisk, B.A., Keenan, M., Schulz, G.L., Kaye, E., Baker, J.N., Mack, J.W., & DuBois, J.M. (2022). Interdependent functions of communication with adolescents and young adults in oncology. *Pediatric Blood and Cancer, 69*(4), e29588. https://doi.org/10.1002/pbc.29588

Sisk, B.A., Schulz, G.L., Blazin, L.J., Baker, J.N., Mack, J.W., & DuBois, J.M. (2021). Parental views on communication between children and clinicians in pediatric oncology: A qualitative study. *Supportive Care in Cancer, 29*(9), 4957–4968. https://doi.org/10.1007/s00520-021-06047-6

Sisk, B.A., Schulz, G.L., Mack, J.W., Yaeger, L., & DuBois, J. (2019). Communication interventions in adult and pediatric oncology: A scoping review and analysis of behavioral targets. *PLOS ONE, 14*(8), e0221536. https://doi.org/10.1371/journal.pone.0221536

Smith, L.A.M., Critoph, D.J., & Hatcher, H.M. (2020). How can health care professionals communicate effectively with adolescent and young adults who have completed cancer treatment? A systematic review. *Journal of Adolescent and Young Adult Oncology, 9*(3), 328–340. https://doi.org/10.1089/jayao.2019.0133

Sørensen, K., Makaroff, L.E., Myers, L., Robinson, P., Henning, G.J., Gunther, C.E., & Roediger, A.E. (2020). The call for a strategic framework to improve cancer literacy in Europe. *Archives of Public Health, 78*, 60. https://doi.org/10.1186/s13690-020-00441-y

Spine, K., Skwira-Brown, A., Schlifke, D., & Carr, E. (2022). Clinical oncology nurse best practices: Palliative care and end-of-life conversations. *Clinical Journal of Oncology Nursing, 26*(6), 612–620. https://doi.org/10.1188/22.CJON.612-620

Srinivas, M., Kaye, E.C., Blazin, L.J., Baker, J.N., Mack, J.W., DuBois, J., & Sisk, B.A. (2023). Advice to clinicians on communication from adolescents and young adults with cancer and parents of children with cancer. *Children, 10*(1), 7. https://doi.org/10.3390/children10010007

Vicente, R.S., Freitas, A.R., Ferreira, R.M.A., Prada, S.P., Martins, T.S., Martins, T.C., ... Barbosa, M. (2023). Communication preferences and perceptions of cancer patient during their first medical oncology appointment. *Psycho-Oncology, 32*(11), 1702–1709. https://doi.org/10.1002/pon.6220

CHAPTER 10

Navigating Each Phase of the Patient Journey

Claudia T. Miller, BSN, RN, OCN®, ONN-CG,
and Deborah M. Christensen, MSN, APRN, AOCNS®

> **KEY TOPICS**
> cancer care continuum, care coordination, nursing process

Overview

The oncology nurse navigator (ONN) is an integral member of the cancer care team, guiding patients and their loved ones through distinct phases of the cancer care continuum: prevention, early detection, diagnosis, treatment, survivorship, palliative care, and end of life. The main objective of oncology navigation is to develop a personalized strategy with each patient to overcome barriers and improve access to timely care and patient outcomes (Chan et al., 2023). Although navigation can occur anywhere along the cancer care continuum, ONNs need a solid understanding of each phase to develop a personalized care plan for each patient. The care plan should be patient centric and evidence based.

It is important to recognize that a universal oncology navigation process cannot adequately address the varying needs of diverse populations across different settings throughout the cancer care continuum. However, navigators share common goals of assessing and addressing barriers to care, coordinating care and care transitions, providing phase-specific education and psychosocial support, and advocating for patients' goals and needs (Gentry, 2021). These principles, along with the concepts from the Oncology Nursing Society's *Oncology Navigation Standards of Professional Practice* and the *Oncology Nurse Navigator Competencies*, create a framework for ONN interventions. It is essential to ask patients about their goals and priorities frequently, as these can change at any time along the cancer care continuum.

This chapter will establish the importance of the ONN role, present phase-specific navigation interventions, and review real-world evidence supporting navigation within the context of cancer care continuum phases.

Prevention and Screening

Prevention and early diagnosis of cancer offer the best opportunity for positive outcomes. The first recognized oncology navigation program started with prevention and screening. Over the years, the value of navigating patients at this stage of the cancer care continuum continues to be recognized, especially in underserved populations (Dwyer et al., 2022; Freeman et al., 1995). Systemic and structural barriers faced by racial and ethnic minority groups also contribute to cancer screening disparities. Oncology navigators and community health services working in rural, impoverished areas of the United States identified mistrust of the healthcare system, poor health literacy, language barriers, and lack of transportation as common obstacles during this phase of cancer care (Hallgren et al., 2023). Language and cultural barriers, lack of health insurance, and limited access to specialty care also present significant barriers to care (American Association for Cancer Research, 2024; Bhatia et al., 2022).

Evaluating social determinants of health, the conditions in which people are born, grow, live, work, and age, can help identify additional barriers that can be addressed on an individual and community basis. Examples of these determinants are neighborhood environment, healthcare availability, social engagement, education, and financial stability. Health-related social needs, such as food resources, housing, utilities, and transportation options, can also affect equitable access to cancer prevention programs and screening services (American Association for Cancer Research, 2024; Haines et al., 2024; Tucker-Seeley et al., 2024).

Given the existing disparities in healthcare access, not all populations receive equal benefits from prevention efforts, with systemic and structural barriers faced by racial and ethnic minority groups contributing to cancer screening inequalities (American Association for Cancer Research, 2024). ONNs are uniquely positioned to address these inequities. Local community health centers, cancer coalitions, and national organizations such as the Cancer Prevention and Control Research Network (www.cpcrn.org) and the Centers for Disease Control and Prevention (www.cdc.gov/cancer) often provide location-specific programs and materials for cancer prevention and screening, local initiatives, and community resources. These resources can prepare ONNs to make a positive impact throughout the cancer prevention and screening phase of cancer care.

Gallup's 2023 Honesty and Ethics poll identified nurses as the most trusted medical professionals (American Nurses Association, 2024). ONNs may have an advantage in addressing skepticism and mistrust issues identified among people of color and ethnic minority groups.

Oncology Nurse Navigator Interventions Within Prevention and Screening

During the prevention and screening phases, ONNs can perform the following (Oncology Nursing Society & Oncology Nursing Certification Corporation, 2024):

- Assess social determinants of health and include this assessment in care interventions.
- Evaluate health literacy, learning readiness, and learning preferences.
- Streamline the process for identifying high-risk individuals.
- Facilitate referrals to genetic counselors as needed.
- Connect patients with transportation, financial assistance, and psychosocial resources.
- Empower patients by providing education and checking for understanding.

The involvement of navigators not only benefits patients but may also generate financial advantages for healthcare institutions by improving patient retention and facilitating ancillary testing. Additionally, ONN interventions may indirectly lower overall treatment costs by addressing issues early. This comprehensive approach ultimately reduces health disparities and promotes better health equity within communities (Kline et al., 2019).

Real-World Evidence: Navigating Breast, Colorectal, and Cervical Cancer Screenings

Nelson et al. (2020) conducted a meta-analysis to determine the effectiveness of oncology navigation in improving screening rates for breast, colorectal, and cervical cancer in disparaged populations. The analysis included three studies with multiple cancer types and 4, 11, and 28 studies for cervical, breast, and colorectal cancers, respectively. Navigation services included outreach education, appointment reminders, interpretive services, education on preparing for the screening test, and assistance with travel. Results indicated that oncology navigation (Nelson et al., 2020):
- Improved adherence to breast screening in previously nonadherent patients
- Increased screening rates in mixed populations of adherent and nonadherent patients
- Generated higher cervical cancer screening rates compared to patients who did not receive navigation services
- Boosted colorectal cancer screening in all patient populations in 23 of the studies

Despite variability in the navigation interventions and study populations, navigation interventions contributed to increases in cancer screening—one of the major initiatives in the 2022 revival of the Cancer Moonshot initiative (The White House, 2022).

Diagnosis

When patients are diagnosed with cancer, it is a significant and life-changing event. This point of care may mark the beginning of the navigator–patient–family relationship or continue the relationship developed during the prevention and screening phase of the cancer care continuum. Patients and their families are often filled with anxiety and fear about the uncertainty of their situation. Waiting for additional appointments and staging can be exceptionally difficult, and communication is essential to help minimize anxiety and provide reassurance. Providing patients with accurate and reasonable timelines also helps manage their anxieties and expectations (Chan et al., 2023).

Oncology Nurse Navigator Interventions at Diagnosis

Assessment is foundational in health care. As an initial step, ONNs introduce themselves and their role, evaluate patient understanding of the diagnosis, and address any misunderstandings. People hear information differently, and this assessment will help ONNs identify knowledge gaps and help patients understand their diagnosis and next steps. Assessing social determinants of health and potential barriers should occur throughout the cancer care continuum, as patients' situations can change during their cancer experience (Hughes Halbert, 2022; Tucker-Seeley et al., 2024).

Cross-cultural issues, such as language, ethnicity, race, and religion, can influence how patients and their families perceive illness, cope, and respond psychologically to a cancer diagnosis. ONNs can use assessment tools such as the National Comprehensive Cancer Network Distress Thermometer, Patient-Reported Outcomes Measures (PROMIS), and Patient Health Questionnaire-9 (PHQ-9) to identify and address distress and depression (Neal et al., 2021).

ONNs can advise patients on the risks of relying on unverified online sources, especially those promoting unproven treatments or therapies that can be harmful. Validating and honoring patients' lived experiences can build trust and set the stage for a therapeutic relationship. Supporting patients' wishes, such as seeking a second opinion, exemplifies the ONN's role as a patient educator and advocate. ONNs may be asked to answer questions about genetic testing, clinical trials, work or school concerns, disability benefits, and child or elder care. Anticipating and proactively addressing patients' and loved ones' immediate concerns is a primary theme throughout the diagnostic and staging phase of cancer care.

Although survivorship is a recognized phase of the cancer care continuum, survivorship planning essentially begins at diagnosis and includes patients' inner circle of family and friends (Austin et al., 2021). ONNs can help patients understand the role of exercise, nutrition, pain management, and psychosocial support to prepare them for the next phase of their cancer journey.

The integration of precision oncology and biomarker testing can influence treatment selection. Delays in ordering testing and sending tumor specimens to external laboratories can lead to delays in treatment. Given the recommendations from organizations such as the National Comprehensive Cancer Network, ONNs can ensure that patients receive timely and appropriate testing. Keeping up with the latest biomarker testing guidelines, understanding laboratory processes, and collaborating with pathologists, oncologists, and laboratory personnel are ways ONNs can support biomarker testing.

The involvement of ONNs during the diagnostic phase enhances patient experiences and adds value to the healthcare system. Models such as the Centers for Medicare and Medicaid Services' Oncology Care Model and the Centers for Medicare and Medicaid Innovation's Enhancing Oncology Model recognize navigation as a critical component for reimbursement. In today's healthcare landscape, where plans aim for efficiency and bundled services, studies have indicated that navigation can be a cost-effective intervention, contributing to improved outcomes and potentially reducing overall costs (Lopez et al., 2019).

Real-World Evidence: Precision Oncology Stewardship

In 2021, Sanford Health, a large rural health system in the Midwest, piloted the role of Oncology Nurse Navigator, Genomics (ONNG) to address common challenges and improve coordination in biomarker testing. This specialized ONNG role included the following responsibilities (Association of Community Cancer Centers, 2022):
- Acting as a central liaison for the healthcare team
- Explaining the clinical importance of biomarker testing to patients
- Addressing access barriers (e.g., insurance coverage)
- Tracking the testing process through completion
- Educating staff on precision oncology
- Keeping patients and their families informed
- Completing key performance indicator reports

As of 2023, Sanford Health was looking to expand the role to all of its sites or use telehealth to centralize the stewardship role (Association of Community Cancer Centers, 2023).

Treatment

One of the most important ONN roles during the treatment phase is proactively identifying and addressing any known or potential barriers to care that may impede adherence to treatment. Barriers can be structural, cultural, or related to individual circumstances, such as limited knowledge, fewer financial resources, and lack of health insurance coverage. Moreover, living far away from care providers and lacking access to community resources can add to these challenges (Chan et al., 2023).

Ensuring that patients understand their treatment plans and providing support to enhance adherence is crucial for achieving better health outcomes. The transition from *compliance* to *adherence* represents a more patient-centered approach, recognizing that individual preferences and circumstances can significantly impact patients' ability to follow a treatment regimen. This shift fosters a partnership between healthcare providers and patients, promoting shared decision-making and greater engagement (Mir, 2023).

As precision oncology and the use of oral agents in cancer treatment become more prevalent, the importance of treatment adherence grows. The complexity of modern treatment plans, which often involve multimodal regimens, necessitates frequent clinical interventions to address emerging barriers. Research has shown that navigation can positively influence various aspects of cancer care, including treatment initiation, adherence, quality of care, and patient satisfaction—particularly among vulnerable populations (Chan et al., 2023; Chen et al., 2024).

Given that national spending on cancer care in the United States is estimated to be $200 billion annually and continues to rise, financial toxicity has become a pressing issue. Many patients face difficult decisions between paying for essential living expenses and affording life-sustaining cancer treatments (Smith et al., 2022).

Oncology Nurse Navigator Interventions During Active Treatment

Once the treatment plan is established, ONNs can collaborate with financial navigators (when available) who can help determine patients' financial obligations, potential grant opportunities, and co-pay assistance programs. Case managers within private insurance companies can be another significant patient resource. ONNs work with the treatment team to coordinate care, reinforce education, and assist with any medical or personal equipment needed during treatment (i.e., cold caps, head coverings, prosthetics, specialized clothing). Additional considerations for individual populations may include addressing body image and sexuality, discussing fertility preservation options, and referring to genetic counseling.

ONNs can encourage patients who have employment to contact their human resources department to determine if they are eligible for disability benefits. If patients are likely to become unemployed while on treatment, ONNs should ensure they understand their options for continued health coverage if they carry health insurance and that family members understand how to apply for the Family and Medical Leave Act to help care for their loved ones.

As patients and their families navigate cancer treatment, ONNs should stay in regular contact with their patients to ensure that no new barriers have emerged. Friends, family members, and neighbors are often willing to help by providing transportation, child care, elder care, or meals. ONNs can encourage patients to accept this support. In addition, many national and community resources are available to support patients during treatment, such as the American Cancer Society's Road to Recovery and Hope Lodge programs, which help address transportation and lodging needs. Organizations dedicated to specific cancer types also can provide patient education materials and other resources (see Chapter 18).

The role of the ONN is pivotal in enhancing treatment adherence and managing financial toxicity, ultimately leading to improved health outcomes and a more supportive care environment for patients navigating their cancer journeys.

Real-World Evidence: Treatment Plan Adherence

Chen et al. (2024) reviewed 17 research articles examining the impact of oncology navigation on patient adherence to treatment plans and scheduled appointments. Significant improvements in treatment adherence were noted in multiple cancer groups, including breast (five), cervical (three), osteosarcoma (one), lymphoma (one), and mixed studies (two). One cervical cancer study noted that the percentage of patients completing a minimum of five cycles of carboplatin was 93% in navigated patients compared to 74% in those who did not receive navigation services (Dessources et al., 2020). Patient no-show rates decreased in navigated patients compared with controls in gastrointestinal (9.6% vs. 12.5%), head and neck (4.3% vs. 11.9%), and hematologic malignancies (9.2% vs. 14.7%) (Percac-Lima et al., 2015).

Survivorship

The number of cancer survivors in the United States is expected to continue growing and is projected to reach 22.5 million by 2032 (National Cancer Institute, 2024a). In response to a growing cancer survivor population, health care must shift some focus from the diagnostic and treatment delivery phase to survivorship care. The question becomes: Why treat the cancer and create cancer survivors if we are not going to support them post-treatment?

During the treatment phase, patients have become accustomed to being seen at regular intervals, providing a sense of security. When treatment ends, patients transition to a surveillance plan where they have less frequent contact with their treatment team and are expected to go live their "new normal" life. If patients are not educated on the late and long-term side effects that cancer treatments can produce, their health outcomes will suffer (Pratt-Chapman et al., 2011).

Financial toxicity remains a critical concern during survivorship. While patients prioritize survival during active treatment, financial considerations often take a backseat. However, the economic burden of cancer extends well beyond treatment, with financial strain frequently intensifying during survivorship. Survivors face both direct costs, such as ongoing medical care, and indirect costs, which tend to have a more substantial impact. These include reduced employment, job loss, depleted savings, or inadequate insurance coverage—all of which significantly affect patients' economic well-being during survivorship (Scheidegger et al., 2023).

Addressing financial toxicity early in the cancer care continuum is vital to ensuring cancer survivors can thrive. By raising awareness and offering support at the outset, healthcare providers can help mitigate long-term financial challenges and empower survivors to achieve a higher quality of life (QoL) post-treatment. Chapter 8 provides vital information and interventions related to financial toxicity.

Oncology Nurse Navigator Interventions in Survivorship

ONNs can assist patients in survivorship by starting the conversation prior to the end of treatment to prepare them for this transition. They may also perform a needs assessment to determine if any barriers impede ongoing care, such as housing, transportation, lack of finances, and access to a primary care physician. This assessment is vital and will help ensure that patients are able to attain the highest QoL possible in survivorship.

Following active treatment, ONNs can provide patients with information about self-care, the long-term and late side effects of treatment, and appropriate surveillance recommendations, as well as help them understand the impact of cancer treatment on their overall well-being. Motivational interviewing techniques, such as open-ended questions, can help patients make realistic goals and choices as they move beyond treatment. ONNs can continue to address any psychosocial issues and advocate for appropriate support services.

ONN care coordination among oncology, primary care providers, and other specialists is critical to optimal survivorship care (Alfano et al., 2022). Suboptimal coordination may lead to both the primary care physician and oncology provider believing the other is taking charge of critical aspects of the patient's post-treatment care. This can result in missed screenings, delayed detection of recurrence, or inadequate management of patients' ongoing health needs (Alfano et al., 2022).

While supporting patients during this phase, ONNs can discuss recommendations for healthy living, such as weight management, exercise, or smoking cessation programs, and offer referrals to community and national resources. Fatigue, shortness of breath, lymphedema, and peripheral neuropathy are potential physical issues that may arise after active treatment, and patients may need a referral to a rehabilitation specialist (Alfano et al., 2022). If patients have been on disability leave, ONNs should ensure that they understand their rights as they transition back to work. Several national organizations provide employment and legal advice for patients with cancer (see Chapter 18).

Real-World Evidence: Survivorship Navigation Outcomes

Ramirez et al. (2020) compared the effect of enhanced patient navigation with usual patient navigation among Latina breast cancer survivors, hypothesizing that females receiving enhanced patient navigation would rate their QoL higher than those in the navigation-only control group. Navigators in the study were proficient in Spanish and included one community health worker and two oncology nurses. Sequential randomization was used to stratify into two groups of 60 females. Functional Assessment of Cancer Therapy questionnaires (FACT–General and FACT–Breast) were used to evaluate QoL. Participants in the patient navigation cohort received a study fact sheet with the navigator's contact information. Unless contacted directly by the participant, the navigators only met with patients during the assessments. Participants in the enhanced patient navigation cohort received culturally crafted education materials in Spanish or English, along with consistent, personalized assistance, including regular phone contact, reminder calls, transportation assistance, and education on community resources such as exercise classes and support groups. No significant differences existed between cohorts at baseline. At six months, the control group's FACT scores worsened. In contrast, the enhanced patient navigation groups noted improvements in all scores except the FACT–General physical well-being subscale, suggesting that enhanced navigation in survivorship can enhance QoL in specialized groups of patients.

Advanced, Metastatic, and Recurrent Disease

Advances in medicine have led to the development of newer drugs with improved side effect profiles and better response rates, allowing patients with advanced or metastatic cancer to live longer and more fulfilling lives, even when their disease remains incurable. As a result, ONNs play a vital role in guiding these patients through the complexities of their care. The considerations that apply during the diagnostic and treatment phase continue to be relevant for patients with recurrent or advanced and metastatic cancer.

However, an additional aspect that becomes especially important in this phase is the discussion around advance directives and end-of-life planning. ONNs must ensure these conversations are initiated early, as making decisions about end-of-life care can significantly reduce the emotional burden on patients and their families. Addressing these sensitive topics before a crisis arises provides patients with a sense of control and helps families feel more prepared, ultimately leading to better emotional and psychological outcomes.

Some patients are diagnosed with advanced cancer from the outset, meaning the disease has already spread beyond its original site at the time of diagnosis. This can often occur with cancers that do not show early symptoms or are difficult to detect.

Oncology Nurse Navigator Interventions for Patients With Advanced and Metastatic Disease

ONNs caring for patients during this stage of the cancer care continnum must rely on their clinical knowledge to provide emotional support and clarify potential options. Communication within the healthcare team is critical so patients do not receive conflicting information. These patients may present with unique needs because of the advanced stage of their disease. Patients will have new treatment decisions ranging from ongoing treatment to comfort care. Active listening and validation are beneficial skills during this phase of care. In the advanced and metastatic phase of the continuum, it is essential to balance hope with reality. See Chapter 9 for additional communication skills.

For newly diagnosed patients with advanced cancer, the issues highlighted in the diagnosis phase apply. Patients with a prior cancer diagnosis may be facing cancer treatment effects and persistent financial challenges, including depleted retirement funds and difficulties paying monthly bills. ONNs can address these issues by advocating for referrals to rehabilitation or home health and providing information on financial assistance programs. Patients with late-stage disease also need substantial emotional or spiritual support as they adjust to living with cancer as a chronic disease or transition toward end-of-life care.

Oncology social workers and spiritual care specialists can provide valuable support. Patients may not always realize how these professionals can help. If patients or their loved ones hesitate to use these services, ONNs can discuss their concerns and address misunderstandings (Chan et al., 2023).

For patients who choose symptom management rather than active treatment, ONNs can coordinate care between oncology, palliative care, and hospice while helping patients and their loved ones understand their options and what each service provides.

Real-World Evidence: Complex Care Navigation

In 2021, a randomized controlled trial was conducted to determine whether the addition of navigation interventions increased supportive care interventions, advance directive completion, and QoL (Soto-Perez-de-Celis et al., 2021). Patients with metastatic cancer (N = 134) were randomly assigned to one of two groups. Group one (n = 67) received personalized support from an oncology navigator, and those from group two (n = 67) received usual care, with oncologists referring patients to supportive care services as needed. At 12 weeks, 74% of navigated patients (group 1) received supportive care, and 48% completed advance directives. In contrast, in the usual care cohort (group 2), only 24% received supportive care, and none completed advance directives (Soto-Perez-de-Celis et al., 2021).

End of Life

Initiating a discussion about end-of-life care can be challenging, but it is an essential part of providing comprehensive support to patients with advanced or terminal illnesses. ONNs may need to act as intermediaries between patients, families, and providers to ensure this vital conversation takes place. In some cases, ONNs may need to bring up the subject themselves, which requires sensitivity, empathy, and strong communication skills.

It is equally important for ONNs to reflect on their perspectives surrounding life and death, as personal biases can unintentionally affect the tone and outcome of these discussions. By being self-aware and prepared, ONNs can approach the topic with professionalism and compassion.

Many patients and family members may struggle with feelings of "giving up" when transitioning from curative treatment to comfort care or hospice. During this emotionally complex time, ONNs must clearly understand the patient care goals and ensure that those goals are communicated effectively to the entire healthcare team. This helps ensure that patient wishes remain at the forefront of all decisions.

Acting as a patient advocate at the end of life means more than just facilitating medical decisions—it involves helping patients and their families navigate this transition with dignity. This advocacy may also include assisting patients to plan their lasting legacy, giving them a sense of control and purpose during a vulnerable time. The ONN's role is to ensure that patient values and desires are respected, providing emotional support and guidance throughout the final stages of care (National Cancer Institute, 2024b).

The unpredictability of living with and navigating a cancer diagnosis can be accompanied by grief and loss long before actual physical death occurs. Conversations about death are complex and rooted in personal histories of loss, experiences of the dying process, and the family dynamic (Mackenzie & Lasota, 2020).

Oncology Nurse Navigator Interventions at the End of Life

ONNs are uniquely positioned to help facilitate end-of-life education. Even though beginning these conversations can be challenging and uncomfortable, talking about goals of care helps clarify patients' priorities and values and should be initiated early. Unfortunately, these discussions often occur during emergency decision points (e.g., need for life-sustaining treatment) or when patients are within a few days to weeks of dying (Mackenzie & Lasota, 2020). When ONNs have had conversations about advance directives early in the cancer continuum, they can approach these conversations with added confidence and unreserved compassion.

When patient-centered communication occurs between ONNs, patients, and families, it becomes therapeutic, fostering trust and addressing patients' and caregivers' needs, concerns, and preferences. ONNs can balance clinical knowledge of the disease complexities, patient and caregiver stressors, and the death and dying process with compassion. Many ONN interventions discussed throughout this chapter, such as active listening, validation, and compassionate care, are also effective during end-of-life care.

The SPIKES and PEWTER communication models (see Chapter 9) outline the following steps for having difficult conversations (Kumar & Sarkhel, 2023):
- Locate a quiet and private setting for the conversation to take place.
- Prepare participants for a sensitive conversation.
- Assess the patient's and family's prior experience with death and dying.
- Respect patient preferences for the amount of information they prefer.
- Use simple language balancing honesty with compassion.
- Summarize and answer questions.

Kwame and Petruka (2021) proposed a four-tiered process for patient-centered care and communication (PC4). Although not explicitly designed for end-of-life care, its application is an example of why patient-centered communication is vital to the success of end-of-life conversations. The lowest tier of PC4 consists of task-oriented communication, process-oriented communication, and patient-centered communication. In the final phase of the cancer care continuum, task-oriented communication occurs between medical professionals, medical terms are used, and tasks are accomplished. Patients and families may be part of process-oriented conversations about the death and dying process or how hospice functions in the home setting. The conversation is more directed at patients in an informational way. Patient-centered communication occurs when patients and caregivers are seen as partners in the care process, and the relationship between the care provider (ONN) and receiver (patients and their families) becomes more interactive. This leads to a mutual and ongoing negotiation between both parties.

Building strong, trusting relationships with patients allows ONNs to navigate sensitive discussions organically, ensuring that patients' needs and wishes are fully understood and respected. Patient-centered communication skills are essential in helping patients and their families make informed decisions about end-of-life care. Additionally, ONNs must prioritize self-care to maintain well-being and provide the highest level of care, acknowledging the emotional toll of losing patients to cancer (Mackenzie & Lasota, 2020).

Real-World Evidence: Research Gap in Navigation at the End of Life

A noticeable gap in research persists within oncology navigation focusing on end-of-life care, signifying the need for studies examining the effect of navigator interventions during the final stage of the cancer care continuum. Potential research opportunities that align with the Oncology Nursing Society's *Oncology Nurse Navigator Competencies* and *Oncology Navigation Standards of Professional Practice* and the Academy of Oncology Nurse and Patient Navigators' *Navigation Metrics Toolkit* include measuring the impact of ONNs in supporting smooth transitions to hospice care, preparing patients and families for signs and symptoms experienced at the end of life, facilitating referrals to hospice care, and implementing best practices for end-of-life care (Academy of Oncology Nurse and Patient Navigators & American Cancer Society, 2020; Oncology Nursing Society & Oncology Nursing Certification Corporation, 2024; Professional Oncology Navigation Task Force, 2022).

Additional research should include ONN knowledge of the dying process and skills for managing moral distress when working with patients in hospice care.

Summary

Oncology navigation is a dynamic process that occurs at defined phases of the cancer care continuum and as patient situations and needs change. ONNs address known and potential barriers to care, including financial constraints, lack of access to transportation, language barriers, and limited health literacy. They provide personalized education, facilitate shared decision-making, and advocate for patient referrals to specialists and supportive care programs. ONNs can learn skills to engage in conversations about end-of-life care preferences and support patients and their families in making these critical decisions. ONN interventions such as these have led to increased rates of breast, colorectal, and cervical cancer screening and reduced time from suspicious findings to diagnosis and subsequent treatment. Better biomarker testing coordination and patient adherence to treatment plans and follow-up appointments are additional benefits noted in the diagnostic and treatment phases of care. Patients with navigation support show enhanced QoL, earlier referrals to palliative care services, and completion of advance directives. Continued research into the benefits of oncology navigation is needed, especially at the end of life.

ONNs need to stay flexible and adaptable as they navigate the complexities of cancer care. The considerations discussed in this chapter can serve as guideposts for ONNs who must be prepared to navigate challenges as they arise across the cancer care continuum and provide the most comprehensive support for patients.

The authors would like to acknowledge Lori McMullen, MSN, RN, and Sharon Cavone, BSN, RN, OCN®, for their contribution to this chapter that remains unchanged from the previous edition of this book.

References

Academy of Oncology Nurse and Patient Navigators & American Cancer Society. (2020). *Navigation metrics toolkit*. American Cancer Society. https://www.aonnonline.org/images/resources/navigation_tools/2020-AONN-Navigation-Metrics-Toolkit.pdf

Alfano, C.M., Oeffinger, K., Sanft, T., & Tortorella, B. (2022). Engaging TEAM medicine in patient care: Redefining cancer survivorship from diagnosis. *American Society of Clinical Oncology Educational Book, 42,* 1–11. https://doi.org/10.1200/EDBK_349391

American Association for Cancer Research. (2024). *AACR cancer disparities progress report 2024.* https://cancerprogressreport.aacr.org/wp-content/uploads/sites/2/2024/05/AACR_CDPR__2024.pdf

American Nurses Association. (2024, January 22). *America's most trusted: Nurses continue to rank the highest*. https://www.nursingworld.org/news/news-releases/2024/americas-most-trusted-nurses-continue-to-rank-the-highest

Association of Community Cancer Centers. (2022). *Precision medicine stewards: A case study from Sanford Health*. https://www.accc-cancer.org/docs/documents/oncology-issues/articles/2022/v37-n6/v37-n6-precision-medicine-stewards-a-case-study-from-sanford-health.pdf

Association of Community Cancer Centers. (2023). *Precision medicine stewards: Applying precision principles to biomarker testing processes to improve patient access*. https://www.accc-cancer.org/docs/projects/precision-medicine/precisionmedicine_biomarkertesting_article_032123.pdf

Austin, J.D., Allicock, M., Fernandez, M.E., Balasubramanian, B.A., & Lee, S.C. (2021). Understanding the delivery of patient-centered survivorship care planning: An exploratory interview study with complex cancer survivors. *Cancer Control, 28*. https://doi.org/10.1177/10732748211011957

Bhatia, S., Landier, W., Paskett, E.D., Peters, K.B., Merrill, J.K., Phillips, J., & Osarogiagbon, R.U. (2022). Rural–urban disparities in cancer outcomes: Opportunities for future research. *Journal of the National Cancer Institute, 114*(7), 940–952. https://doi.org/10.1093/jnci/djac030

Chan, R.J., Milch, V.E., Crawford-Williams, F., Agbejule, O.A., Joseph, R., Johal, J., ... Hart, N.H. (2023). Patient navigation across the cancer care continuum: An overview of systematic reviews and emerging literature. *CA: A Cancer Journal for Clinicians, 73*(6), 565–589. https://doi.org/10.3322/caac.21788

Chen, M., Wu, V.S., Falk, D., Cheatham, C., Cullen, J., & Hoehn, R. (2024). Patient navigation in cancer treatment: A systematic review. *Current Oncology Reports, 26*(5), 504–537. https://doi.org/10.1007/s11912-024-01514-9

Dessources, K., Hari, A., Pineda, E., Amneus, M.W., Sinno, A.K., & Holschneider, C.H. (2020). Socially determined cervical cancer care navigation: An effective step toward health care equity and care optimization. *Cancer, 126*(23), 5060–5068. https://doi.org/10.1002/cncr.33124

Dwyer, A.J., Staples, E.S., Harty, N.M., LeGrice, K.E., Pray, S.L.H., & Risendal, B.C. (2022). What makes for successful patient navigation implementation in cancer prevention and screening programs using an evaluation and sustainability framework. *Cancer, 128*(Suppl. 13), 2636–2648. https://doi.org/10.1002/cncr.34058

Freeman, H.P., Muth, B.J., & Kerner, J.F. (1995). Expanding access to cancer screening and clinical follow-up among the medically underserved. *Cancer Practice, 3*(1), 19–30.

Gentry, S. (2021, December 3). The journey of oncology navigation. *American Nurse.* https://www.myamericannurse.com/the-journey-of-oncology-navigation

Haines, E., Shelton, R.C., Foley, K., Beidas, R.S., Dressler, E.V., Kittel, C.A., ... Rendle, K.A. (2024). Addressing social needs in oncology care: Another research-to-practice gap. *JNCI Cancer Spectrum, 8*(3), pkae032. https://doi.org/10.1093/jncics/pkae032

Hallgren, E., Yeary, K.H.K., DelNero, P., Johnson-Wells, B., Purvis, R.S., Moore, R., ... McElfish, P.A. (2023). Barriers, facilitators, and priority needs related to cancer prevention, control, and research in rural, persistent poverty areas. *Cancer Causes and Control, 34*(12), 1145–1155. https://doi.org/10.1007/s10552-023-01756-1

Hughes Halbert, C. (2022). Social determinants of health and cancer care: Where do we go from here? *Journal of the National Cancer Institute, 114*(12), 1564–1566. https://doi.org/10.1093/jnci/djac175

Kline, R., Rocque, G.B., Rohan, E.A., Blackley, K.A., Cantril, C.A., Pratt-Chapman, M.L., ... Shulman, L.N. (2019). Patient navigation in cancer: The business case to support clinical needs. *Journal of Oncology Practice, 15*(11), 585–590. https://doi.org/10.1200/JOP.19.00230

Kumar, V., & Sarkhel, S. (2023). Clinical practice guidelines on breaking bad news. *Indian Journal of Psychiatry, 65*(2), 238. https://doi.org/10.4103/indianjpsychiatry.indianjpsychiatry_498_22

Kwame, A., & Petrucka, P.M. (2021). A literature-based study of patient-centered care and communication in nurse-patient interactions: Barriers, facilitators, and the way forward. *BMC Nursing, 20*(1), 158. https://doi.org/10.1186/s12912-021-00684-2

Lopez, D., Pratt-Chapman, M.L., Rohan, E.A., Sheldon, L.K., Basen-Engquist, K., Kline, R., ... Flores, E.J. (2019). Establishing effective patient navigation programs in oncology. *Supportive Care in Cancer, 27*(6), 1985–1996. https://doi.org/10.1007/s00520-019-04739-8

Mackenzie, A.R., & Lasota, M. (2020). Bringing life to death: The need for honest, compassionate, and effective end-of-life conversations. *American Society of Clinical Oncology Educational Book, 40,* 1–9. https://doi.org/10.1200/EDBK_279767

Mir, T.H. (2023). Adherence versus compliance. *HCA Healthcare Journal of Medicine, 4*(2), 219–220. https://doi.org/10.36518/2689-0216.1513

National Cancer Institute. (2024a, May 9). *Cancer statistics.* https://www.cancer.gov/about-cancer/understanding/statistics

National Cancer Institute. (2024b, May 9). *Planning the transition to end-of-life care in advanced cancer (PDQ®)–Health professional version.* https://www.cancer.gov/about-cancer/advanced-cancer/planning/end-of-life-hp-pdq

Neal, J.W., Roy, M., Bugos, K., Sharp, C., Galatin, P.S., Falconer, P., ... Ramchandran, K. (2021). Distress screenings through Patient-Reported Outcomes Measurement Information System (PROMIS) at an academic cancer center and network site: Implementation of a hybrid model. *JCO Oncology Practice, 17*(11), e1688–e1697. https://doi.org/10.1200/op.20.00473

Nelson, H.D., Cantor, A., Wagner, J., Jungbauer, R., Fu, R., Kondo, K., ... Quiñones, A. (2020). Effectiveness of patient navigation to increase cancer screening in populations adversely affected by health disparities: A meta-analysis. *Journal of General Internal Medicine, 35*(10), 3026–3035. https://doi.org/10.1007/s11606-020-06020-9

Oncology Nursing Society & Oncology Nursing Certification Corporation. (2024). *Oncology nurse navigator competencies.* https://www.ons.org/oncology-nurse-navigator-competencies

Percac-Lima, S., Cronin, P.R., Ryan, D.P., Chabner, B.A., Daly, E.A., & Kimball, A.B. (2015). Patient navigation based on predictive modeling decreases no-show rates in cancer care. *Cancer, 121*(10), 1662–1670. https://doi.org/10.1002/cncr.29234

Pratt-Chapman, M., Simon, M.A., Patterson, A.K., Risendal, B.C., & Patierno, S. (2011). Survivorship navigation outcome measures: A report from the ACS patient navigation working group on survivorship navigation. *Cancer, 117*(15, Suppl.), 3573–3582. https://doi.org/10.1002/cncr.26261

Professional Oncology Navigation Task Force. (2022). Oncology navigation standards of professional practice. *Clinical Journal of Oncology Nursing, 26*(3), E14–E25. https://doi.org/10.1188/22.CJON.E14-E25

Ramirez, A.G., Muñoz, E., Long Parma, D., Perez, A., & Santillan, A. (2020). Quality of life outcomes from a randomized controlled trial of patient navigation in Latina breast cancer survivors. *Cancer Medicine, 9*(21), 7837–7848. https://doi.org/10.1002/cam4.3272

Scheidegger, A., Bernhardsgrütter, D., Kobleder, A., Müller, M., Nestor, K., Richle, E., & Baum, E. (2023). Financial toxicity among cancer survivors: A conceptual model based on a feedback perspective. *Supportive Care in Cancer, 31*(10), 618. https://doi.org/10.1007/s00520-023-08066-x

Smith, G.L., Banegas, M.P., Acquati, C., Chang, S., Chino, F., Conti, R.M., ... Yabroff, K.R. (2022). Navigating financial toxicity in patients with cancer: A multidisciplinary management approach. *CA: A Cancer Journal for Clinicians, 72*(5), 437–453. https://doi.org/10.3322/caac.21730

Soto-Perez-de-Celis, E., Chavarri-Guerra, Y., Ramos-Lopez, W.A., Alcalde-Castro, J., Covarrubias-Gomez, A., Navarro-Lara, Á., ... Goss, P.E. (2021). Patient navigation to improve early access to supportive care for patients with advanced cancer in resource-limited settings: A randomized controlled trial. *Oncologist, 26*(2), 157–164. https://doi.org/10.1002/onco.13599

The White House. (2022, February 2). *Fact sheet: President Biden reignites Cancer Moonshot to end cancer as we know it* [Fact sheet]. https://bidenwhitehouse.archives.gov/briefing-room/statements-releases/2022/02/02/fact-sheet-president-biden-reignites-cancer-moonshot-to-end-cancer-as-we-know-it

Tucker-Seeley, R., Abu-Khalaf, M., Bona, K., Shastri, S., Johnson, W., Phillips, J., ... Hinyard, L. (2024). Social determinants of health and cancer care: An ASCO policy statement. *JCO Oncology Practice, 20*(5), 621–630. https://doi.org/10.1200/op.23.00810

CHAPTER 11

Unique Navigation Issues

Rachel Brody, PhD(c), MSN, RN

> **KEY TOPICS**
> community, outreach, collaboration, barriers to care

Overview

Navigation is an ever-evolving process, and oncology nurse navigators (ONNs) adapt to patient and caregiver needs throughout the cancer journey. Whether in an urban, suburban, or rural area, obstacles and barriers to oncology care, treatment, and support persist despite dedicated efforts to minimize their impact in countless demographics. Addressing barriers, overcoming obstacles, and finding solutions for patients with cancer requires creativity, perseverance, and the desire to learn from every patient and fellow ONNs.

This chapter will examine different settings where ONNs practice and address barriers to quality care access. It includes complex navigation case studies emphasizing unique issues, barriers, and interventions. These cases demonstrate the importance of collaboration and resource awareness in distinctive situations.

Navigating Diverse Environments

Academic medical centers located in resource-rich environments offer extensive oncologic options for care. Within these environments, patients with cancer have access to specialists from a wide array of clinical backgrounds. These include specific diagnostics, surgery options, radiation and medical oncologists, geneticists, oncology disease-specific subspecialists, clinical trial options, and support groups. ONNs navigate these options to facilitate accurate and timely referrals.

Patients initially diagnosed with cancer in an environment with fewer resources, such as in a rural community setting, may be referred to a more resource-rich environment for their cancer treatment. In these scenarios, travel, housing accommodations, financial implications, and changes to psychosocial support structures can become a significant concern, as patients may miss work because of travel time and distance. They may also be separated from those who usually provide consistent emotional and psychological support from home. The more complex the oncology diagnosis and treatment plan, the more critical it is for ONNs to facilitate access to care that addresses patients' needs. ONNs must be aware of and current on available resources in their geographic areas, as they can change over time.

Some navigation barriers, such as transportation and appointment scheduling, are apparent and easy to identify. Potentially less obvious issues include the following (American Association for Cancer Research, 2024):
- Distrust of medical care and the healthcare system
- Language, health, and digital literacy barriers
- Nonadherence to treatment
- Housing and food insecurities
- Immigration or residency status
- Financial or healthcare insurance insufficiency
- Cultural belief barriers
- Racial and sexual orientation marginalization

Outcome variance for patients with cancer of different racial backgrounds has been found in survival rates, comorbidities, and access to care—even more notable during the COVID-19 pandemic (American Association for Cancer Research, 2024; Fu et al., 2022).

As a critical component of the oncology care team, ONNs must be sensitive to racial, cultural, sexual, educational, geographical, and financial disparities and barriers when working with patients with cancer and their caregivers (Professional Oncology Navigation Task Force, 2022).

Case Studies Depicting Unique Navigation Issues

The *Oncology Nurse Navigator Competencies* from the Oncology Nursing Society and the Oncology Nursing Certification Corporation (2024) outline essential knowledge, skills, and abilities that ONNs use to effectively identify and address barriers to quality oncology care. The following case studies demonstrate how the ONN competencies guide navigation interventions. Each case highlights distinctive patient issues, barriers and interventions, and system connections that require collaboration across geography and systems.

Case Study 1: Limited English Proficiency, Undocumented Immigrant

Carmen, a 40-year-old Hispanic woman, discovers a lump in her left breast. She has no insurance, speaks with limited English proficiency (LEP), and lives in a remote part of the county. She contacts a community health center, is connected with a Spanish-speaking community health worker, and learns she qualifies for a no-cost mammogram. The community health worker contacts Karen, a mobile mammography breast ONN. Using a Spanish-speaking interpreter, Karen schedules Carmen for a mammogram. Karen reviews Carmen's pre-screening questionnaire, noting that Carmen's mother and sister died from ovarian and breast cancer, respectively. Carmen is an undocumented immigrant, so Karen contacts the nearest nonprofit hospital, helps her schedule an appointment with a genetic counselor, and provides her with the hospital's financial assistance application in Spanish. She ensures that Carmen has reliable transportation and gives her the contact information for a bilingual breast navigator in the hospital-associated cancer center.

Carmen's mammogram identifies a suspicious mass; a subsequent biopsy indicates triple-negative breast cancer, and germline testing is *BRCA1* positive. Cascade germline testing is recommended for her three daughters—all U.S. citizens—to assess hereditary cancer risk.

Identified Barriers and Interventions

The navigators in this scenario anticipated, assessed, and addressed potential and realized barriers to care: LEP, no insurance, and undocumented immigration status. They provided instructions and information in Carmen's preferred language and connected her to essential financial assistance resources.

More than 25 million individuals with LEP live in the United States (Chen et al., 2023). Although many hospital systems use interpretive services, patients with LEP still face significant barriers to accessing care. In an audit study of 144 hospitals in 12 states with demographic diversity, trained investigators, simulating the role of English-, Spanish-, or Mandarin-speaking patients, called the hospital information line and, using a standardized script, requested instructions on how to access lung, thyroid, or colon cancer care. The resulting analysis demonstrated that 93.5% of English speakers received instructions versus 37.7% of Spanish-speaking and 27.5% of Mandarin-speaking callers (Chen et al., 2023).

Connections and Competencies

The collaborative relationship between public health staff and the nonprofit organization was central to coordinating care transitions from the community center to the mobile mammography unit and ultimately to the nonprofit hospital for further care. Karen's awareness of and connection with state and grant funding programs provided Carmen with timely access to genetic counseling and mammography services.

Navigator interventions and connections addressing diversity and equity are imperative and must consider the cultural and linguistic needs of patients and their families (Oncology Nursing Society & Oncology Nursing Certification Corporation, 2024).

Case Study 2: Comorbidities, Caregiver Responsibilities, Genetic Risk

Joe, a 42-year-old White man, is visiting a health fair sponsored by a local academic medical center. He stops by the cancer center display and tells an ONN, Kelli, that people in his family are "cancer magnets." His sister and paternal uncle died of gastric cancer, and his estranged brother is in treatment for colon cancer. Joe is worried about his health, has a history of hypertension and type 1 diabetes, and is on disability for ankylosing spondylitis, a chronic inflammatory disease that affects the spine. No polyps were seen on a recent colonoscopy, and his primary care provider referred him to a genetic counselor. However, he was told his insurance would not pay for testing unless he had a cancer diagnosis. He lost his wife two years ago and cares for his older adult mother and a son with special needs.

Joe's family history is suspicious for Lynch syndrome (hereditary nonpolyposis colorectal cancer). Kelli gives Joe information on a public health program with grant funding that covers the cost of medically indicated single-site gene testing for qualifying individuals. She also offers to connect him directly with the program director. She directs him to other organizations at the health fair, including the senior center for information on respite care, The Arc of the United States (a community-based advocacy group for people with disabilities), and the American Diabetes Association.

Identified Barriers and Interventions

By participating in health fairs and other community-based events, navigators can educate and connect people to applicable resources. Kelli identified and proactively addressed the barriers affecting Joe's desire to improve his and his family's health: poorly controlled diabetes, caregiver fatigue, and insurance denial for genetic testing.

Connections and Competencies

Navigators can further raise awareness of community resources and programs by forming connections with personnel within the respective programs. These connections can help ensure that people take advantage of the resources provided. With Joe's permission, Kelli collaborated with the genetics program manager to ensure that Joe received testing.

Case Study 3: Transgender, Social Stigma, Distrust in Medical System

Gerry is a 50-year-old Black transgender woman who underwent gender-affirming surgery in 2021 and has been taking hormone therapy in the form of testosterone blockers since 2020. Gender-affirming surgery maintains the prostate. Earlier prostate cancer screening at age 40–45 years is recommended for higher-risk patients, which includes Black and cisgender men (Lillard et al., 2022). Gerry's primary care physician is aware of Gerry's retention of her prostate. That knowledge, in combination with her race and age, prompted Gerry's primary care physician to recommend checking her prostate-specific antigen levels. When the prostate-specific antigen levels came back elevated, Gerry's primary care physician referred her to an oncologist knowledgeable about transgender-specific oncologic needs. Genetic testing was recommended for *BRCA2*, and a biopsy confirmed *BRCA2*-negative, stage IIA prostate cancer.

Providing effective care to transgender patients with cancer requires not only expert, patient-specific clinical competency but also the skills to offer transgender-competent emotional support when needed. ONNs can play a critical role in emotionally and logistically supporting transgender patients with cancer as they navigate complex decisions.

Although transgender patients represent a relatively small proportion of the worldwide population, approximated to be 0.4%–1.3% in 2023 (Nik-Ahd et al., 2023), or about 1.5 million in the United States, ONNs will likely interact with transgender patients with cancer during their careers. Lauren, an ONN, learned that Gerry felt comfortable sharing her prostate cancer diagnosis with select close friends, as she felt those individuals would maintain confidentiality and offer the best support. Gerry expressed interest in being connected with transgender cancer support groups, and Lauren facilitated those connections.

Identified Barriers and Interventions

Transgender individuals have historically been marginalized, but efforts in the United States have facilitated productive dialogue and positive support because of heightened awareness and education on transgender concerns, including gender dysphoria (when biological sex does not match gender identity). ONNs and other healthcare professionals need to be aware that gender dysphoria has been well documented to increase risks of self-harm and suicide (Kidd et al., 2023; Kirakosian et al., 2023).

Transgender patients have unique oncology considerations, including experiencing a cancer diagnosis of an organ (such as the prostate) that is not removed as part of gender-affirming care. These patients may also face difficult choices in terms of altering or discontinuing hormone therapy during cancer treatment. This aspect is essential to consider when confronting a hormone-sensitive cancer, such as prostate, breast, or ovarian. Alterations in hormone therapy and concerns about gender dysphoria compound the overall stress patients face about their diagnosis and present unknowns in terms of treatment recommendations from a lack of available data.

Specific cancer diagnoses, including prostate cancer, bladder cancer, and non-Hodgkin lymphoma, are associated with poorer survival outcomes for transgender patients than for cisgender patients (Jackson et al., 2021). One of the most significant risk factors for transgender patients with cancer is the delay in accessing cancer screening and treatment because of fear of stigma and discrimination in the healthcare environment (Haviland et al., 2020). Cancer screening guidelines specific to transgender patients have not been standardized, reinforcing perceived and real obstacles and simultaneously disempowering patients and providers (Schmidt et al., 2019). These significant obstacles to care result in delays in cancer diagnosis and treatment and lead to poorer outcomes overall.

As researchers and clinicians work toward developing comprehensive cancer screening guidelines for transgender patients, ONNs should be mindful of the following factors:
- Genetic testing for *BRCA1* and *BRCA2* in transgender men due to increased risk of breast cancer (Schmidt et al., 2019)
- Genetic testing for *BRCA2* in transgender women due to increased risk of prostate cancer (Nik-Ahd et al., 2023)

- Biomarker testing for prostate-specific antigen in transgender women (Nik-Ahd et al., 2023)
- CA-125 biomarker testing in transgender men retaining female reproductive organs (Schmidt et al., 2019)
- Human papillomavirus (HPV) testing for transgender men due to the risk of HPV-mediated cervical, anal, and other cancers
- HPV screening for transgender women at risk of HPV-mediated anal and other cancers
- The use of hormone therapy when treating hormone-sensitive cancers (Schmidt et al., 2019)
- Fertility preservation during anticancer treatment (Schmidt et al., 2019)
- The incorporation of transgender cancer screening guidelines into the primary care setting (Haviland et al., 2020)
- Increased risk for mood imbalances in the setting of a cancer diagnosis in combination with hormone discontinuation and increased risk for gender dysphoria (Kidd et al., 2023)

Connections and Competencies

ONNs can provide transgender awareness and education to referring primary care physician practices, as a lack of knowledge about transgender patients contributes to lower cancer screening rates for this population. ONNs can use distress screening tools, such as the National Comprehensive Cancer Network Distress Thermometer, to determine the levels and sources of distress at various points during the cancer journey. Psychological screening and support are critically important aspects of providing culturally competent care for transgender patients facing cancer diagnoses. The ability of ONNs to connect transgender patients with appropriate care teams and other transgender patients experiencing a cancer diagnosis will provide additional layers of support during a challenging time. If resources are limited within a geographic area, connecting patients with virtual resources for support may be invaluable.

Case Study 4: Incarceration, Homelessness, Lack of Social Support

Jesse is a formerly incarcerated 67-year-old man who had experienced abdominal discomfort, characterized by bloating and cramping, for at least three months prior to his release from prison. Although he had not previously experienced symptoms such as this during his four-year sentence, he thought it was most likely caused by prison food. Jesse was also disinclined to mention that he was not feeling well to anyone in prison, including the nurse, because he thought it would make him look vulnerable and weak. He was aware that he was being released soon, so he decided to follow up on the outside.

Unfortunately, when Jesse sees his primary care provider and receives a colonoscopy, several worrisome lesions are biopsied. Pathology reveals stage IIIA colorectal cancer. Complicating matters more, when Jesse was released from prison, he was unable to secure stable housing. Not having stable housing is common for formerly incarcerated individuals. It is a significant stressor for a healthy individual, but for someone undergoing surgery and adjuvant chemotherapy, it quickly becomes nearly impossible to navigate.

Cancer is the leading cause of death for incarcerated individuals aged 45 years or older (Aziz et al., 2021). Research from Yale University extracted tumor registry and demographic data for incarcerated and formerly incarcerated individuals between 2005 and 2016. The analyses revealed that incarcerated individuals are less likely to be diagnosed with cancer than the general population; however, the rate of cancer diagnosis is higher among recently released, formerly incarcerated individuals than the general population (Aminawung et al., 2023). The authors postulated that screening for breast, prostate, and colorectal cancers may not be regularly incorporated into prison healthcare models, and valuable time is lost while individuals remain incarcerated. Early diagnosis of cancers and reduced time to treatment start are important predictors of outcome and survival.

Oncology nurses and ONNs working in prisons and with formerly incarcerated individuals are critical in aiding the coordination of cancer screening and facilitating access to necessary treatment options for this vulnerable patient population. For Jesse, the ONN in the community, Dave, is connected with various nonprofits working with formerly incarcerated individuals. After completing several housing applications, Dave was able to secure housing for Jesse for one year within proximity to the local cancer center where he is receiving treatment.

Identified Barriers and Interventions

Incarcerated and formerly incarcerated individuals are a particularly vulnerable subset of patients with cancer. Cancer-directed screening, treatment, and follow-up are ad hoc and inconsistent in the prison system. For formerly incarcerated individuals with unstable employment, finances, housing, insurance, and transportation, the ability to navigate a cancer diagnosis becomes nearly impossible without the assistance of skilled ONNs working within a dedicated oncology care team.

ONNs facilitate essential referrals to community-based organizations and social workers for assistance with housing, insurance, transportation, and employment opportunities. They ensure that access and care are optimized by identifying barriers as they arise throughout the oncology journey for individuals facing the dual stressors of incarceration and a cancer diagnosis.

Connections and Competencies

ONNs must be aware that incarceration presents additional barriers to access to screening, cancer care, and follow-up. To optimize care interventions, ONNs can identify appropriate points of contact within the prison, such as a nurse. Similarly, ONNs should coordinate efforts with social workers and case managers for formerly incarcerated individuals so that barriers are identified and addressed early.

> **Case Study 5: Natural Disaster, Limited Access, Complex Care Transitions**
>
> Tonya is a 35-year-old with stage IIIB breast cancer living in a rural area more than 100 miles from the closest cancer treatment center. Wildfires destroyed the center where she was receiving her chemotherapy infusions. Compounding her limited access are her challenges of being a single parent with young children at home.
>
> Her ONN, Mandy, contacts Tonya despite cell phone service outages and variable internet support due to the wildfires. Mandy is her lifeline, communicating and reassuring Tonya that her treatments will not be interrupted. The connections Mandy has with other infusion facilities within the same healthcare system can accommodate Tonya. The distance to the new facility is 250 miles round trip; however, infusion nurses can access all of Tonya's records via her electronic health record. Tonya is able to maintain contact via video visits with her medical oncologist and attend virtual support groups for young women.

Identified Barriers and Interventions

Disasters, both natural and man-made, include wildfires, weather-related floods, tornadoes, hurricanes, biological disasters, and accidents. Emergency departments and hospitals may be closed or low on resources. ONNs can be a critical conduit to assure patients and families that care coordination, although challenging, remains a primary focus. Communication between healthcare system navigators and other cancer care providers is challenged beyond capacity at times. Knowing how and where to identify resources during disasters is imperative. Often, oncology staff have lost their own homes permanently or temporarily, and recovery takes time. ONNs have the skills and competencies to help transcend disasters and overcome barriers (Fadadu et al., 2024).

Connections and Competencies

As part of community and healthcare system policy, emergency preparedness lists should be provided to patients and families year-round. Navigators can help ensure these lists include essential elements, such as personal documents, contact lists of family members and friends, nonperishable food, medications, and emergency equipment (e.g., flashlights, batteries, solar charging lights, first aid kits) (Fadadu et al., 2024).

Medical staff can encourage patient enrollment in local emergency alert systems. Whenever possible, key communication tools are electronic health records and virtual visits. Encouraging patients and families to use these applications is essential for healthcare communication between patients and providers.

Summary

Unique navigation issues are encountered and addressed every day in hospitals, community centers, and public health centers as well as during communications among organizations and providers. A critical part of being an ONN is evaluating each patient as an individual and being appropriate yet creative in response. It also is a fluid process in which ONNs help to connect the threads through collegiality, evidence-based practices, continuing education, and participation in national organizations. ONNs work to support each other and their patients. Recognizing the limitations of the system or community and collaborating with others are essential to support patients. Each navigation issue is unique and can benefit from a multiple resources approach. ONNs must facilitate connections among patients, caregivers, and care facility systems to maximize the use of resources in the most effective manner.

The author would like to acknowledge Alice S. Kerber, MN, APRN, ACNS-BC, AOCN®, AGN-BC, for her contribution to this chapter that remains unchanged from the previous edition of this book.

References

American Association for Cancer Research. (2024). *AACR cancer disparities progress report 2024: Achieving the bold vision of health equity.* https://www.cancerdisparitiesprogressreport.org

Aminawung, J.A., Soulos, P.R., Oladeru, O.T., Lin, H.-J., Gonsalves, L., Puglisi, L.B., ... Gross, C.P. (2023). Cancer incidence among incarcerated and formerly incarcerated individuals: A statewide retrospective cohort study. *Cancer Medicine, 12*(14), 15447–15454. https://doi.org/10.1002/cam4.6162

Aziz, H., Ackah, R.L., Whitson, A., Oppong, B., Obeng-Gyasi, S., Sims, C., & Pawlik, T.M. (2021). Cancer care in the incarcerated population: Barriers to quality care and opportunities for improvement. *JAMA Surgery, 156*(10), 964–973. https://doi.org/10.1001/jamasurg.2021.3754

Chen, D.W., Banerjee, M., He, X., Miranda, L., Watanabe, M., Veenstra, C.M., & Haymart, M.R. (2023). Hidden disparities: How language influences patients' access to cancer care. *Journal of the National Comprehensive Cancer Network, 21*(9), 951–959. https://doi.org/10.6004/jnccn.2023.7037

Fadadu, R.P., Solomon, G., & Balmes, J.R. (2024). Wildfires and human health. *JAMA, 332*(12), 1011–1012. https://doi.org/10.1001/jama.2024.13600

Fu, J., Reid, S.A., French, B., Hennessy, C., Hwang, N., Gatson, N.T., ... Shah, D.P. (2022). Racial disparities in COVID-19 outcomes among black and white patients with cancer. *JAMA Network Open, 5*(3), e2224304. https://doi.org/10.1001/jamanetworkopen.2022.4304

Haviland, K.S., Swette, S., Kelechi, T., & Mueller, M. (2020). Barriers and facilitators to cancer screening among LGBTQ individuals with cancer. *Oncology Nursing Forum, 47*(1), 44–55. https://doi.org/10.1188/20.ONF.44-55

Jackson, S.S., Han, X., Mao, Z., Nogueira, L., Suneja, G., Jemal, A., & Shiels, M.S. (2021). Cancer stage, treatment, and survival among transgender patients in the United States. *Journal of the National Cancer Institute, 113*(9), 1221–1227. https://doi.org/10.1093/jnci/djab028

Kidd, J.D., Tettamanti, N.A., Kaczmarkiewicz, R., Corbeil, T.E., Dworkin, J.D., Jackman, K.B., ... Meyer, I.H. (2023). Prevalence of substance use and mental health problems among transgender and cisgender U.S. adults: Results from a national probability sample. *Psychiatry Research, 326*, 115339. https://doi.org/10.1016/j.psychres.2023.115339

Kirakosian, N., Stanton, A.M., McKetchnie, S.M., King, D., Dolotina, B., O'Cleirigh, C., ... Batchelder, A.W. (2023). Suicidal ideation disparities among transgender and gender diverse compared to cisgender community health patients. *Journal of General Internal Medicine, 38*(6), 1357–1365. https://doi.org/10.1007/s11606-022-07996-2

Lillard, J.W., Jr., Moses, K.A., Mahal, B.A., & George, D.J. (2022). Racial disparities in Black men with prostate cancer: A literature review. *Cancer, 128*(21), 3787–3795. https://doi.org/10.1002/cncr.34433

Nik-Ahd, F., Jarjour, A., Figueiredo, J., Anger, J.T., Garcia, M., Carroll, P.R., ... Freedland, S.J. (2023). Prostate-specific antigen screening in transgender patients. *European Urology, 83*(1), 48–54. https://doi.org/10.1016/j.eururo.2022.09.007

Oncology Nursing Society & Oncology Nursing Certification Corporation. (2024). *Oncology nurse navigator competencies.* https://www.ons.org/oncology-nurse-navigator-competencies

Professional Oncology Navigation Task Force. (2022). Oncology navigation standards of professional practice. *Clinical Journal of Oncology Nursing, 26*(3), E14–E25. https://doi.org/10.1188/22.CJON.E14-E25

Schmidt, M., Ditrio, L., Shute, B., & Luciano, D. (2019). Surgical management and gynecologic care of the transgender patient. *Current Opinion in Obstetrics and Gynecology, 31*(4), 228–234. https://doi.org/10.1097/GCO.0000000000000553

CHAPTER 12

Personalized Medicine and Novel Therapies

Deborah M. Christensen, MSN, APRN, AOCNS®

> **KEY TOPICS**
> precision oncology, biomarker testing, targeted therapy, cell-based therapy

Overview

Personalized medicine signifies a transformative paradigm shift where medical decisions are based on the patient's genetic makeup, environment, and lifestyle (National Human Genome Research Institute, n.d.). Although often used synonymously, personalized medicine and precision medicine emphasize slightly different aspects of cancer management, with both approaches seeking to enhance response to therapy, reduce side effects, conserve organ function, and ultimately improve quality of life (Baird et al., 2023). Precision oncology, as a subset of personalized medicine, focuses on leveraging genomic variations and advanced molecular profiling to develop targeted therapies that address the unique biology of each patient's tumor. This chapter uses the term precision oncology to highlight the integration of genomic insights and novel therapeutic strategies in modern oncology care.

As critical facilitators in the healthcare journey, oncology nurse navigators (ONNs) are instrumental in helping patients navigate the complexities of oncology care. Their role in precision oncology can include identifying individuals at high risk for cancer and providing education on lifestyle risks, environmental carcinogens, and the significance of biomarker testing. Genetic (inherited) and genomic (acquired) biomarkers can be predictive, prognostic, and diagnostic. They can be measured over time to assess the status of a disease and monitor treatment effects (Oncology Nursing Society [ONS], n.d.-c).

Other ONN responsibilities may include helping patients access biomarker testing, explaining cancer biomarker reports, monitoring adherence to targeted therapies, and discussing clinical trials using novel therapies. As precision oncology advances, ONNs must stay current on the emerging science, taxonomy, and technology used in precision oncology. To help meet this need, ONS developed the Genomics and Precision Oncology Learning Library (www.ons.org/genomics-and-precision-oncology-learning-library), which includes a biomarker database, genomics taxonomy, clinical practice resources, patient education material, and other precision oncology assets (ONS, n.d.-b).

Historically, cancer diagnoses and treatments were based on the histologic origin of the cancer cells. Over time, clinical trials showed that particular drugs were more effective for specific sites of origin, leading to the development of disease-specific standards of care (Zhong et al., 2021). Although still used today, general cytotoxic drugs have given way to more targeted medications as biomarker testing identifies pathologic variants within the cellular makeup. These newer drugs are designed to target cancer cells while leaving healthy cells unharmed, resulting in highly effective treatments with fewer toxic side effects than traditional chemotherapy (Shuel, 2022; Zhong et al., 2021).

This chapter will explore advances in precision oncology, consider how pathologic variants guide treatment options, discuss the importance of biomarker testing, review targeted and cell-based therapies, and consider precision oncology implications for ONNs.

Targeting the Hallmarks of Cancer Development

Cancer is a genetic disease caused by cancer-associated gene alterations resulting in the activation of oncogenes and inactivation of tumor suppressor genes (Boussios et al., 2023). These changes include sporadic genomic variants that develop over time (somatic) and heredity genetic variants (germline) that are inherited from parent sperm and egg cells (Friend & Mahon, 2023). Messenger RNA (mRNA) can also mutate or fuse, affecting protein synthesis and leading to uncontrolled cell proliferation and tumor development. Targeted therapies can disrupt these specific pathways by inhibiting the proteins produced by these genetic changes, thereby preventing the progression and spread of cancer (American Association for Cancer Research, 2023; Sarhadi & Armengol, 2022). In other cases, the microenvironment around the tumor—which includes blood vessels, immune cells, and other cell types—can influence abnormal behavior in cancer cells (Boussios et al., 2023). Targeted therapies can also be developed to intervene in these situations. For example, trastuzumab is designed to block the signals from overexpressed HER2 on cancer cells (Waarts et al., 2022). Bevacizumab inhibits the excess vascular endothelial growth factor proteins produced by tumors to help them develop new blood vessels. By inhibiting vascular endothelial growth factor proteins, bevacizumab disrupts the tumor's blood supply, which is necessary for growth (Shuel, 2022). Immune checkpoint inhibitors are an example of a targeted therapy that interacts with the tumor microenvironment, blocking immune checkpoints responsible for turning "off" the immune system (Hanahan, 2022; Shuel, 2022). Therapies targeting the fundamental characteristics of cancer development and proliferation continue to be developed and studied in clinical trials (Hanahan, 2022).

Diagnostic and Biomarker Testing Techniques

Advancements in biotechnology led to the discovery of other unique biologic features associated with cancer development. These features can be detected using DNA profiling, immune marker identification, and RNA analyses (Tsimberidou et al., 2020). Using this information, clinicians can optimize cancer treatments for each patient. Overall, biomarker testing has unveiled a complex reality regarding malignancies, necessitating a shift in therapy from histology-driven to gene- and immune-directed therapy based on biomarker analysis (Tsimberidou et al., 2020).

Significant progress in identifying biomarkers has aided in the development and approval of novel and targeted treatments. Various techniques have been used to identify biomarkers, each serving a specific clinical purpose (Ritterhouse, n.d.). Table 12-1 provides examples of commonly used biomarker testing techniques, including details on their specific applications.

TABLE 12-1. Examples of Testing Methods Used in Precision Oncology

Test	Method/Result
Polymerase chain reaction (PCR)	Amplifies DNA sequences to detect genetic changes
Real-time quantitative reverse transcription polymerase chain reaction (qRT-PCR)	Allows for the reliable detection and measurement of products generated during each cycle of the PCR process
Immunohistochemistry	Detects specific proteins in cells of a tissue section
Fluorescence in situ hybridization (FISH)	Uses fluorescent probes that only attach to parts of chromosomes to identify chromosomal abnormalities and gene variants
Next-generation sequencing (NGS)	Allows for a broader examination of the genome to detect known and unknown variants across multiple genes simultaneously
Sanger sequencing	Amplifies DNA strands using fluorescent-tagged dideoxy terminators, sorted by size, and sequenced nucleotide by nucleotide
Comparative genomic hybridization (CGH)	Assesses copy number changes across the genome

Note. Based on information from Sarhadi & Armengol, 2022.

Initially, Sanger sequencing was the gold standard for DNA sequencing, and real-time quantitative reverse transcription polymerase chain reaction (qRT-PCR) was preferred for RNA sequencing. Next-generation sequencing is now the preferred method for both DNA and RNA sequencing because of its ability to sequence large genomes and transcriptomes quickly and affordably, providing a more comprehensive analysis (Nikanjam et al., 2022; Slatko et al., 2018).

Tumor tissue and body fluids containing malignant cells can be used to identify germline and somatic pathogenic variants, as well as to monitor for treatment response and disease progression. The tissue or fluid sample choice used for molecular tumor testing depends on several factors, such as cancer type, location, accessibility, and clinical stage (Lin et al., 2021; Nikanjam et al., 2022). However, the quality and quantity of the tissue or liquid sample can significantly affect the reliability of the test results (Nikanjam et al., 2022). ONNs can help patients and their families understand the sample needed for testing and why the test is being performed, assisting them in making informed decisions.

Cancer Biomarker Identification and Application

The National Comprehensive Cancer Network (NCCN) guidelines endorse targeted biomarker testing for prevalent cancers, such as lung, breast, colorectal, melanoma, and leukemia (NCCN, 2025a, 2025c, 2025d, 2025e, 2025f). Patients with advanced stages of cancer or with rare cancer types (e.g., biliary tract cancers, sarcomas, cancer of unknown primary) should also receive biomarker testing to tailor treatment plans effectively (NCCN, 2025b, 2025g, 2025h). Biomarker testing panels may identify a pathogenic variation in a gene linked to a hereditary cancer syndrome. In these situations, referral to a genetic professional is indicated. For females with epithelial ovarian cancer, American Society of Clinical Oncology guidelines recommend paired germline and somatic biomarker testing (Mahon, 2020b). Additional scenarios where paired biomarker testing might be recommended include patients with a family history of a known hereditary cancer syndrome (e.g., breast, ovarian, pancreatic, colon, endometrial), a history of multiple primary cancers, and specific tumor characteristics such as triple-negative breast cancer and prostate cancer with a Gleason score higher than 7 (Mahon, 2020b).

Biomarkers and genetic alterations in tumor cells can provide valuable information about cancer risk, offer prognostic insights, enable accurate diagnoses, and help determine treatment options (Mahon, 2020a). Cancer biomarker identification also drives new prognostic-, diagnostic-, and treatment-related discoveries (Rulten et al., 2023). Microsatellite instability–high (MSI-H), mismatch repair deficiency (dMMR), and tumor molecular burden–high (TMB-H) are examples of tumor agnostic biomarkers. Tumors expressing these biomarkers may be eligible for targeted therapy regardless of the histologic origin of the cancer. Examples include poly (ADP-ribose) polymerase (PARP) inhibitors for dMMR or *BRCA* variants and pembrolizumab for tumors expressing MSI-H or dMMR (Rulten et al., 2023).

Targeted Cancer Therapy

Targeted therapies fall into two main categories: small molecules and immunomodulatory drugs, namely monoclonal antibodies (mAbs). Antibody–drug conjugates (ADCs) are a novel class of mAbs linked with a chemotherapy agent. This approach merges the precise targeting of cancer cells with a powerful ability to destroy them. ADC research and development has emerged as a critical focus in creating and studying new cancer treatments (Fu et al., 2022; Marei et al., 2022). Cell- and gene-based therapies are an emerging field of immunomodulatory treatments (Wang et al., 2023).

Small Molecule Therapy

The principle of small molecule targeted compounds in cancer treatment is based on targeting the specific aspects of molecular biology that lead to cancer development (tumorigenesis). These compounds are designed to interact with and regulate the activity of specific proteins in the body or affect pathways involved in the growth and spread of cancer cells. Enzymes and receptors are the main protein targets for these compounds (Waarts et al., 2022).

Enzyme and Receptor Targets

Enzymes are proteins that facilitate biochemical reactions in the body, and their dysregulation can contribute to cancer. Small molecule inhibitors counteract cancerous processes by interrupting the activity of enzymes. Receptors, conversely, are proteins typically found on cell surfaces that receive and respond to signals from the body or the environment (Sun et al., 2021). When small molecule compounds attach to receptors, they can act as agonists or antagonists. Agonists are compounds that activate the receptor, mimicking the effect of the natural signaling molecule. Antagonists block the receptor, preventing the biologic signaling molecule from activating it. By modulating these receptors, the compounds can influence cellular behaviors critical in cancer development, such as cell growth, division, and survival (Sun et al., 2021).

Pathway Targets

Beyond the well-studied kinase pathways, several non-kinase pathways are considered actionable for therapeutic intervention. One important pathway is the DNA damage response pathway, which is responsible for repairing DNA damage that occurs throughout a person's lifetime. Preventing cancer cells from repairing DNA single-strand breaks leaves them susceptible to DNA damage and eventual cell death (Liu et al., 2022; Sun et al., 2021).

Another pathway target is the hormone pathway, which is commonly used in the treatment of prostate cancer and hormone receptor–positive breast and ovarian cancer. Hormone receptor antagonists block the action of hormones, whereas drugs that reduce androgen levels can also effectively treat these types of cancer (Choi & Chang, 2023). Additional pathways targeted in precision oncology are blocking metabolic pathways, developing blood vessels (angiogenesis), and modifying immune checkpoints (Liu et al., 2022; Sun et al., 2021). Examples of drugs used to target these pathways are displayed in Table 12-2. Table 12-3 provides examples of additional pathway targets and U.S. Food and Drug Administration–approved therapies.

TABLE 12-2. Examples of Cancer Hallmarks and Accompanying Targeted Therapies

Cancer Cell Development Hallmarks	Targeted Therapy Classification	Targeted Drug Examples
Maintaining ongoing cell growth signals	Epidermal growth factor inhibitors	Cetuximab Erlotinib Panitumumab
Dodging factors that suppress growth	Cyclin-dependent kinase inhibitors	Abemaciclib Palbociclib Ribociclib
Escaping destruction by the immune system	Cytotoxic T-lymphocyte antigen 4 monoclonal antibodies	Ipilimumab Tremelimumab
Granting continuous cell division	Telomerase inhibitors	Imetelstat (granted Fast Track designation by the U.S. Food and Drug Administration in August 2023)
Fostering inflammation that leads to tumors	Selective anti-inflammatory drugs	Celecoxib
Initiating the spread and colonization of new areas in the body	Hepatocyte growth factor/cellular-mesenchymal epithelial transition factor receptor tyrosine kinase (c-Met) inhibitors	Cabozantinib Crizotinib (for non-small cell lung cancer) Tivantinib
Encouraging the formation of new blood vessels	Vascular endothelial growth factor signaling inhibitors	Bevacizumab Pazopanib Sunitinib
Causing continuous genetic changes and variants	Poly (ADP-ribose) polymerase inhibitors	Niraparib Olaparib Talazoparib
Defying the natural process of cell death	Proapoptotic BH3 mimetics	ABT-737 Navitoclax (ABT-263) Obatoclax
Disrupting the normal energy processing in cells	Aerobic glycolysis inhibitors	Some approved chemotherapies have an effect. Research is ongoing.

Note. Based on information from Hanahan, 2022.

TABLE 12-3. Examples of Targetable Pathways and U.S. Food and Drug Administration–Approved Therapies

Pathway	Inhibits	Targeted Therapy
Hormone	Estrogen receptor signaling	Tamoxifen, fulvestrant
	Androgen receptor signaling	Enzalutamide, abiraterone acetate
DNA damage response	PARP (poly [ADP-ribose] polymerase) on BRCA variant carriers	Olaparib, niraparib, rucaparib
Proteasome	Proteasomes	Bortezomib, carfilzomib
Epigenetic modifiers	Histone deacetylase (HDAC)	Vorinostat, romidepsin, belinostat, panobinostat
	DNA methyltransferase	Azacitidine, decitabine
Metabolic	Folate metabolism	Methotrexate
	Amino acid deprivation or metabolism	Asparaginase
	IDH1 (isocitrate dehydrogenase) and IDH2 (also intersect with epigenetic regulation pathways)	Enasidenib, ivosidenib
Immune checkpoints	Cytotoxic T-lymphocyte antigen 4	Ipilimumab
	Programmed cell death protein 1	Nivolumab, pembrolizumab
	Programmed cell death-ligand 1	Atezolizumab, durvalumab
Apoptosis	BCL-2 family protein	Venetoclax
Angiogenesis	Vascular endothelial growth factor	Bevacizumab, ramucirumab
Signal transduction	Hedgehog signaling	Vismodegib, sonidegib
Cell cycle	Cyclin-dependent kinase inhibitors	Palbociclib, abemaciclib, ribociclib, trilaciclib

Note. Based on information from Liu et al., 2022; Wang et al., 2023.

Immunomodulatory Therapy

Monoclonal Antibodies

The mAbs are specialized proteins created by using mouse or human cells through a process called hybridoma technology. Their role is multifaceted. They can inhibit the binding of signaling molecules to cell receptors, thereby blocking cell signals, and they also contribute to the destruction of cells through mechanisms involving the immune system, such as triggering immune cells to kill the targeted cell (antibody-dependent cellular cytotoxicity) or activating the complement system to assist in cell destruction (complement-mediated cytotoxicity). Additionally, mAbs can fine-tune the immune response by modulating it, which can either ramp up or dampen the immune system's activity to suit therapeutic needs. These properties make mAbs useful as immunomodulatory agents in treating diseases.

Antibody–Drug Conjugates

ADCs were created to bridge the gap between mAbs and cytotoxic drugs by combining the selectivity of mAbs and the efficacy of chemotherapy. ADCs consist of three primary components: an antibody targeting a specific antigen found on the surface of the cancer cells, a linker, and a cytotoxic drug. Once the antibody binds to the antigen, the attached drug is released into the cancer cell, which can kill the cell or stop its growth (Marei et al., 2022; Shastry et al., 2023).

The overall effectiveness of an ADC depends significantly on the specific characteristics and interactions of these components. A critical step in designing an ADC is selecting an appropriate antibody with high specificity for antigens found predominantly on cancer cells rather than healthy cells. This involves identifying cell surface proteins that are abundant in tumor cells but have limited or no expression in noncancerous tissues. By targeting these tumor-specific antigens, ADCs deliver chemotherapy directly to cancer cells, thereby reducing the systemic side effects often associated with conventional chemotherapy. This targeted approach allows ADCs to offer new treatment possibilities for diseases with a poor outlook and limited therapeutic options (Marei et al., 2022).

Bispecific Antibodies

In contrast to mAbs, bispecific antibodies target two different antigens. This dual targeting of cell surface or soluble proteins can occur independently or synergistically (Brinkmann & Kontermann, 2021). Blinatumomab, for example, binds to a tumor-specific antigen on malignant B cells (CD19) and an activating antigen (CD3) on T cells, independently bringing the activated T cells in close proximity to the malignant B cells.

Amivantamab, another bispecific antibody, targets epidermal growth factor receptor (EGFR) and mesenchymal–epithelial transition (MET) in non-small cell lung cancers with an EGFR exon 20 insertion pathologic variant. This synergistic binding inhibits EGFR and MET pathways, downgrades EGFR and MET receptors, and tags malignant cells for destruction (Brazel & Nagasaka, 2021). By the end of 2023, 11 bispecific antibodies had been approved, and many others are being investigated in clinical trials (Klein et al., 2024).

Immune Checkpoint Inhibitors

Cancer cells can develop mechanisms to evade the immune system. One key strategy involves manipulating immune checkpoints—the immune system regulators, which normally prevent the immune system from attacking the body's own cells. Two significant benefits of immune checkpoint inhibitor therapy are restoring the function of the immune system and forming a lasting memory of the antigen. Immune targets include programmed cell death protein 1 (PD-1), programmed cell death-ligand 1 (PD-L1), and cytotoxic T-lymphocyte antigen 4 receptors (CTLA-4) (Sun et al., 2021).

Cell- and Gene-Based Therapies

Cell therapy is the transfer of cellular material, which can be from the same individual (autologous) or a different individual (allogeneic), into a patient for therapeutic purposes. This also includes genetically modified cell therapies, such as chimeric antigen receptor T-cell therapy, where cells are engineered to enhance their therapeutic potential (El-Kadiry et al., 2021). Human gene therapy involves altering the genetic material within a person's cells to treat or prevent disease (Wang et al., 2023).

Autologous and allogeneic stem cell transplantation using stem cells sourced from the bone marrow, peripheral blood, or umbilical cord blood have been used successfully in hematologic malignancies but have not seen the same success in solid tumors (El-Kadiry et al., 2021). Similarly, although chimeric antigen receptor T-cell therapy has shown significant success in treating hematologic malignancies, its effectiveness in solid tumors has been limited, primarily because of the complex and challenging nature of the tumor microenvironment (Kankeu Fonkoua et al., 2022; Wang et al., 2023). Chimeric antigen receptor T-cell therapy use in solid tumors continues to be studied in clinical trials (Lamprecht & Dansereau, 2019).

Other examples of cell-based therapies include antigen-presenting cell–based anticancer vaccines and oncolytic viruses. Antigen-presenting cell vaccines stimulate the immune system to recognize and attack cancer cells by introducing specific antigens to trigger an immune response. Oncolytic viruses use engineered viruses to infect and kill cancer cells while also boosting the immune system's ability to recognize and target cancer (El-Kadiry et al., 2021; Wang et al., 2023).

As new applications and approvals for cell- and gene-based therapies evolve, the oncology treatment landscape increases in complexity, requiring ongoing education and adaptability among healthcare professionals and ONNs to ensure optimal patient care (Sharma et al., 2022).

Overcoming Challenges in Providing Precision Oncology

Precision oncology faces significant obstacles despite the promises and hopes for improved cancer care. Biologic obstacles include a low prevalence of targetable drivers in solid tumors and high levels of variation within a tumor (Mroz & Rocco, 2017). Over time, changes in genes, proteins, and other molecules result in tumor heterogeneity, characterized by different traits and behaviors within the same tumor. Such variability in the tumor and microenvironment enables growth, metastasis, and resistance to therapy (Ramón y Cajal et al., 2020). As such, repeat somatic biomarker testing may be necessary to identify new pathologic variants or changes in the tumor that could affect treatment decisions (Reed et al., 2019).

Practical limitations to precision oncology are linked to a limited understanding of the clinical significance of biomarker tests in guiding patient management and a need for more consensus on the levels of evidence required to validate specific biomarker tests (Lassen et al., 2021). In precision oncology, actionable pathologic variants must be accurately identified and interpreted. However, biomarker testing guidelines are inconsistent across practice settings and tumor types (Sadik et al., 2022). In non-small cell lung cancer, where most patients have tumors with biomarker alterations, many do not receive testing, showing implementation challenges. Quality or sample management issues contribute to over a third of deaths for patients with cancer in the United States. These patients are often missing out on precision oncology treatments despite actionable biomarker results (Martin et al., 2021; Sadik et al., 2022). A consensus does not exist among different stakeholders, including clinicians, patients, testing facilities, and payors, on incorporating biomarker information into patient health records, delivering accessible and affordable testing technologies to patients, and ultimately contributing value for healthcare practitioners and payers (Schroll et al., 2022).

The diversity of terms used in the healthcare setting to describe genetics, genomics, biomarkers, and testing methods can compromise patient and provider communication, ultimately leading to poor comprehension of the significance of biomarker testing in oncology (Martin et al., 2021). Studies show that even among well-educated individuals, genetic literacy is poor (Chapman et al., 2019).

Overcoming the challenges associated with precision oncology will require a collective effort. The ONS Genomics Advisory Board (GAB), established in 2019, brought together genomics nursing experts to identify and address gaps in genomic knowledge. A key initiative was establishing standardized terminology for the evolving genomic landscape. GAB identified essential terms, analyzed current materials, used peer-reviewed definitions, and created supporting graphics and clinical examples, categorizing terms by their practical use. The taxonomy was then peer-reviewed by GAB. The resulting ONS Genomics Taxonomy (www.ons.org/genomics-taxonomy) supports standardized genomic education materials and communication between nurses and when educating patients. ONS collaborated with external entities to develop the Genomics and Precision Oncology Learning Library, which offers many clinical and educational resources for nurses. GAB continues to update these resources to reflect the evolution of precision oncology (ONS, n.d.-b).

Additional interventions can include developing patient education and awareness resources, implementing patient support programs, improving access to genetic counseling, and using interprofessional cancer care teams (Lassen et al., 2021; Schroll et al., 2022). As an integral part of the interprofessional team, ONNs must advocate for patients to receive appropriate biomarker testing and understand how it can influence their treatment options. It is vital that ONNs understand and can effectively discuss tumor biomarker testing methods, common cancer biomarkers, and personalized treatment strategies.

The ONN's role may include assisting patients with access to biomarker-based clinical trials and addressing insurance issues that can occur in this setting. The following case studies (see Figure 12-1) demonstrate the ONN's role in advocating for biomarker testing and clinical trial access and addressing the ethical considerations for targeted therapies and personalized cancer care. The latter studies focus specifically on *KRAS G12V* variants and *NTRK* gene fusions.

FIGURE 12-1 Case Studies

Case Study 1: Biomarker Testing Education and Advocacy

Ginny, a 55-year-old woman, has been diagnosed with colon cancer. She is feeling lost and anxious when she meets with Sarah, her oncology nurse navigator (ONN). Ginny mentions that the only history of cancer in her extended family is her grandfather, who had prostate cancer. Sarah explains that somatic biomarker testing can also identify predictive variants associated with hereditary cancers and how germline testing is typically performed on blood or saliva.

Ginny's report identifies two pathologic variants (epidermal growth factor receptor [EGFR] and *BRCA2*) and three variants of unknown significance. Because Sarah prepared Ginny for this potential result, Ginny understands why she is referred to a genetic counselor to discuss cascade testing and potential implications for her family.

Ginny's case demonstrates the essential role of ONNs in educating patients about the intricacies involved in somatic and germline biomarker testing. ONNs can use the Oncology Nursing Society (ONS) Biomarker Database (www.ons.org/clinical-tools/biomarkers; registration required) to learn about individual biomarkers associated with specific malignancies and targeted therapies. The database also includes testing guidelines, implications for patient care, and additional considerations, including clinical trials, for each biomarker (ONS, n.d.-a).

Case Study 2: Advocating for a Biomarker Testing Protocol

Jane, an RN and the director of oncology nurse navigation at an urban cancer center, initiates an interprofessional team to develop a standardized process for ordering biomarker testing and ONN follow-up. The team uses the ONS Biomarker Database and National Comprehensive Cancer Network guidelines to identify and tag cancer types for biomarker testing in the electronic health record. ONNs are responsible for educating patients on biomarker testing, verifying that the test was ordered, and confirming that the test results were available for review at the patient's follow-up appointment. If test results are delayed, the scheduling team calls the patient and reschedules their appointment.

Results from a pre- and post-implementation survey show that patients better understand the importance and reasons for biomarker testing and how the results can affect treatment options. Thanks to the efforts of the ONNs, patients receive their biomarker test results during their next oncology visit, eliminating the need for an additional office visit.

(Continued on next page)

FIGURE 12-1 Case Studies *(Continued)*
Case Study 3: Facilitating Clinical Trials for *KRAS* G12V Pathogenic Variant in Pancreatic Cancer Michael is diagnosed with early-stage pancreatic cancer at age 63 years. Genetic testing does not reveal any germline variants. He completes neoadjuvant therapy, surgical resection, and four additional cycles of chemotherapy. Michael has a locally advanced recurrence eight months later, and biomarker testing results indicate a *KRAS* G12V pathologic variant. Laura, an ONN, explains the variant's implications and the possibility of clinical trials targeting *KRAS* G12V. Laura further coordinates with the clinical trials team, and Michael is evaluated and eligible for a clinical trial using a tyrosine kinase inhibitor in combination with gemcitabine.   This case study highlights the role of ONNs in simplifying biomarker testing and empowering patients to make informed treatment decisions.

Case Study 4: Navigating Insurance Denial for *NTRK* Fusion Medication
 	
In a challenging case, Emily, an ONN, faces some ethical and policy issues surrounding biomarker testing and insurance denial. Her patient, Tom, is diagnosed with a rare cancer featuring an *NTRK* gene fusion. However, his insurance company denies coverage for a promising U.S. Food and Drug Administration–approved targeted therapy.
    Emily works to understand the intricacies of an *NTRK* fusion and the associated targeted therapy. Meanwhile, Tom's oncologist uses NCCN guidelines and its Biomarkers Compendium to file a second appeal. Emily updates Tom on the appeals process and proactively encourages him to complete a patient access form for co-pay assistance through the pharmaceutical manufacturer. Tom's insurance company finally approves the medication, and soon after, he receives the needed co-pay assistance.
    Emily's story highlights the role of ONNs in navigating the complex intersection of patient care, ethics, and healthcare policies.

Summary

Precision oncology is an essential part of modern cancer care. It involves personalized treatment based on an individual's genetic makeup, environment, and lifestyle. Next-generation sequencing and other biotechnologies led to the development of targeted therapies, such as small molecules and mAbs. New advancements, such as cell- and gene-based therapies and ADCs, have added complexity to oncology care.

ONNs are becoming increasingly vital, as they advocate for essential biomarker testing, explain targeted and immunomodulatory treatment implications, and help patients and their loved ones understand and navigate personalized care plans that stem from precision oncology. The ONS Genomics and Precision Oncology Learning Library provides comprehensive resources, including a biomarker database, genomics taxonomy, clinical practice guidelines, and patient education materials, that can assist oncology nurses in learning and staying current on precision testing and treatment options (ONS, n.d.-b). ONNs can anticipate the increasing benefits of precision oncology by staying updated on the latest advancements, ensuring patients receive personalized, evidence-based support to optimize outcomes throughout their cancer journey.

The author would like to acknowledge Debra Wujcik, PhD, RN, AOCN®, FAAN, for her contribution to this chapter that remains unchanged from the previous edition of this book.

References

American Association for Cancer Research. (2023). *AACR cancer progress report 2023.* https://cancerprogressreport.aacr.org/progress

Baird, A.-M., Westphalen, C.B., Blum, S., Nafria, B., Knott, T., Sargeant, I., ... Wong-Rieger, D. (2023). How can we deliver on the promise of precision medicine in oncology and beyond? A practical roadmap for action. *Health Science Reports, 6*(6), e1349. https://doi.org/10.1002/hsr2.1349

Boussios, S., Sanchez, E., & Sheriff, M. (2023). Frontiers of molecular biology of cancer. *International Journal of Molecular Sciences, 24*(24), 17187. https://doi.org/10.3390/ijms242417187

Brazel, D., & Nagasaka, M. (2021). Spotlight on amivantamab (JNJ-61186372) for EGFR exon 20 insertions positive non-small cell lung cancer. *Lung Cancer: Targets and Therapy, 12,* 133–138. https://doi.org/10.2147/LCTT.S337861

Brinkmann, U., & Kontermann, R.E. (2021). Bispecific antibodies. *Science, 372*(6545), 916–917. https://doi.org/10.1126/science.abg1209

Chapman, R., Likhanov, M., Selita, F., Zakharov, I., Smith-Woolley, E., & Kovas, Y. (2019). New literacy challenge for the twenty-first century: Genetic knowledge is poor even among well educated. *Journal of Community Genetics, 10*(1), 73–84. https://doi.org/10.1007/s12687-018-0363-7

Choi, H.Y., & Chang, J.-E. (2023). Targeted therapy for cancers: From ongoing clinical trials to FDA-approved drugs. *International Journal of Molecular Sciences, 24*(17), 13618. https://doi.org/10.3390/ijms241713618

El-Kadiry, A.E.-H., Rafei, M., & Shammaa, R. (2021). Cell therapy: Types, regulation, and clinical benefits. *Frontiers in Medicine, 8,* 756029. https://doi.org/10.3389/fmed.2021.756029

Friend, P., & Mahon, S.M. (2023). How did the variant get its name? Understanding gene and variant nomenclature. *Clinical Journal of Oncology Nursing, 27*(3), 251–254. https://doi.org/10.1188/23.CJON.251-254

Fu, Z., Li, S., Han, S., Shi, C., & Zhang, Y. (2022). Antibody drug conjugate: The "biological missile" for targeted cancer therapy. *Signal Transduction and Targeted Therapy, 7*(93). https://doi.org/10.1038/s41392-022-00947-7

Hanahan, D. (2022). Hallmarks of cancer: New dimensions. *Cancer Discovery, 12*(1), 31–46. https://doi.org/10.1158/2159-8290.CD-21-1059

Kankeu Fonkoua, L.A., Sirpilla, O., Sakemura, R., Siegler, E.L., & Kenderian, S.S. (2022). CAR T cell therapy and the tumor microenvironment: Current challenges and opportunities. *Molecular Therapy Oncolytics, 25,* 69–77. https://doi.org/10.1016/j.omto.2022.03.009

Klein, C., Brinkmann, U., Reichert, J.M., & Kontermann, R.E. (2024). The present and future of bispecific antibodies for cancer therapy. *Nature Reviews Drug Discovery, 23,* 301–319. https://doi.org/10.1038/s41573-024-00896-6

Lamprecht, M., & Dansereau, C. (2019). CAR T-cell therapy: Update on the state of the science. *Clinical Journal of Oncology Nursing, 23*(2, Suppl.), 6–12. https://doi.org/10.1188/19.CJON.S1.6-12

Lassen, U.N., Makaroff, L.E., Stenzinger, A., Italiano, A., Vassal, G., Garcia-Foncillas, J., & Avouac, B. (2021). Precision oncology: A clinical and patient perspective. *Future Oncology, 17*(30), 3995–4009. https://doi.org/10.2217/fon-2021-0688

Lin, D., Shen, L., Luo, M., Zhang, K., Li, J., Yang, Q., ... Zhou, J. (2021). Circulating tumor cells: Biology and clinical significance. *Signal Transduction and Targeted Therapy, 6*(1), 404. https://doi.org/10.1038/s41392-021-00817-8

Liu, G.-H., Chen, T., Zhang, X., Ma, X.-L., & Shi, H.-S. (2022). Small molecule inhibitors targeting the cancers. *MedComm, 3*(4), e181. https://doi.org/10.1002/mco2.181

Mahon, S.M. (2020a). Shifting to a biomarker paradigm across cancer care. *Clinical Journal of Oncology Nursing, 24*(6), 633–634. https://doi.org/10.1188/20.CJON.633-634

Mahon, S.M. (2020b). Tumor genomic testing: Identifying characteristics associated with germline risk for developing malignancy. *Clinical Journal of Oncology Nursing, 24*(6), 623–626. https://doi.org/10.1188/20.CJON.623-626

Marei, H.E., Cenciarelli, C., & Hasan, A. (2022). Potential of antibody–drug conjugates (ADCs) for cancer therapy. *Cancer Cell International, 22*, 255. https://doi.org/10.1186/s12935-022-02679-8

Martin, N.A., Tepper, J.E., Giri, V.N., Stinchcombe, T.E., Cheng, H.H., Javle, M.M., & Konnick, E.Q. (2021). Adopting consensus terms for testing in precision medicine. *JCO Precision Oncology, 5*, 1563–1567. https://doi.org/10.1200/PO.21.00027

Mroz, E.A., & Rocco, J.W. (2017). The challenges of tumor genetic diversity. *Cancer, 123*(6), 917–927. https://doi.org/10.1002/cncr.30430

National Comprehensive Cancer Network. (2025a). *NCCN Clinical Practice Guidelines in Oncology: (NCCN Guidelines®): Acute myeloid leukemia* [v.2.2025]. https://www.nccn.org

National Comprehensive Cancer Network. (2025b). *NCCN Clinical Practice Guidelines in Oncology: (NCCN Guidelines®): Biliary tract cancers* [v.1.2025]. https://www.nccn.org

National Comprehensive Cancer Network. (2025c). *NCCN Clinical Practice Guidelines in Oncology: (NCCN Guidelines®): Breast cancer* [v.3.2025]. https://www.nccn.org

National Comprehensive Cancer Network. (2025d). *NCCN Clinical Practice Guidelines in Oncology: (NCCN Guidelines®): Colon cancer* [v.2.2025]. https://www.nccn.org

National Comprehensive Cancer Network. (2025e). *NCCN Clinical Practice Guidelines in Oncology: (NCCN Guidelines®): Melanoma: Cutaneous* [v.2.2025]. https://www.nccn.org

National Comprehensive Cancer Network. (2025f). *NCCN Clinical Practice Guidelines in Oncology: (NCCN Guidelines®): Non-small cell lung cancer* [v.3.2025]. https://www.nccn.org

National Comprehensive Cancer Network. (2025g). *NCCN Clinical Practice Guidelines in Oncology: (NCCN Guidelines®): Occult primary* [v.2.2025]. https://www.nccn.org

National Comprehensive Cancer Network. (2025h). *NCCN Clinical Practice Guidelines in Oncology: (NCCN Guidelines®): Soft tissue sarcoma* [v.5.2024]. https://www.nccn.org

National Human Genome Research Institute. (n.d.). *Talking glossary of genomic and genetic germs*. https://www.genome.gov/genetics-glossary

Nikanjam, M., Kato, S., & Kurzrock, R. (2022). Liquid biopsy: Current technology and clinical applications. *Journal of Hematology and Oncology, 15*(1), 131. https://doi.org/10.1186/s13045-022-01351-y

Oncology Nursing Society. (n.d.-a). *Biomarkers*. https://www.ons.org/biomarkers

Oncology Nursing Society. (n.d.-b). *Genomics and precision oncology learning library*. https://www.ons.org/learning-libraries/precision-oncology

Oncology Nursing Society. (n.d.-c). *Next-generation sequencing toolkit*. https://www.ons.org/toolkits/next-generation-sequencing-toolkit

Ramón y Cajal, S., Sese, M., Capedevila, C., Aasen, T., De Mattos-Arruda, L., Diaz-Cano, S., ... Castellvi, J. (2020). Clinical implications of intratumor heterogeneity challenges and opportunities. *Journal of Molecular Medicine, 98*(2), 161–177. https://doi.org/10.1007/s00109-020-01874-2

Reed, E.K., Steinmark, L., Seibert, D.C., & Edelman, E. (2019). Somatic testing: Implications for targeted treatment. *Seminars in Oncology Nursing, 35*(1), 22–23. https://doi.org/10.1016/j.soncn.2018.12.009

Ritterhouse, L.L. (n.d.). *Use of next-generation sequencing in oncology*. Personalized Medicine in Oncology. https://www.personalizedmedonc.com/supplements/faculty-perspectives-next-generation-sequen cing-testing-in-oncology-part-4-of-a-4-part-series/26564:use-of-next-generation-sequencing-in-oncology

Rulten, S.L., Grose, R.P., Gatz, S.A., Jones, J.L., & Cameron, A.J.M. (2023). The future of precision oncology. *International Journal of Molecular Sciences, 24*(16), 12613. https://doi.org/10.3390/ijms241612613

Sadik, H., Pritchard, D., Keeling, D.-M., Policht, F., Riccelli, P., Stone, G., ... Munksted, S. (2022). Impact of clinical practice gaps on the implementation of personalized medicine in advanced non–small-cell lung cancer. *JCO Precision Oncology, 6,* e2200246. https://doi.org/10.1200/PO.22.00246

Sarhadi, V.K., & Armengol, G. (2022). Molecular biomarkers in cancer. *Biomolecules, 12*(8), 1021. https://doi.org/10.3390/biom12081021

Schroll, M.M., Agarwal, A., Foroughi, O., Kong, E., Perez, O., Pritchard, D., ... Gustavsen, G.G. (2022). Stakeholders perceptions of barriers to precision medicine adoption in the United States. *Journal of Personalized Medicine, 12*(7), 1025. https://doi.org/10.3390/jpm12071025

Sharma, A., Farnia, S., Otegbeye, F., Rinkle, A., Shah, J., Shah, N.N., ... Maus, M.V. (2022). Nomenclature for cellular and genetic therapies: A need for standardization. *Transplantation and Cellular Therapy, 28*(12), 795–801. https://doi.org/10.1016/j.jtct.2022.08.029

Shastry, M., Gupta, A., Chandarlapaty, S., Young, M., Powles, T., & Hamilton, E. (2023). Rise of antibody-drug conjugates: The present and future. *American Society of Clinical Oncology Educational Book, 43,* e390094. https://doi.org/10.1200/EDBK_390094

Shuel, S.L. (2022). Targeted cancer therapies. *Canadian Family Physician, 68*(7), 515–518. https://doi.org/10.46747/cfp.6807515

Slatko, B.E., Gardner, A.F., & Ausubel, F.M. (2018). Overview of next-generation sequencing technologies. *Current Protocols in Molecular Biology, 122*(1), e59. https://doi.org/10.1002/cpmb.59

Sun, G., Rong, D., Li, Z., Sun, G., Wu, F., Li, X., ... Sun, Y. (2021). Role of small molecule targeted compounds in cancer: Progress, opportunities, and challenges. *Frontiers in Cell and Developmental Biology, 9,* 694363. https://doi.org/10.3389/fcell.2021.694363

Tsimberidou, A.M., Fountzilas, E., Nikanjam, M., & Kurzrock, R. (2020). Review of precision cancer medicine: Evolution of the treatment paradigm. *Cancer Treatment Reviews, 86,* 102019. https://doi.org/10.1016/j.ctrv.2020.102019

Waarts, M.R., Stonestrom, A.J., Park, Y.C., & Levine, R.L. (2022). Targeting mutations in cancer. *Journal of Clinical Investigation, 132*(8), e154943. https://doi.org/10.1172/JCI154943

Wang, L., Liu, G., Zheng, L., Long, H., & Liu, Y. (2023). A new era of gene and cell therapy for cancer: A narrative review. *Annals of Translational Medicine, 11*(9), 321. https://doi.org/10.21037/atm-22-3882

Zhong, L., Li, Y., Xiong, L., Wang, W., Wu, M., Yuan, T., Yang, W., ... Yang, S. (2021). Small molecules in targeted cancer therapy: Advances, challenges, and future perspectives. *Signal Transduction and Targeted Therapy, 6*(201). https://doi.org/10.1038/s41392-021-00572-w

CHAPTER 13

Spiritual Considerations

Katie L. Fanslau, DNP, RN

> **KEY TOPICS**
> spirituality, spiritual care, nurse well-being

Overview

No standard definition of *spirituality* exists in the context of health care; however, it is acknowledged as an important factor in whole-person care (de Brito Sena et al., 2021; Hu et al., 2019; Murgia et al., 2020; Syamsiah et al., 2020). The COVID-19 pandemic magnified the necessity of spiritual nursing care. The nursing profession has long been associated with spirituality and religion as a calling vocation to fulfill God's will, live a meaningful life, and contribute to the well-being of society (Kallio et al., 2022). Nurses serve as advocates for and nurture therapeutic bonds with patients and families. For more than 20 years, Americans have ranked nurses as the most ethical and trustworthy among all professionals (American Nurses Association [ANA], 2023). Oncology nurse navigators (ONNs) excel at connecting with patients, honoring their beliefs and goals, and enhancing their quality of care. Although they often prioritize the needs of patients, nurses also need to tend to their spiritual health to maintain well-being and reaffirm their purpose within the nursing profession.

This chapter will explore the relationship between spirituality and religion, focusing on their distinctions and unique overlaps. Spiritual care is discussed as it pertains to nursing theory, nursing education, and workplace training. Special emphasis is placed on the intersection of ONNs and spiritual nursing care. Finally, strategies to foster workplace well-being through spirituality will be discussed.

Spirituality Versus Religion

Spirituality is difficult to define because it is a dynamic, complex, and fluid concept. In general terms, it is our ability to connect meaningfully in some way to the world around us (Ramachenderan, 2023). Our individual interpretations of spirituality help us make sense of our lives and our purpose. Brené Brown, a renowned research professor, expresses:

> Spirituality is recognizing and celebrating that we are all inextricably connected to one another by a power greater than all of us, and that our connection to that power and to one another is grounded in love and belonging. Practicing spirituality brings a sense of perspective, meaning, and purpose to our lives (Brown, 2015, p.10).

A 2023 study by the Pew Research Center found that 83% of adults in the United States believed that people have a soul or spirit along with a physical body (Alper et al., 2023). For some, spirituality may be related to religion or a higher power. In contrast, others may identify a spiritual connection to nature, music, art, or other everyday experiences that give their lives purpose and contentment. About half of all Americans believe that animals have a spirit or soul and that spirits reside in nature and places for memorials, such as cemeteries (Alper et al., 2023). Our experiences with and expressions of spirituality are as unique as each person; therefore, a universally accepted definition of spirituality is unlikely (Saad & de Medeiros, 2021). The concept of spirituality has evolved and can be dependent on cultural settings and individual perception (Murgia et al., 2020). However, many common patterns and terms are associated with spirituality, such as *connection, meaning, values, transcendence,* and *humanism* (Saad & de Medeiros, 2021). Spiritual health is an essential part of overall wellness, which directly correlates to one's ability to cope with challenges and overcome adversity (Hu et al., 2019).

One expression of spirituality is a connection with religion. In the past, the term *spirituality* was used to describe how people practice their faith and participate in religious services (de Brito Sena et al., 2021). Although the words *spirituality* and *religiosity* may still be used interchangeably, *spirituality* is a broad concept involving individuals, whereas *religiosity* pertains to faith-based communities. *Religion* is associated with groups that share a set of beliefs, rituals, and ceremonies that are often developed as traditions and practiced within families and congregations (De Diego-Codero et al., 2022). Religious institutions tend to be organized and hierarchical, with clearly defined rules and predetermined beliefs (Murgia et al., 2020). Religious doctrine provides a framework for a person's faith and belief system, whereas spirituality affords space for a person to develop their values and meaningful connections regardless of religious belief.

In 2022, the Public Religion Research Institute (PRRI, 2023) conducted a survey that found that 42% of respondents were White Americans who were Christian, 25% were people of color who were Christian, 26.8% had no religious affiliation, 1.9% were Jewish, and 0.6% were Muslim. Less than 1% of Americans identified as Buddhist, Hindu, or Universalist (PRRI, 2023). The 2023 Pew Research Center survey also showed that approximately 22% of U.S. adults described themselves as spiritual but not religious (Alper et al., 2023). Furthermore, the PRRI survey revealed that younger Americans are more likely to be unaffiliated with any religion or identify with a non-Christian faith. A growing number of younger Americans favor a mix of spiritual components and practices instead of identifying with one organized religion (Alper et al., 2023).

Spiritual well-being and religious practice have several health implications that nurses must consider. Idler (2021) posited that religion should be included as a social determinant of health, as it is often related to the circumstances in which one is born and intersects with other social determinants. Children born into religious households are connected to their faith's practices and norms early, which may influence health behaviors such as diet, smoking, sexual activity, and alcohol and drug use. People who regularly attend religious services also report better health outcomes than their nonreligious peers. Overall, regardless of faith, active participation in a religion has a protective effect on the health of individuals, in part, because of the social nature of religious communities (Idler, 2021).

Spiritual beliefs and practices favorably affect health as well, such as lower rates of substance misuse and deaths by suicide, fewer hospitalizations, better treatment adherence, and lower rates of depression (de Brito Sena et al., 2021). Additionally, spiritual practices are often integrated with the treatment of substance misuse (Idler, 2021). Conversely, some religious beliefs may be at odds with healthcare recommendations and public health initiatives. Health issues such as family planning and fertility, abortion, immunizations, gender identity, and end-of-life decisions may be seen through a medical, faith-based, and political lens, which can inform and complicate shared decision-making (Idler, 2021). Furthermore, religious beliefs can affect decisions on resuscitation efforts and life-prolonging treatments (Wirpsa et al., 2019).

Nursing Care and Spirituality

Health care and spirituality have been closely linked throughout time, as spiritual leaders were often viewed as healers (Saad & de Medeiros, 2021). Even Florence Nightingale, a pioneer of secular nursing, believed that spirituality was an inherent resource within all individuals that allowed them to thrive and cope (De Diego-Codero et al., 2022). In the United States, Catholic sisters contributed to the development of nursing schools and nursing as a profession. Between 1886 and 1915, Catholic sisters were credited with establishing 220 nursing schools that enrolled both sisters and laywomen (Wall, 2001). The Catholic sisters are said to have instilled many of the altruistic values and underpinnings of professional nursing, such as ministry to those in need and care for a patient's spiritual health (Wall, 2001). ANA (2015) maintains many of these tenets as described in the *Code of Ethics for Nurses With Interpretive Statements*. In Provision 6, the code delineates that nurses are held to a higher moral standard, which is necessary to promote human dignity, respect, transparency, and a caring environment. Provision 5 advocates for nurses to set aside time for self-care and wellness by maintaining personal relationships, hobbies, and religious or spiritual practices (ANA, 2015).

Holistic nursing care encompasses the physical, emotional, social, and spiritual components of a person's well-being. Nurses must attain a comprehensive knowledge and understanding of humanity and the world (Henderson, 2006).

Harnessing education and compassion, nurses develop caring relationships with patients as an integral part of their role. Many nursing theorists address the spiritual aspects of nursing care by emphasizing the importance of the nurse–patient connection as well as the nurse's focus on whole-person care. Watson (2020) described her theory of Unitary Caring Science as a framework to preserve human caring and dignity and to nurture the human spirit by way of authentic presence and sacred activism, a blend of compassion, courage, and nursing science in action. Nurses must maintain this critical part of their work despite advances in technology and growing complexity in health care, which can take the focus away from holistic nursing care. Professional nurses are called to be moral leaders and address healthcare and societal challenges by respecting human dignity and rights in an increasingly unjust world.

Virginia Henderson's (2006) Nursing Need theory emphasizes the nursing role in helping patients toward independence and focuses on patients' basic human needs. Her theory stresses the importance of a nursing assessment and process that includes evaluating patients based on 14 components of human needs (Henderson, 2006):
- Breathe normally.
- Eat and drink adequately.
- Eliminate body waste.
- Move and maintain a desirable posture.
- Sleep and rest.
- Select suitable clothes.
- Maintain body temperature.
- Keep the body clean.
- Avoid dangers.
- Communicate with others.
- Worship according to one's faith.
- Work in a way that feels satisfactory.
- Participate in various forms of recreation.
- Learn, discover, or satisfy curiosity.

Henderson believed that the physical, psychological, and social components of well-being should all be addressed to maintain health. Her theory acknowledges that patients must be free to practice their faith, find meaning in their lives, and openly communicate their needs and feelings.

Although the theory does not explicitly mention spirituality, the inclusion of faith, focus on mental health, and the importance of the nurse caring for the whole person highlights many aspects of spiritual care (Panczyk et al., 2021). Henderson's 1977 concept of nursing also identifies a need for nurses to have an appreciation for people of all cultures, creeds, and socioeconomic backgrounds to care for a variety of patients. Furthermore, Henderson stated that nursing care is open ended and that the quality of care provided is "limited only by the imagination and competence of the nurse who interprets it" (Henderson, 2006, p. 26). This highlights a nurse's autonomy in crafting their blend of the science and art of nursing based on their education and experience, which is relevant when incorporating spiritual care.

Nursing education incorporates training on evidence-based practice (EBP) and cultural humility—both of which include elements of spiritual care. EBP and cultural humility emphasize the importance of meeting patients where they are and including them as part of the healthcare team. Although healthcare providers contribute expertise in medical care, patients are the experts on themselves. EBP is a clinical decision-making process that uses the best practice evidence, clinical knowledge, assessment, and patient values and preferences to inform care (Panczyk et al., 2021). Cultural humility is a lifelong process of committed learning and self-reflection; the nurse focuses on each patient to learn about their beliefs and values as they pertain to their care (Loue, 2017; Murray-García et al., 2021). To practice cultural humility means to be open and nonjudgmental about a patient's beliefs and values and understand how race, ethnicity, spirituality and religion, gender identity, sexual orientation, and all the dimensions of identity inform their decisions (Loue, 2017). Using EBP and cultural humility enhances the whole-person care nurses provide to their patients by honoring their innate worth and values.

Spiritual Care Training

Healthcare providers must continually hone their spiritual care skills to meet the needs of patients. A study by Green et al. (2020) on nurses' perception of spiritual care competence revealed that only 40% of participants recall learning about spiritual care in nursing school, and 30% reported receiving spiritual care training from their employer. The study also indicated that nurses were performing aspects of spiritual care but struggled when documenting their interventions (Green et al., 2021). In reference to the COVID-19 pandemic, Ferrell et al. (2020) stated that "we have seen that spiritual care is not a luxury, it is a necessity for any system that claims to care for people—whether the people are in the bed or draped in protective gear" (p. e8).

In a 2023 TEDx Talk, palliative care physician Jonathan Ramachenderan described the spiritual dimension of medicine as the most important in all facets of health care. He stressed how our spiritual identity is the foundation of our physical and psychological existence. Furthermore, patients in spiritual distress will experience amplified side effects such as pain and nausea. Spiritual distress occurs when a person experiences psychological suffering because of their inability to find meaning and purpose in their lives and may question their beliefs and values (Roze des Ordons et al., 2020). Spiritual distress is shared across all illnesses and in all cultures. Studies show that up to 96% of patients report spiritual distress at some point in their lives; therefore, addressing spiritual distress is an essential part of patient care (Puchalski et al., 2020).

Nurses are well positioned to assess the spiritual health of patients, as they often spend more time with patients than other healthcare professionals. Nurses serve as the first line of assessment for clinical, psychological, and spiritual distress and provide interventions to alleviate distress independently and in collaboration with the interprofessional team. Nurses are likely to address patients' spiritual care needs without directly acknowledging them. Hawthorne and Gordon (2020) described the "invisibility of spiritual nursing care" as it pertains to holistic care. Spiritual care nursing involves incorporating a patient's culture, values, and goals into their care, as well as providing education and support to facilitate shared decision-making. Characteristics of spiritual care include patient-centered interventions, a healing presence, and the creation of a nurturing environment (Yildirim & Ertem, 2022). Early in their education, nurses are taught the concepts of therapeutic use of self, healing presence, and active listening (Syamsiah et al., 2020). These components of spiritual care are interwoven into nursing practice and inform all nursing interactions with patients.

Implementation of spiritual care practices in nursing is largely dependent on the nurse providing care, as well as their understanding of and attitude toward spirituality. Studies have shown a close connection between a nurse's spiritual health and the spiritual care the nurse provides to their patients (Hu et al., 2019). Nurses may decide not to incorporate spiritual care assessments and interventions because of their personal feelings about spirituality (Murgia et al., 2020). Other barriers to providing spiritual care include fear of unintentionally enforcing their beliefs onto a patient, fear of being too vulnerable with a patient, and fear of feeling unprepared to provide spiritual care (Hawthorne & Gordon, 2020). Also, nurses may find it difficult to separate religion from spirituality because of elusive and overlapping terminology (Hawthorne & Gordon, 2020). A study by Syamsiah et al. (2020) revealed that nurses newer to practice were not as confident in providing spiritual care compared with their more experienced peers.

Spiritual care training starts with a focus on nurses' spiritual health and personal growth. Nurses who nurture their spiritual health, strengthen their coping skills, and find meaning in their lives are better able to tend to the spiritual needs of patients (Syamsiah et al., 2020). Hu et al. (2019) conducted a 12-month nonrandomized study to pilot a spiritual care training program at a hospital in China. Clinical nurses completed a baseline survey and were assigned to either the study group or the control group. The study group completed spiritual care training, which included lectures, case conferences, group discussions, and individual psychological counseling. A large portion of the training was focused on self-reflection and personal development, as well as learning about the spiritual needs of patients. The control group attended monthly lectures on nursing research about common psychological issues among patients with cancer. After the 12-month period ended, each group completed a Spiritual Health Scale and the Chinese version of the Spiritual Care Competency Scale (Hu et al., 2019). Overall, spiritual health and spiritual care competency proved to be higher in the intervention group. Additionally, the researchers observed a therapeutic effect from the intervention group discussions whereby the nurses provided support to one another.

In addition to fostering nurses' spiritual and personal growth, nursing education stresses the development of excellent communication skills and the use of EBP in patient care. EBP is a reminder of how important it is to involve patients in all aspects of their care. Nurses serve as the connection between patients and the interprofessional team and are often advocates for incorporating patient perspectives into the plan of care.

Panczyk et al. (2021) studied the intersection of EBP, communication skills, and spiritual nursing care by surveying undergraduate and postgraduate nursing students in Poland. The students completed the Evidence-Based Practice Competence Questionnaire, the Spirituality and Spiritual Care Rating Scale, and the Communication Skills Attitude Scale (Panczyk et al., 2021). The study showed the importance of the nurses' mindset on spiritual care, the nurses' perceived competence in their communication skills, and the active participation of patients to include spirituality in EBP successfully. It also highlighted that a nurse's age and life experience positively affected their perception of integrating EBP, effective communication, and spiritual care into practice. The experienced nurses showed a favorable attitude toward evidence-based assessment and spiritual care while also indicating a need to improve their communication skills. It was also observed that nurse leadership and the work culture within the nursing team had a direct effect on individual nurses' attitudes regarding improved communication skills and the use of EBP and spiritual care. The study highlighted the importance of balancing the hard and soft skills in nursing education and the need for continuing education throughout a nurse's career.

The COVID-19 pandemic signified the need for increased spiritual care personnel, training, and resources within healthcare settings. Because of the limited resources and risks involved during the COVID-19 pandemic, patients admitted to hospitals were frequently without spiritual care providers (Ferrell et al., 2020).

Aliabadi et al. (2021) completed a descriptive correlation study on nurses caring for patients with the COVID-19 virus in three Iranian hospitals to evaluate the association of spiritual intelligence, empathy, and resilience of nurses. *Spiritual intelligence* refers to one's self-awareness, life purpose, and ability to adapt and cope with stressors (Aliabadi et al., 2021). Spiritual intelligence in nursing care refers to incorporating spirituality and empathy into work to improve the quality of life for patients and nurses alike. Aliabadi et al. (2021) used the Jefferson Scale of Empathy questionnaire and the Spiritual Intelligence Questionnaire to evaluate 338 nurses caring for patients with the COVID-19 virus. They found a positive correlation between spiritual intelligence and empathy in the context of respecting patient rights. The authors noted that empathy scores differed based on the acuity of the patients. Lower empathy scores from the higher acuity facilities were associated with compassion fatigue and burnout. The pandemic reinforced the reality that patients, nurses, and healthcare workers require additional spiritual care support in times of crisis to maintain hope and empathy. Spiritual care training in nursing schools and healthcare organizations is crucial to support nurses' spiritual health and well-being throughout their careers.

A spiritual care training program called the Interprofessional Spiritual Care Education Curriculum is available to healthcare providers seeking additional education in spiritual assessment and interventions (Puchalski et al., 2020). This course is available as an online, self-paced curriculum or an in-person classroom training course. The goal of the course is to train interprofessional teams to provide spiritual assessment and intervention. Clinical teams are trained to work collaboratively with chaplains and spiritual care specialists. The teaching materials include case-based learning, videos, virtual presentations, and reading assignments (Puchalski et al., 2020). Learning topics include spiritual distress, whole-person assessment, holistic treatment, and essential communication skills for spiritual care (Ferrell et al., 2020).

Spiritual Care Assessment Tools and Frameworks

Validated spiritual assessment tools are available for use in a variety of healthcare settings. Best practice states that spiritual assessments are needed whenever there is a change in clinical status and throughout the continuum of care (Ferrell et al., 2020). Examples of mnemonic spiritual assessment tools are FICA, FACT, and HOPE. The four domains of spiritual health addressed in the FICA assessment are (Borneman et al., 2010):
- Faith and beliefs
- Importance: the importance of spirituality for the patient and the influence of spirituality on the patient's health
- Community: the patient's spiritual or religious community
- Address: the interventions used to address spiritual needs

The FACT spiritual assessment tool also explores four areas of spirituality (Ross et al., 2022):
- Faith and beliefs
- Active: how active the patient is in their faith and how available their supports are within the community
- Coping and comfort strategies
- Treatment appropriateness

The HOPE spiritual assessment stands for the following (Ross et al., 2022):
- Hope, meaning, and strength
- Organized religion
- Personal spirituality practices
- Effects on health and end-of-life issues

These assessment tools have been used to gauge a patient's spiritual distress and identify interventions to support and comfort them (Celano et al., 2022). Spiritual assessment tools may or may not be available within a standardized nursing assessment, making mnemonics helpful to ensure that nurses remember the domains of spiritual health. Hawthorne and Gordon (2020) advocated for the inclusion of a spiritual health assessment within the electronic health record.

Nurses can provide spiritual care by adopting the spiritual care framework of RSC (religion, spirituality, and culture); healthcare chaplains use this model in their advanced spiritual care training (Donesky et al., 2020). The RSC model conceptualizes the idea that every patient has a culture, and within that culture, a spirituality, and within that spirituality, sometimes a religion (Donesky et al., 2020). The HealthCare Chaplaincy Network has encouraged nurses to view themselves as spiritual care generalists because nurses are often the providers identifying spiritual distress and referring patients to chaplains (Donesky et al., 2020). Chaplains and nurses perform many overlapping and complementary spiritual care interventions, including assessing for spiritual distress, facilitating spiritual care practices, affirming values, and providing supportive listening and empathy. Nurses often perform primary spiritual care interventions, and some may feel comfortable providing higher levels of spiritual care based on their background and education. Nurses refer patients to chaplains and other spiritual care professionals when needed. Partnering with chaplains and using the RSC framework can enrich holistic nursing practice and increase nurses' comfort in offering spiritual care interventions.

Oncology Nurse Navigation and Spiritual Care

ONNs fulfill a unique role within the interprofessional healthcare team. Involvement from ONNs positively affects care coordination, emotional well-being, and patient satisfaction with oncology care (Chan et al., 2022). ONNs serve as liaisons between patients and all members of the healthcare team and provide education, support, care coordination, and timely access to care. They are not only experts in oncology care but also in the respective health systems in which they work. ONNs must maintain relationships with all team members, have access to oncology care resources, and refer patients to appropriate support services throughout the continuum of care.

To fully understand patient needs, ONNs must assess patients for barriers to care and consider their social determinants of health. By using a whole-person assessment, ONNs can address barriers, mitigate potential barriers, facilitate communication between all members of the healthcare team, and contribute favorably to patient outcomes (Perron, 2019). Although some ONNs work with patients face to face, many primarily communicate via phone and messaging through the electronic health record. Despite the lack of face-to-face communication, ONNs must connect with patients and develop a therapeutic relationship. To build trust with patients and caregivers, ONNs go beyond task-oriented interactions, such as confirming appointments, and facilitate rich conversations to learn about patients' lives, values, and goals of care. Each touchpoint is an opportunity to build upon the relationship and better understand the needs of patients and caregivers. Developing a meaningful connection with patients is necessary to care for the whole person, incorporate spiritual considerations into the care plan, and facilitate shared decision-making.

The Supportive Care Framework for Cancer Care is a model used to improve nurse navigation assessment and effectively identify barriers to oncology care (Gamblin & Bickes, 2020). Consistent with Henderson's Nursing Need theory, the framework includes seven domains: physical, informational, emotional, psychological, social, spiritual, and practical. The assessment endorses the need for holistic nursing care from the navigator by considering all facets of the patient's life that would affect their plan of care.

ONNs have the autonomy to incorporate spiritual care into their practice based on their comfort level. Spiritual care assessments can be used in person or when talking to patients on the phone. Interventions include giving emotional support, providing resources for coping, referring to a chaplain or support group, and encouraging patients to practice their spiritual beliefs. A study by Wirpsa et al. (2019) revealed that most chaplains (92%) are eager to participate in shared medical decision-making as part of the interprofessional team; however, only half of the oncology chaplains were directly involved in family meetings and case conferences. As healthcare leaders, ONNs can increase collaboration with chaplains and connect them to patients, families, and oncology care team members. ONNs can refer patients to integrative oncology services to complement their treatment plan. As recommended by the National Comprehensive Cancer Network, many cancer centers offer integrative therapies known to decrease anxiety and depression, such as music therapy, massage, yoga, and meditation (Mao et al., 2022).

ONNs can partner with their social work colleagues to facilitate support groups and workshops. For example, the oncology social work team at Penn Medicine's Abramson Cancer Center offers a variety of support groups and writing workshops that contribute to the spiritual health of patients and caregivers (Penn Medicine, n.d.). The "What's the Meaning of This?" support group creates a safe space for self-reflection and open discussion for patients to find meaning in their cancer experience as well as build connections with other patients. Writing workshops such as "Writing a Life" and "The Legacy Program" allow patients to write stories, poems, or journals as a creative outlet to explore their values and express themselves (Penn Medicine, n.d.). ONNs can work collaboratively with social workers to develop these programs and refer patients to support groups and workshops based on their spiritual care needs.

Emory Saint Joseph's Hospital in Georgia provides another example of integrating spiritual care and nurse navigation. The hospital performed its community assessment and identified several patients with chronic medical conditions at risk for frequent emergency department visits and hospitalizations (Heitkam, 2019). Each patient was paired with a faith community nurse navigator who provided frequent check-ins and care coordination to improve medication adherence and facilitate communication between the patient and multiple care providers. More than 300 nurses volunteered to participate in the project and completed the Foundations in Faith Community Nursing course. The nurse navigators would call patients weekly and, at times, visit their homes and accompany patients to appointments. In addition, the nurse navigators would provide spiritual care and pray with their patients. The project continued for one year. The hospital noted a 79% decrease in 30-day readmissions, a 57.2% decrease in inpatient admissions, and a 13.3% decrease in emergency department visits (Heitkam, 2019). This project highlighted the efficacy of including faith community nursing with nurse navigation to elevate the therapeutic relationship between nurses and their patients.

ONNs offer themselves as a direct resource to patients and families, providing support, compassion, clarity, and education. This human-to-human connection is vital during all phases of oncology care. As the delivery of care becomes more complex and fragmented for both patients and providers, maintaining a connection with the ONN ensures that patients remain at the center of care. ONNs provide spiritual care by maintaining a therapeutic bond, practicing cultural humility, and facilitating shared decision-making. They practice sacred activism when they address patient barriers, both individual and systemic, to improve equity and access to oncology care

(Watson, 2020). By leveraging their knowledge, leadership, and courage, ONNs serve as healers in their healthcare organizations to close gaps in care.

Workplace Well-Being and Spirituality

The well-being of the nurse directly affects the care provided to the patient. Nurses are held to a high moral standard and are committed to improving the lives of their patients and communities. For nurses to achieve these expectations, they must be self-aware, spiritually and emotionally intelligent, empathetic, and resilient.

Resilience

Resilience is "a positive concept that allows nurses to overcome stressful situations and to adapt positively, resulting in the maintenance of their psychological well-being and mental health" (Kim & Chang, 2022, p. 2). It gives nurses the ability to thrive in the face of adversity and has been proposed as an antidote to burnout. Resilience has been shown to decrease nurses' psychological stress and increase their physical and mental health. It can have a mediating effect on the relationship between burnout and physical and mental health (Kim & Chang, 2022).

The Connor-Davidson Resilience Scale measures how well one is equipped to bounce back after trauma, stressful events, and tragedies. One study of nurses in a pediatric intensive care unit demonstrated that staff-designed bundle interventions increased group resilience from a score of 79.9 to 83.4 within six months of bundle implementation. Elements in the resiliency bundle included the following (Davis & Batcheller, 2020, p. 606):
- Ethical issue resolution process
- Mindfulness reminders through cell phone applications
- Patient death process outline
- Case conference discussions
- Structured debriefings with pastoral care
- Discussions with colleagues and supportive staff
- Leadership notification
- Social events
- Host site educational courses aimed at improved well-being
- Employee assistance program

Resilience can decrease the effects of moral distress. Implementing evidence-based interventions to increase resilience, such as the resiliency bundle, can also address burnout.

Burnout

Burnout is described as the "anguish experienced—internal and external as a threat to one's composure, integrity, sense of self, or the fulfillment of expectations" (De

Diego-Codero et al., 2022, p. 612). Burnout is common in health care, particularly with nurses. Up to 70% of nurses are affected by burnout (Roux & Benita, 2020). In 2019, the World Health Organization added *burnout* to the International Classification of Diseases and described it as a workplace occurrence (Moss, 2020). Because *burnout* is defined as a workplace issue and not a work–life balance issue, healthcare organizations must develop strategies to prevent and alleviate the problem (Moss, 2020). A Gallup poll revealed that the top five causes of burnout were unfair treatment in the workplace, unmanageable workload, lack of role clarity, lack of support and communication from superiors, and unreasonable time demands (Moss, 2020).

Burnout is a chronic syndrome resulting from unmanaged stress in the workplace comprised of three dimensions: exhaustion, mental and emotional detachment from work, and decreased professional accomplishment (De Diego-Cordero et al., 2022; Moss, 2020). Physical manifestations of burnout include headaches, fatigue, insomnia, and gastrointestinal distress (Roux & Benita, 2020). Psychological symptoms of burnout are anxiety, hopelessness, and exhaustion (Moss, 2020; Roux & Benita, 2020). Nurses may appear to lack empathy and have a cynical outlook on their work (Moss, 2020). They are highly susceptible to burnout because of their work conditions and ongoing exposure to human suffering. As a chronic phenomenon, burnout develops over time. It may not be identified in the early stages, but left untreated, it will decrease the quality of care and patient satisfaction and may increase patient morbidity and mortality (Roux & Benita, 2020).

A study by Yildirim and Ertem (2022) showed that nurses experiencing high levels of burnout and moderate levels of compassion fatigue reported a disconnect in spiritual beliefs and values. Burnout directly impacts a nurse's desire to work and their ability to provide personalized care and therapeutic communication (Yildirim & Ertem, 2022).

For nurses, perceptions of workplace quality of life are determined by experiences with burnout, compassion fatigue, and compassion satisfaction. Quality of life is a self-reported measure of a person's feelings regarding their satisfaction in all aspects of life as it pertains to expectations, values, goals, and life challenges (Blom et al., 2023). As caregivers, nurses engage in need-based relationships with patients and families, continual demands from physicians and patients, and ongoing expectations for giving of themselves (Roux & Benita, 2020). Nurses may also possess an internal expectation of perfection in their work and a tendency to overcommit to responsibilities as a way of fulfilling their life's purpose of serving others; however, this altruistic predisposition increases the likelihood of burnout (Roux & Benita, 2020). Nurses who feel regularly unsatisfied with the quality of their nursing care are more likely to report burnout and compassion fatigue (Yildirim & Ertem, 2022). Furthermore, nurses who experience burnout have reported an unwillingness to work and insensitive behaviors toward patients (Yildirim & Ertem, 2022).

Assessing for burnout in healthcare professionals can be accomplished using the Maslach Burnout Inventory (MBI), which is a self-assessment questionnaire (Maslach & Leiter, 2021; Roux & Benita, 2020). This assessment was developed in the early 1980s as the first measurement of burnout and continues to be used in research and health and human service professions (Maslach & Leiter, 2021). The MBI is meant to be applied in organizations to benefit employees and improve work culture. Self-care is typically recommended for burnout; however, this places the onus on the nurse rather than the workplace. The MBI provides three scores for each respondent: exhaustion, cynicism, and professional efficacy. It measures each dimension on a frequency scale. Burnout is indicated when all three dimensions have a negative score. Maslach and Leiter (2021) cautioned to use the assessment tool correctly to identify burnout within a healthcare organization. The MBI is not a diagnostic tool for individual health problems but a measure of the workplace culture and its effects on the employees. Healthcare organizations can actively prevent burnout by managing nurse workloads, encouraging nurse autonomy, showing gratitude, and creating a just community (Moss, 2020). Because nurse burnout produces negative outcomes for nurses and patients, healthcare leaders must maintain a culture of wellness within their organizations.

Caring for the Caregiver

Nurses have a responsibility to care for themselves as they would for patients, but their instinct is to put the care of patients and families first. Self-care seems antithetical to the values and mission of the nursing profession to the point where ANA included a code for self-care to remind nurses to prioritize themselves. Nurses must allow themselves grace, self-compassion, and space for reflection to protect against burnout and compassion fatigue. Practicing one's spiritual or religious beliefs can have a protective effect from burnout (De Diego-Cordero et al., 2022). Meditation and prayer, regardless of religious beliefs, were found to have positive effects on nurses' ability to cope with the day-to-day stressors of patient care (De Diego-Cordero et al., 2022). Spiritual quality of life was found to have the greatest influence on caregiver satisfaction compared to other components, and a higher perception of caregiver satisfaction leads to improved mental health and healthy behaviors among caregivers (Blom et al., 2023).

Additionally, in a study by Watson (2024), nurses attributed their ability to cope throughout the COVID-19 pandemic to maintaining connections with their nursing colleagues, loved ones, community, and patients. Nurturing these relationships had a favorable impact on their resilience and intention to stay in the nursing profession. The most important factor in spirituality is the ability to connect meaningfully to the people and things that affirm one's life purpose and bring contentment.

Summary

Spiritual care is essential in healthcare delivery. The importance of humans helping humans to find and maintain purpose and meaning cannot be understated. In Tyler Merritt's (2021) autobiography, *I Take My Coffee Black*, he offered a recipe for "Better Society Gumbo," with ingredients including proximity, honesty, value, and a common goal. Merritt explained that proximity breeds empathy, and honesty fosters vulnerable dialogue. He also stressed the need to value each other's innate worth and to recognize how people are more alike than different and often have common goals. Merritt's observations align with the core values of nursing, sacred activism, cultural humility, and spirituality. Nurses have been serving "Better Society Gumbo" since the days of Nightingale, and this is reflected in the profound impact that nurses have on their patients and families. ONNs can incorporate the elements of spiritual care in their professional and personal lives and serve as leaders in whole-person care in their healthcare organizations.

The author would like to acknowledge Rev. Diane Baldwin, RN, OCN®, CBCN®, for her contribution to this chapter that remains unchanged from the previous edition of this book. This chapter is dedicated to the Abramson Cancer Center's Patient and Family Services Department staff for their tireless efforts in supporting patients affected by cancer.

References

Aliabadi, P.K., Zazoly, A.Z., Sohrab, M., Neyestani, F., Nazari, N., Mousavi, S.H., ... Ferdowsi, M. (2021). The role of spiritual intelligence in predicting the empathy levels of nurses with COVID-19 patients. *Archives of Psychiatric Nursing, 35*(6), 658–663. https://doi.org/10.1016/j.apnu.2021.10.007

Alper, B.A., Rotolo, M., Tevington, P., Nortey, J., & Kallo, A. (2023). *Spirituality among Americans*. Pew Research Center. https://www.pewresearch.org/religion/2023/12/07/spirituality-among-americans

American Nurses Association. (2015). *Code of ethics for nurses with interpretive statements*. https://www.nursingworld.org/practice-policy/nursing-excellence/ethics/code-of-ethics-for-nurses

American Nurses Association. (2023). *Americans continue to rank nurses most honest and ethical professionals* [Press release]. https://www.nursingworld.org/news/news-releases/2022-news-releases/americans-continue-to-rank-nurses-most-honest-and-ethical-professionals

Blom, C., Reis, A., & Lencastre, L. (2023). Caregiver quality of life: Satisfaction and burnout. *International Journal of Environmental Research and Public Health, 20*(16), 6577. https://doi.org/10.3390/ijerph20166577

Borneman, T., Ferrell, B., & Puchalski, C.M. (2010). Evaluation of the FICA tool for spiritual assessment. *Journal of Pain and Symptom Management, 40*(2), 163–173. https://doi.org/10.1016/j.jpainsymman.2009.12.019

Brown, B. (2015). *Rising strong: How the ability to reset transforms the way we live, love, parent, and lead*. Random House.

Celano, T., Harris, S., Sawyer, A.T., & Hamilton, T. (2022). Promoting spiritual well-being among nurses. *Nurse Leader, 20*(2), 188–192. https://doi.org/10.1016/j.mnl.2021.08.002

Chan, R.J., Milch, V.E., Crawford-Williams, F., Agbejule, O.A., Joseph, R., Johal, J., ... Hart, N.H. (2022). Patient navigation across the cancer care continuum: An overview of systematic reviews and emerging literature. *CA: A Cancer Journal for Clinicians, 73*(6), 565–589. https://doi.org/10.3322/caac.21788

Davis, M., & Batcheller, J. (2020). Managing moral distress in the workplace: Creating a resiliency bundle. *Nurse Leader, 18*(6), 604–608. https://doi.org/10.1016/j.mnl.2020.06.007

de Brito Sena, M.A., Damiano, R.F., Lucchetti, G., & Prieto Peres, M.F. (2021). Defining spirituality in healthcare: A systematic review and conceptual framework. *Frontiers in Psychology, 12*, 756080. https://doi.org/10.3389/fpsyg.2021.756080

De Diego-Codero, R., Iglesias-Romo, M., Badanta, B., Lucchetti, G., & Vega-Escaño, J. (2022). Burnout and spirituality among nurses: A scoping review. *Explore, 18*(5), 612–620. https://doi.org/10.1016/j.explore.2021.08.001

Donesky, D., Sprague, E., & Joseph, D. (2020). A new perspective on spiritual care: Collaborative chaplaincy and nursing practice. *Advances in Nursing Science, 43*(2), 147–158. https://doi.org/10.1097/ANS.0000000000000298

Ferrell, B.R., Handzo, G., Puchalski, C., & Rosa, W.E. (2020). The urgency of spiritual care: COVID-19 and the critical need for whole-person palliation. *Journal of Pain and Symptom Management, 60*(3), e7–e11. https://doi.org/10.1016/j.jpainsymman.2020.06.034

Gamblin, K.A., & Bickes, D. (2020). Implementation of a standardized navigation barrier assessment for oncology patients based on a person-centered framework. *Journal of Oncology Navigation and Survivorship, 11*(2). https://jons-online.com/issues/2020/february-2020-vol-11-no-2/2799:implementation-of-a-standardized-navigation-barrier-assessment-for-oncology-patients-based-on-a-person-centered-framewor

Green, A., Kim-Godwin, Y.S., & Jones, C. (2020). Perceptions of spiritual care, education, competence, and barriers in providing spiritual care among registered nurses. *Journal of Holistic Nursing, 38*(1), 41–51. https://doi.org/10.1177/0898010119885266

Hawthorne, D.M., & Gordon, S.C. (2020). The invisibility of spiritual care in clinical practice. *Journal of Holistic Nursing, 38*(1), 147–155. https://doi.org/10.1177/0898010119889704

Heitkam, R. (2019). Reducing hospital readmissions through faith community nursing. *Nursing Management, 50*(8), 26–30. https://doi.org/10.1097/01.numa.0000575312.84044.dc

Henderson, V. (2006). The concept of nursing. 1977. *Journal of Advanced Nursing, 53*(1), 21–34. https://doi.org/10.1111/j.1365-2648.2006.03660.x

Hu, Y., Jiao, M., & Li, F. (2019). Effectiveness of spiritual care training to enhance spiritual health and spiritual care competency among oncology nurses. *BMC Palliative Care, 18*(1), 104. https://doi.org/10.1186/s12904-019-0489-3

Idler, E. (2021). Health and religion. In W.C. Cockerham (Ed.), *The Wiley Blackwell companion to medical sociology* (pp. 370–388). Wiley Blackwell. https://doi.org/10.1002/9781119633808.ch18

Kallio, H., Kangasniemi, M., & Hult, M. (2022). Registered nurses' perceptions of having a calling to nursing: A mixed-method study. *Journal of Advanced Nursing, 78*(5), 1473–1482. https://doi.org/10.1111/jan.15157

Kim, E.Y., & Chang, S.O. (2022). Exploring nurse perceptions and experiences of resilience: A meta-synthesis study. *BMC Nursing, 21*(1), 26. https://doi.org/10.1186/s12912-021-00803-z

Loue, S. (2017). *Handbook of religion and spirituality in social work practice and research*. Springer.

Mao, J.J., Pillai, G.G., Andrade, C.J., Ligibel, J.A., Basu, P., Cohen, L., ... Salicrup, L.A. (2022). Integrative oncology: Addressing the global challenges of cancer prevention and treatment. *CA: A Cancer Journal for Clinicians, 72*(2), 144–164. https://doi.org/10.3322/caac.21706

Maslach, C., & Leiter, M.P. (2021). Health and behavioral science: How to measure burnout accurately and ethically. *Harvard Business Review*. https://hbr.org/2021/03/how-to-measure-burnout-accurately-and-ethically

Merritt, T. (2021). *I take my coffee black: Reflections on Tupac, musical theatre, faith, and being Black in America*. Worthy Publishing.

Moss, J. (2020). Rethinking burnout: When self-care is not the cure. *American Journal of Health Promotion, 34*(5), 565–568. https://doi.org/10.1177/0890117120920488b

Murgia, C., Notarnicola, I., Rocco, G., & Stievano, A. (2020). Spirituality in nursing: A concept analysis. *Nursing Ethics, 27*(5), 1327–1343. https://doi.org/10.1177/0969733020909534

Murray-García, J., Ngo, V., Marsh, T., Pak, T., Ackerman-Barger, K., & Cavanagh, S.J. (2021). Cultural humility meets antiracism in nurse leader training. *Nurse Leader, 19*(6), 608–615. https://doi.org/10.1016/j.mnl.2021.08.017

Panczyk, M., Iwanow, L., Musik, S., Wawrzuta, D., Gotlib, J., & Jaworski, M. (2021). Perceiving the role of communication skills as a bridge between the perception of spiritual care and acceptance of evidence-based nursing practice—Empirical model. *International Journal of Environmental Research and Public Health, 18*(23), 12591. https://doi.org/10.3390/ijerph182312591

Penn Medicine. (n.d.). *Abramson Cancer Center: Support groups and workshops*. https://www.pennmedicine.org/cancer/navigating-cancer-care/support-services/support-groups-and-workshops

Perron, M. (2019). The growing importance of cancer care navigation. *Oncology Times, 41*(7), 1, 16. https://doi.org/10.1097/01.cot.0000557599.61162.2c

Public Religion Research Institute. (2023). *2022 PRRI census of American religion: Religious affiliation updates and trends.* https://www.prri.org/spotlight/prri-2022-american-values-atlas-religious-affiliation-updates-and-trends

Puchalski, C., Jafari, N., Buller, H., Haythorn, T., Jacobs, C., & Ferrell, B. (2020). Interprofessional spiritual care education curriculum: A milestone toward the provision of spiritual care. *Journal of Palliative Medicine, 23*(6), 777–784. https://doi.org/10.1089/jpm.2019.0375

Ramachenderan, J. (2023, August). *The spiritual dimension of medicine* [Video]. Tedx Talks. https://www.youtube.com/watch?v=1cvTnvcnQHk

Ross, L., Grimwade, L., & Eagger, S. (2022). Spiritual assessment. In C.C.H. Cook & A. Powell (Eds.), *Spirituality and psychiatry* (2nd ed., pp. 23–48). Cambridge University Press.

Roux, N., & Benita, T. (2020). Self-care for nurses: Best practices for burnout self-care. *Nursing Management, 51*(10), 31–35. https://doi.org/10.1097/01.numa.0000698116.82355.0d

Roze des Ordons, A.L., Stelfox, H.T., Sinuff, T., Grindrod-Millar, K., Smiechowski, J., & Sinclair, S. (2020). Spiritual distress in family members of critically ill patients: Perceptions and experiences. *Journal of Palliative Medicine, 23*(2), 198–210. https://doi.org/10.1089/jpm.2019.0235

Saad, M., & de Medeiros, R. (2021). Spirituality and healthcare—Common grounds for secular and religious worlds and its clinical implications. *Religions, 12*(1), 22. https://doi.org/10.3390/rel12010022

Syamsiah, N., Rahma, M., & Hassan, H.C. (2020). The relation between knowledge and attitudes with behavior of nurse in providing spiritual care. *Enfermería Clínica, 30*(55), 196–201. https://doi.org/10.1016/j.enfcli.2019.11.053

Wall, B.M. (2001). "Definite Lines of Influence": Catholic sisters and nurse training schools, 1890–1920. *Nursing Research, 50*(5), 314–321. https://doi.org/10.1097/00006199-200109000-00010

Watson, A.L. (2024). Connections ease nurses' burdens. *American Nurse, 19*(2), 26–31 https://doi.org/10.51256/anj022426

Watson, J. (2020). Nursing's global covenant with humanity—Unitary caring science as sacred activism. *Journal of Advanced Nursing, 76*(2), 699–704. https://doi.org/10.1111/jan.13934

Wirpsa, M.J., Johnson, R.E., Bieler, J., Boyken, L., Pugliese, K., Rosencrans, E., & Murphy, P. (2019). Interprofessional models for shared decision making: The role of the health care chaplain. *Journal of Health Care Chaplaincy, 25*(1), 20–44. https://doi.org/10.1080/08854726.2018.1501131

Yildirim, J.G., & Ertem, M. (2022). Professional quality of life and perceptions of spirituality and spiritual care among nurses: Relationship and affecting factors. *Perspectives in Psychiatric Care, 58*(2), 438–447. https://doi.org/10.1111/ppc.12794

SECTION IV

Personalized Care for Unique Populations

Chapter 14. Survivorship Navigation
Chapter 15. Mental Health Issues
Chapter 16. Gero-Oncology Considerations
Chapter 17. Pediatrics, Adolescents, and Young Adults
Chapter 18. Navigation Resources

CHAPTER 14

Survivorship Navigation

Tara Sweeney, BSN, RN, CHPN, OCN®, and Darcy Burbage, DNP, RN, AOCN®, CBCN®

> **KEY TOPICS**
> cancer survivors, symptom management, surveillance

Overview

The National Coalition for Cancer Survivorship (2014, para. 2) defines *survivorship* as "living with, through, and beyond a cancer diagnosis" and recognizes family, friends, and caregivers as part of the experience. Survivorship also acknowledges the physical, psychosocial, spiritual, financial, and employment effects that a cancer diagnosis has on patients with cancer and their loved ones (Tonorezos et al., 2024).

With evolving guidelines and care models shifting to promote personalized survivorship care from diagnosis, the terms *survivor* and *survivorship* do not always resonate with patients, caregivers, or interprofessional care team members and do not always translate to other languages (Miller et al., 2022).

An estimated 18 million cancer survivors were living in the United States as of January 2022; that number is expected to reach 26 million by 2040. Statistics show that 70% of cancer survivors are alive 5 years beyond diagnosis, 47% at 10 years or more, and 19% at 20 years or more (Tonorezos et al., 2024).

As survivorship is multidimensional and encompasses the cancer care continuum, oncology nurse navigators (ONNs) are well-positioned to support and provide individualized survivorship care to a variety of patient populations in various settings in health care (Oncology Nursing Society [ONS] & Oncology Nursing Certification Corporation [ONCC], 2024). ONN interventions improve patients' access to care, reduce the barriers and disparities common to those experiencing the cancer journey, and enhance cancer survivors' knowledge, satisfaction, and quality of life (Chan et al., 2023).

This chapter will explore the stages and components of cancer survivorship, including its long-term and late effects, psychosocial needs, sexual side effects, and financial challenges. It will also discuss the role of ONNs in survivorship and future opportunities for improving cancer survivorship care.

Stages of Survivorship

In 1985, Fitzhugh Mullan's essay *Seasons of Survival: Reflections of a Physician With Cancer* explored and acknowledged survivorship as a unique process for a person diagnosed with cancer. Just as cancer is defined in stages to support treatment guidelines and care planning, Mullan identified three separate stages of survivorship: acute, extended, and permanent (Mullan, 1985).

The acute stage is the initial phase of survivorship, encompassing diagnosis through active treatment. The focus is often on the cancer diagnosis and treatment, including immediate physical changes that occur and the experience of new symptoms or side effects (Koczwara et al., 2023; Mullan, 1985; Sheikh-Wu et al., 2023).

Extended survivorship begins at the end of active treatment and continues through active surveillance. The focus shifts from treating the disease to reducing the risk of recurrence, using possible maintenance therapies, and promoting healthy living. As medical visits become less frequent, survivors may experience increased anxiety and varied mental, physical, social, and emotional stressors (Koczwara et al., 2023; Mullan, 1985; Sheikh-Wu et al., 2023).

The permanent or long-term stage of survivorship begins when a cancer recurrence is less likely. Often starting five years after diagnosis, this phase continues until the end of life. The focus is primarily on the long-term or secondary effects of cancer and ongoing risk reduction, prevention, and screening (Koczwara et al., 2023; Mullan, 1985; Sheikh-Wu et al., 2023).

These stages broadly classify care for survivors diagnosed with early-stage cancer; however, survivors living with advanced or metastatic cancer identify similar needs and parallel experiences across these stages. The metastatic or chronic stage of survivorship often includes a focus on patient-specific goals of care, management of ongoing treatment, palliative care, and end-of-life care considerations (Lai-Kwon et al., 2023; Sheikh-Wu et al., 2023).

Psychosocial, physical, financial, spiritual, and interpersonal factors can affect health outcomes and quality of life throughout each survivorship stage. Understanding common themes and key components of care within each stage can help ONNs enhance survivorship care. Similar to how interprofessional teams use cancer staging, ONNs can tailor care based on the survivorship stage, engage in conversations with survivors, support awareness and education related to survivorship stages and resources, and further identify and address care needs across the continuum (see Figure 14-1).

Components of Survivorship Care

With each stage of care comes a unique set of potential physical changes, along with a very personal, social, and emotional journey. Recognizing key components to improve survivors' outcomes continues to be an expanding focus in cancer care and research (Mollica et al., 2024).

FIGURE 14-1. Stages of Survivorship Across the Continuum of Cancer Care

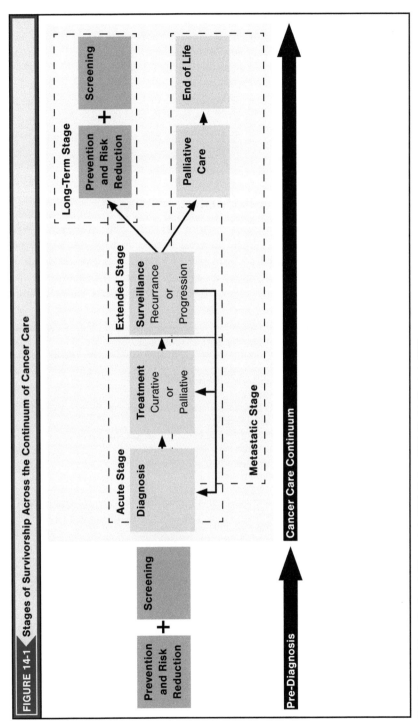

Note. Based on information from Lai-Kwon et al., 2023; Mullan, 1985; Sheikh-Wu et al., 2023.

The National Comprehensive Cancer Network (NCCN) and the European Society for Medical Oncology have identified essential components of quality survivorship care. ONNs can educate survivors and collaborate with care teams on components of quality survivorship care as outlined in Figure 14-2 (NCCN, 2025d; Vaz-Luis et al., 2022). Depending on the survivor, the diagnosis, the extent of the disease, and treatment toxicities, survivorship care can include a combination of each component throughout the continuum to support the individual. ONNs can use these components to guide personalized survivorship care and to evaluate opportunities for survivorship program development.

Long-Term and Late Effects of Treatment

Cancer and subsequent treatments result in survivors often experiencing physical, functional, emotional, social, and spiritual distress. In addition, many experience financial and spiritual effects. The type of symptoms and potential effects can vary based on the treatment course, along with patient and diagnostic factors, such as age, comorbidities, cancer type, and stage. These effects can range from

---

FIGURE 14-2 Components of Quality Survivorship Care

- Providing surveillance and follow-up care
  - Ongoing surveillance for recurrence or metastasis
  - Screening for secondary cancers
  - Performing follow-up visits to assess, address, and plan ongoing survivorship care
- Promoting health and disease prevention
  - Offering prevention and screening for late effects of cancer and therapies
  - Performing screening for new cancers
  - Providing surveillance and management of chronic conditions
  - Promoting overall health and well-being
- Assessing and addressing care needs
  - Monitoring and managing cancer-related side effects, including physical, psychosocial, immunologic, and financial effects
  - Recurring assessment of symptoms and care needs
  - Identifying and providing resources and referrals for specialized interventions as indicated
- Educating and empowering survivors
  - Determining the frequency and role of surveillance, screening, and follow-up care
  - Providing information on cancer, treatments, and acute, long-term, and late treatment-related side effects
  - Educating and promoting recommendations for healthy behaviors
- Care planning and coordination
  - Coordinating care between the oncology care team, specialists, and primary care providers
  - Delineating the roles of healthcare providers
  - Providing interventions to support the impact related to cancer and treatment

Note. Based on information from National Comprehensive Cancer Network, 2024d; Vaz-Luis et al., 2022.

manageable to permanent or even debilitating and impact quality of life (Miller et al., 2022).

An evolving model to reduce morbidity from treatment is cancer prehabilitation. Rock et al. (2022) defined *prehabilitation* as a proactive approach to cancer treatment that uses baseline assessments to guide interventions and improve short- and long-term outcomes. Because ONNs are often the first clinicians to meet with newly diagnosed patients, they can identify those who might benefit from prehabilitation. This may lead to reduced unplanned hospital admissions, decreased costs, and improved patient outcomes (Rock et al., 2022).

Prehabilitation can also be considered a strategy to mitigate the cardiovascular risk and toxicity associated with cancer care. A survivor's cardiovascular risk can increase over time and after receiving certain treatments, such as anthracyclines and radiation therapy to the chest. Several shared risk factors are associated with cardiovascular disease and cancer, including hypertension, dyslipidemia, nicotine use, obesity, and diabetes (Bisceglia et al., 2023). Strategies for ONNs to help with prehabilitation include a thorough assessment of survivors' comorbidities, nutritional status, functionality, and emotional state. ONNs can identify support systems and offer referrals to smoking cessation, counseling, and financial assistance programs.

ONNs can assist survivors in understanding common side effects by providing evidence-based education about their diagnosis and treatments received, discussing recommendations for monitoring and management, and offering resources or referrals as needed (Kozul et al., 2020). They can empower survivors by using their preferred language and learning styles and ensuring they know who to contact with changes or concerns at each survivorship stage. The American Cancer Society, American Society of Clinical Oncology, National Coalition for Cancer Survivorship, and many nationally known advocacy organizations offer free or reduced-cost evidence-based education materials (see Table 14-1).

Symptom Clusters

Identifying symptom clusters can help ONNs tailor survivorship education and interventions. According to Lee et al. (2020), symptom clusters are two or more individual symptoms that coexist. Distinct symptom clusters can occur at each survivorship stage and with differing levels of severity. Studies have shown that survivors can experience 8–15 symptoms during their survivorship journey, with 40% reporting a symptom cluster of fatigue, pain, and sleep disturbances (Lee et al., 2020; Sheikh-Wu et al., 2020; Wu et al., 2023). In a systematic review by Sheikh-Wu et al. (2023), massage, exercise (movement), and behavioral therapy were helpful for this symptom cluster.

Assessing and evaluating survivors at regular intervals for ongoing symptoms can help address potential long-term and late effects of treatment. Assessment intervention resources are available from ONS (www.ons.org/survivorship-learning-library) and NCCN (www.nccn.org).

TABLE 14-1. Resources for Cancer Survivorship

Resource	Website
General Information and Advocacy	
American Cancer Society Survivorship: During and After Treatment	www.cancer.org/cancer/survivorship.html
National Coalition for Cancer Survivorship	www.canceradvocacy.org
Oncology Nursing Society Survivorship Learning Library	www.ons.org/survivorship-learning-library
Guidelines, Assessments, and Program Development	
American Society of Clinical Oncology Survivorship Compendium	www.asco.org/news-initiatives/current-initiatives/cancer-care-initiatives/prevention-survivorship/survivorship-compendium
George Washington University's National Cancer Survivorship Resource Center	https://cancercontroltap.org/news/national-cancer-survivorship-resource-center
National Cancer Institute National Standards for Cancer Survivorship Care	www.cancercontrol.cancer.gov/ocs/special-focus-areas/national-standards-cancer-survivorship-care
National Comprehensive Cancer Network Clinical Practice Guidelines in Oncology	www.nccn.org/guidelines/category_1
Survivorship Care Plan Templates	
American Society of Clinical Oncology Cancer Treatment and Survivorship Care Plans	www.cancer.net/survivorship/follow-care-after-cancer-treatment/asco-cancer-treatment-and-survivorship-care-plans
OncoLink Survivorship Care Plan	https://oncolife.oncolink.org
Care Planning Tools for Survivors	
Cancer Support Community *Coping With Cancer Resources*	www.cancersupportcommunity.org/coping-cancer
Exercise is Medicine® *Moving Through Cancer*	www.exerciseismedicine.org/eim-in-action/moving-through-cancer
National Cancer Institute *Facing Forward: When Someone You Love Has Completed Cancer Treatment*	https://cancerhelpessentiahealth.org/ebooks/Facing_Forward_WSYL_from_BR.html
National Cancer Institute *Making Future Plans With Advanced Cancer*	www.cancer.gov/about-cancer/advanced-cancer/planning
National Coalition for Cancer Survivorship *Cancer Survivorship Checklist: Finished With Treatment*	www.canceradvocacy.org/wp-content/uploads/Survivorship-Checklist-Finished-Treatment.pdf

(Continued on next page)

TABLE 14-1	Resources for Cancer Survivorship *(Continued)*
Resource	Website
Care Planning Tools for Survivors *(Cont.)*	
National Coalition for Cancer Survivorship *Cancer Survivorship Checklist: Living With Advanced and Metastatic Cancer*	www.canceradvocacy.org/wp-content/uploads/Survivorship-Checklist-Living-with-Advanced-Cancer.pdf
National Coalition for Cancer Survivorship *Self-Advocacy: A Cancer Survivor's Handbook*	www.canceradvocacy.org/resources/publications/self-advocacy

Questions that ONNs can ask to assess and address survivors' symptom burden include the following:
- Are these common or uncommon for the treatment, type, and stage of cancer the survivor had/has?
- What is the survivor's baseline?
- What other health conditions or comorbidities does the survivor have?
- How do these symptoms affect other areas of the survivor's life?
- What interventions are available to support or alleviate this symptom/symptom cluster (e.g., pharmacologic, nonpharmacologic, education, internal or external resources, referrals)?

Physical Needs

The physical effects of cancer and treatments can affect overall well-being. Survivors share feelings of anxiety and stress when physical change occurs. ONNs can help survivors recognize potential symptoms and set expectations for common physical changes and timelines (Ross et al., 2022). Common cancer-related physical effects are fatigue, pain, neuropathy, and cognitive changes.

Fatigue

Cancer-related fatigue can be physical, emotional, or cognitive and is one of the most common and persistent side effects, with up to 50% of long-term survivors reporting fatigue years after completing treatment (NCCN, 2025b). Fatigue assessments or scales are resources to monitor trends throughout survivorship. Fatigue can also be related to a secondary cause. Performing a focused history and physical review can aid ONNs in identifying potential contributing factors, such as anemia, new medications, pain, or other concurrent symptoms (Worrell et al., 2021).

Strategies for fatigue prevention include education on healthy lifestyles and exercise opportunities (at least 150 minutes of activity weekly). ONNs can collaborate with the oncology care team when concerns or contributing factors are identified and explore management interventions, including energy conservation strategies, cognitive and supportive therapies, cancer rehabilitation programs, and nutrition counseling (Worrell et al., 2021).

Pain

Pain is another commonly reported symptom throughout survivorship. It can be categorized in several ways, including acute, intractable, and chronic. Cancer-related pain can be complex and related to the location of cancer, treatment side effects, recurrence, or progression. It can manifest physically and psychosocially and, if untreated or undertreated, significantly impact quality of life (Aman et al., 2021; Miller et al., 2022). Pain management strategies include combining pharmacologic or nonpharmacologic interventions, such as integrative physical and cognitive modalities (e.g., mindfulness, massage, spiritual care) (Sheikh-Wu et al., 2020). ONNs can assist patients and care teams by exploring pain-related concerns shared by survivors and identifying barriers to management or care. They can empower survivors and caregivers throughout survivorship by offering education and self-monitoring strategies on potential symptoms based on cancer diagnosis and treatment (Franklin et al., 2022). Expansive tools and evidence-based resources to aid in the assessment and education of survivors for pain management and potential interventions are shown in Table 14-1.

Neuropathy

Neuropathy or neuropathic pain is an example of pain occurring from cancer treatments, including surgery, radiation therapy, and chemotherapy (e.g., taxanes, platinum-based drugs). It can be acute or chronic and lead to safety concerns related to sensory and strength changes from nerve damage, resulting in changes to balance, gait, and dexterity (Loprinzi et al., 2020). Survivor-specific risk can depend on the type, duration, or dosing of treatments, along with considerations such as age, prior history of neuropathy, or diabetes. Limited evidence is available to support the recommendation of both prescription and over-the-counter pharmacologic agents to prevent chemotherapy-induced peripheral neuropathy. Duloxetine is one option with evidence to support its use (Loprinzi et al., 2020).

ONNs can be integral in the care of survivors who experience neuropathy. Strategies include educating on safety considerations (e.g., exercise adaptations) if neuropathy affects balance or using resistance bands instead of free weights (NCCN, 2025a). ONNs can also collaborate on treatment planning to support the palliation of physical effects. Survivors often share concerning changes with ONNs. For example, a survivor might report worsening neuropathic pain accompanied by new back pain. ONNs can advocate for assessment by the oncology provider and coordinate care for earlier surveillance imaging because of new symptoms. They can also engage patients and caregivers in fall safety awareness. Referrals to cancer rehabilitation for physical or occupational therapy or integrative therapies (e.g., acupuncture) may also be helpful (Loprinzi et al., 2020; NCCN, 2025a).

Cognitive Changes

A history of cancer is associated with a 30%–60% increase in self-reported memory problems (Schagen et al., 2022). *Cognitive dysfunction, memory problems, chemobrain,* and *chemo fog* are terms that survivors use to describe changes in cognition, learning, or memory that may occur because of cancer treatment. However, causes other than chemotherapy may contribute to cognitive issues, such as stress, fatigue, other medications, or a combination of these factors. Survivors with brain metastasis or those who have received cranial irradiation or high-dose chemotherapy are at increased risk for cognitive changes. ONNs can support awareness and early identification of symptoms, including forgetfulness, word finding, impaired concentration, decreased attention, difficulty with multitasking, or short-term memory changes. They can also validate symptoms and offer strategies, including using notes and reminders, encouraging exercise, avoiding alcohol use, cognitive training with brain games or puzzles, and offering referrals to integrative therapies, such as yoga, mindfulness, or cognitive rehabilitation pending severity (Worrell et al., 2021).

Immune-Related Adverse Effects

Immunotherapy treatments, such as immune checkpoint inhibitors (e.g., ipilimumab, pembrolizumab) or chimeric antigen receptor T-cell therapies, are expanding the cancer care landscape. Immunotherapies are offered as treatment options across many cancer types and stages. For survivors treated with immunotherapy, ongoing surveillance for immune-related adverse effects during and after treatment is essential to overall health (NCCN, 2025c; Schagen et al., 2022). Common immune-related adverse effects are rash, hyperglycemia, endocrinopathies (e.g., hypothyroidism), fatigue, diarrhea, colitis, pancreatitis, and pneumonitis.

Strategies for ONNs to support survivors include providing education on the differences between immunotherapy and other therapies and engaging survivors in the awareness of potential immune-related adverse effects. The long-term and late effects of immunotherapy are still being researched, but the overall impact on survivors is unknown (Patel et al., 2021). Survivors should be encouraged to inform all healthcare providers that they have received immunotherapy treatment. ONNs should reinforce with patients and caregivers the importance of contacting their oncology care team during and after treatment about new or worsening symptoms for tailored assessment and management.

Psychosocial Needs

Assessing and addressing an individual's mental, social, emotional, and spiritual health throughout survivorship is an important aspect of care. As difficult as it may be to predict which survivors will develop physical effects from cancer and treatment, it can be even more challenging to anticipate the psychosocial effects. A diagnosis of cancer is a life-changing experience, and each experience is unique. Psychosocial needs can be multidimensional and impact survivors' well-being and quality of life. Across the stages of survivorship, survivors might experience vast emotions, such as joy, loss, fear, and uncertainty. Employment issues, financial concerns, social isolation, and changes in social or family dynamics can also occur. Survivors might explore their spiritual beliefs and life meaning or purpose. Psychosocial distress can influence the physical health of survivors by manifesting as physical symptoms, such as pain, fatigue, and sleep disturbances (Ross et al., 2022; Sheikh-Wu et al., 2023).

Not all survivors can self-identify feelings or know to contact their oncology care team with psychosocial concerns. ONNs can acknowledge survivors' personalized experiences and provide education to support early recognition of potential mental or emotional symptoms that could impact their lives. Using open communication and active listening skills, ONNs can provide psychosocial support to patients and caregivers, share coping strategies, and identify potential barriers to care. ONNs can also refer survivors to local and community resources to assist with psychosocial care when needs are identified (Chan et al., 2023; Franklin et al., 2022). Common psychosocial effects related to cancer are fear of recurrence, anxiety, depression, distress, and sexual health.

Fear of Recurrence

For up to 80% of survivors, fear of recurrence or progression is a commonly expressed concern throughout survivorship. After a cancer diagnosis, there is a sense of the unknown. Feelings of fear and uncertainty can amplify at different time points across survivorship. Survivors may become hypervigilant about symptom checking, especially when each new physical symptom experienced is accompanied by fear of cancer recurrence. They also might share increased worry or anxiety around cancer anniversaries, at clinic visits, or with surveillance imaging (often referred to as *scanxiety*). Although fear of recurrence is a commonly reported concern, it is frequently found to be an unmet need. Fear can span from intermittent to debilitating and be associated with a higher risk for depression, anxiety, and poor quality of life for survivors (Peerenboom et al., 2022; Reb et al., 2023).

To assist survivors in recognizing these feelings, ONNs can provide education on common signs or symptoms of emotions, such as fear. Although fear is a common experience for survivors, each of their journeys is uniquely their own. ONNs can engage in open communication with survivors and encourage the sharing of experiences and feelings with supportive friends, family, and the oncology care team. Fear of recurrence can also affect about 50% of caregivers throughout survivorship, often triggered by medical or testing appointments and a lack of knowledge about potential signs and risks of recurrence (Smith et al., 2022). ONNs can involve caregivers in the plan of care and share information on monitoring for potential physical and psychosocial effects to help manage expectations (Smith et al., 2022).

Distress, Anxiety, and Depression

Emotional distress is one of the most common side effects of cancer and cancer treatment, with all survivors experiencing some distress and up to 60% experiencing significant levels depending on the stage and type of cancer (Miller et al., 2022). Survivors are found to be at greater risk for anxiety, depression, and other mental health concerns. Distress can present as a range of emotions, from feelings of worry during a commercial for a new cancer therapy to experiencing debilitating panic attacks or clinical depression. Distress can occur throughout survivorship and has been reported up to 10 years after diagnosis (Gulliver et al., 2023).

Survivors with unmanaged distress are less likely to engage in health promotion activities and are at risk for nonadherence to cancer care (Jacobs et al., 2020). ONNs can recognize risk factors, such as a history of substance misuse or mental illness, and collaborate with the interprofessional care team on individualized care needs. To further explore psychosocial needs, ONNs can regularly screen for distress across survivorship, providing early identification and management of concerns. Distress assessment tools and guidelines are available for ONNs, including NCCN guidelines (www.nccn.org/guidelines). Management strategies can include personalized resources and referrals to psychological interventions, such as coping strategies, support groups, social workers, psychiatrists, or individual counseling (Franklin et al., 2022; Smith et al., 2022).

Sexual Health: Intimacy, Sexuality, and Fertility

Both physical and psychological factors can impact the sexual health of cancer survivors. They might experience functional changes secondary to cancer therapies, fatigue, or pain. Medications used to treat cancer or manage side effects can cause physical changes, such as erectile dysfunction following radiation therapy to the pelvis or endocrine therapy–induced menopausal symptoms. Changes in body image may interfere with sexual desire, such as having an ostomy or implantable port, experiencing weight changes, having new scars or implants after surgery, or receiving radiation tattoos. Psychosocial distress can also contribute to sexual health concerns. As cancer treatment may affect fertility for certain survivors, options surrounding fertility preservation and sexual activity considerations should be discussed prior to initiating treatment and throughout survivorship (Lambertini et al., 2023).

Concerns related to intimacy, sexuality, and fertility can occur in phases throughout survivorship. Relationship dynamics often change after a cancer diagnosis. Some couples find that a partner who is a cancer survivor wants to return to a sense of normalcy, whereas the survivor feels differently, or the inverse can occur. Survivors who are single when diagnosed also face challenges, such as when to tell a potential partner. Survivors can find it difficult to discuss sexual health concerns with their providers. ONNs can assist survivors in discussing sexual health concerns by using the

PLISSIT (Permission, Limited Information, Specific Suggestions, Intensive Therapy) or BETTER (Bring, Explain, Tell, Timing, Educate, Record) models to assess survivors to determine areas of concern and offer specific management strategies (Kaplan, 2021). Additional resources include using validated assessments for assistance in the identification and management of sexual dysfunction, such as the Brief Sexual Symptom Checklist for Women or the Managing Male Sexual Issues Related to Cancer, as this is a vital component of survivorship care (Kaplan, 2021; Lambertini et al., 2023).

Financial and Time Toxicity

For many survivors, the physical and psychosocial effects of cancer diagnosis and treatment are concurrently impacted by the financial burden of care. *Financial toxicity* is a term used to describe the financial burden or sacrifice that survivors face throughout survivorship (Abrams et al., 2021). Some survivors use retirement savings or borrow money to pay high out-of-pocket costs, whereas others accumulate large amounts of medical debt or may need to declare bankruptcy. Financial toxicity can also affect adherence to treatment or follow-up care. Survivors and caregivers also take time away from work for appointments or treatments and are burdened with indirect costs, such as transportation fees (Han et al., 2020). According to Fardell et al. (2023), symptoms can influence the ability to work, with 17% of survivors who experienced pain, cognitive changes, and emotional effects reporting limitations, including reduced hours or decreased engagement. Survivors might need considerations for returning to work, financial planning, or disability support. ONNs can engage in early awareness of the potential for financial concerns, assess survivors for financial toxicity throughout survivorship, and refer to social work or financial counseling for assistance as barriers are identified. Financial toxicity is covered in more detail in Chapter 8.

As patients with cancer express concerns about the financial burden of care, the time spent receiving cancer treatments may affect their income. A relatively new term in cancer care, *time toxicity*, has been described as the time individuals with cancer spend undergoing cancer-related medical care (Gupta et al., 2022). Researchers are just beginning to study this concept (Gupta et al., 2022). ONNs can support survivors with coordinated care, minimizing time away from work or home by clustering imaging studies or other care needs.

The Role of the Oncology Nurse Navigator in Survivorship Care

Across many oncology care models, the role of the ONN begins at the time of diagnosis and continues through the start of survivorship. ONNs serve as a point of contact across the cancer care continuum for patients and caregivers, educating on diagnosis and treatment plans, breaking down barriers to care, coordinating care with the interprofessional team, and addressing physical and psychosocial care needs with resources and referrals (Franklin et al., 2022; ONS & ONCC, 2024). ONNs are central in providing and advocating for coordinated and comprehensive survivorship care for survivors. Survivorship includes an expansive scope of physical and psychosocial healthcare needs. The role of the ONN is to provide holistic care throughout the continuum of care.

ONNs can use disease- and treatment-specific evidence-based strategies to personalize recommendations throughout the stages of survivorship (see Figure 14-3). The following case study outlines strategies for ONNs to expand their role and assist survivors throughout the stages of survivorship (Chan et al., 2023; Lai-Kwon et al., 2023; Mullan, 1985).

Case Study: Colorectal Cancer

Kyle is a 56-year-old married father of two who was diagnosed with stage IIIB (T2N2aM0) colorectal cancer. He presents with rectal bleeding and persistent abdominal pain. A colonoscopy reveals a 5 cm mass in the descending colon, confirmed as adenocarcinoma upon biopsy. Computed tomography scans show no distant metastases. His family history is negative for cancer, and biomarker testing was negative. He is seen by the interprofessional team, who recommend surgical resection with an ostomy, followed by adjuvant chemotherapy with FOLFOX (folinic acid, 5-fluorouracil, and oxaliplatin).

During this acute stage of survivorship, the ONN, Cheryl, meets with Kyle and his family during his initial appointment and provides the following services and support:
- Details education on the diagnosis and recommended treatments, including potential side effects of FOLFOX
- Coordinates appointment with the ostomy nurse and oncology dietitian
- Refers to physical/occupational therapy for baseline assessment and further education to help minimize the fatigue and neuropathy that may occur as a result of treatment
- Assesses psychosocial concerns using the NCCN Distress Thermometer
- Discusses the role of and schedules an appointment with the oncology social worker to assist Kyle in completing Family and Medical Leave of Absence paperwork
- Provides information on cancer psychology and the therapist's role in helping patients and families cope with a new cancer diagnosis and upcoming treatments

Cheryl visits Kyle during inpatient hospitalization after surgical resection and, through open communication, identifies his desire to connect with others who have a similar diagnosis. She refers him to supportive resources, including the health system's Colorectal Cancer Support Group and the Colorectal Cancer Alliance Buddy Program.

Kyle completes chemotherapy and experiences neuropathy, a common side effect of oxaliplatin. Cheryl meets with Kyle to discuss the long-term and late effects of treatment, provide surveillance guidelines, assess for psychosocial issues, and delineate evidence-based management strategies to address his concerns (NCCN, 2025d). In this extended phase of survivorship, health promotion is also included as part of the education provided to Kyle by Cheryl, and the following additional recommendations are shared:
- Details education on recognizing potential long-term and late effects of cancer treatment and who to contact if there are any new or ongoing symptoms unresolved by current treatment

- Discusses the importance of ongoing surveillance and follow-up care, including regular examinations every three to six months for the first three years, every six months until the fifth year, and then annually thereafter. Imaging, blood tests, and colonoscopy are recommended according to NCCN guidelines (2025d).
- Talks about the importance of minimizing personal risk factors, such as ceasing tobacco use, limiting alcohol intake, and using sunscreen
- Addresses information on ongoing medical, dental, and vision care to identify and treat any age-related conditions
- Discusses healthy behaviors, including nutrition and exercise guidelines, and refers to physical/occupational therapy and oncology dietitian for management of ongoing neuropathy, fatigue management, and adequate nutrition because of Kyle's ostomy and healthy lifestyle goals
- Assesses and addresses physical and psychosocial concerns using the NCCN Distress Thermometer and coordinates appointments for Kyle to the following support services:
  - Health psychology to discuss his body image and intimacy concerns
  - A support group and caregiver support for his spouse and children
  - Oncology social worker to discuss how to manage returning to work and any potential adjustments that may need to be made

A survivorship care plan outlining a treatment summary and individualized recommendations for follow-up care is prepared by Cheryl and shared with Kyle and his oncologists, specialists, and primary care providers to aid in ongoing care coordination. The ONN reinforces her role as Kyle's contact person for any questions or concerns that he or his family may have throughout the many years after his initial diagnosis and treatment have ended.

Kyle continues surveillance visits with the interprofessional clinic. During the long-term stage of survivorship, Cheryl explains that although the risk for cancer recurrence may diminish over time, it is not uncommon for survivors to experience long-term or late effects of treatment, including fears of recurrence. The ONN also says that she will continue to be available to support and assist Kyle in transitioning his care to non-oncology providers. Kyle inquires about his children's risk of developing colon cancer and when they should begin screening examinations because of his diagnosis. Cheryl discusses current screening recommendations and the role of genetic counseling and testing.

Although not addressed in this case study, survivors living with advanced or metastatic cancer face the challenges of navigating disease uncertainty, adapting to evolving treatments, and managing both the physical and psychological aspects of care. Strategies can include acute- and extended-stage components along with goals of care discussions and advance care planning, including palliative care for complex symptom management and hospice for end-of-life care.

Coordination of holistic care with the interprofessional team is paramount to mitigate unmet needs across metastatic survivorship. This may involve providing ongoing education related to prognosis, treatment benefits and risks, costs of care, and evaluating physical and psychosocial needs. Health inequities for survivors and caregivers can also compound throughout metastatic survivorship, including greater challenges related to financial and time toxicity along with gaps in insurance and disability coverage (Lai-Kwon et al., 2023).

Chapter 14. Survivorship Navigation ◀ **203**

FIGURE 14-3. Strategies for Oncology Nurse Navigators Across the Stages of Survivorship

Acute Stage
- Educate on cancer diagnosis, treatments, and recognizing acute side effects.
- Educate on disease and personal risk factors, as well as genetic counseling.
- Assist in coordination of patient-centered care.
- Assess and address physical and psychosocial concerns.
- Consider barriers to care and personal factors, including health literacy, finances, goals of care, and social relationships.
- Consider nutrition and exercise recommendations based on diagnosis, treatment, and survivorship goals.
- Collaborate with interprofessional team to address needs, providing resources and referrals. Examples include:
  – Physical therapy for lymphedema management
  – Psychology for recurrent feelings of isolation and anxiety
  – Oncology social worker for caregiver support group

Extended Stage
- Assist in coordination of patient-centered care and identify team member roles and responsibilities in extended survivorship.
- Communicate importance of ongoing surveillance and follow-up care, including frequency and which providers to contact.
- Educate on recognizing potential long-term and late effects of cancer treatment.
- Educate on prevention and detection of new or recurrence of cancers.
- Educate on personal risk factors, screening recommendations, and prevention opportunities such as ceasing tobacco use, limiting alcohol intake, and using sunscreen.
- Discuss health behaviors, including exercise guidelines, and consider referrals to resources as needed.
- Collaborate with interprofessional team to address needs, providing resources and referrals. Examples include:
  – Oncology nutritionist for weight gain after treatment
  – Sexual health specialist for intimacy concerns following mastectomy
  – Referral to community organization for integrative therapy
- Encourage and educate self-advocacy skills for survivors and caregivers.

Long-Term Stage
- Reinforce education on recognizing potential long-term and late effects.
- Assess and address physical and psychosocial concerns, providing referrals as needed.
- Provide ongoing education of screening, follow-up care, and prevention.
- Provide continued education of healthy behaviors.
- Assist in coordination or transition of care to non-oncology providers as needed.

Prevention and Risk Reduction + Screening

Diagnosis → Treatment Curative or Palliative → Surveillance Recurrence or Progression → Palliative Care → End of Life

Metastatic Stage
- Incorporate strategies from acute stage and extended stage survivorship at diagnosis and throughout active treatment.
- Consider goals of care discussions and advance care planning.
- Prepare patients and caregivers for signs and symptoms of progression and end of life.
- Collaborate with interprofessional team to address acute and chronic care needs, providing resources and referrals. Examples include:
  – Physical therapy for cancer-related fatigue
  – Palliative care for complex symptom management
  – Financial counselor for disability

Cancer Care Continuum

Note. Based on information from Chan et al., 2023; Franklin et al., 2022; Koczwara et al., 2023; Lai-Kwon et al., 2023; Mullan, 1985; Oncology Nursing Society & Oncology Nursing Certification Corporation 2024; Sheikh-Wu et al., 2023; Vaz-Luis et al., 2022.

Resources to Assist in the Care of Survivors

Cancer care is complex; it can be challenging to assess, address, educate, and support the holistic health of each survivor throughout their survivorship trajectory. Coordination of patient-centered care is essential during this time and is one of the core competencies of ONNs (ONS & ONCC, 2024). Multiple models have been developed to meet the needs of this growing subspecialty, as no one-size-fits-all model of survivorship care exists (see Table 14-2). In each of these models, ongoing communication among all healthcare providers involved in the care of a survivor is paramount in ensuring the delivery of seamless, coordinated, and individualized survivorship care. ONNs can support this process, as they possess the clinical expertise, knowledge of available resources, and flexibility to meet the needs of this unique population.

As models of survivorship care are explored, the role of primary care providers and specialists in survivorship care is also expanding to manage cancer-related side effects,

TABLE 14-2. Models of Survivorship Care

Features	Embedded	Consultative	Multidisciplinary Clinic	Integrated Care
Individualized and personalized care and resources	x	x	x	x
On-site consultation at time of scheduled appointments to avoid travel to multiple locations at different times	x			
Point of contact for questions or concerns post-treatment	x			x
Impromptu referrals	x			
Comprehensive physical examination performed by a mid-level provider of the survivor's primary oncology team		x	x	x
Multiple providers are available and provide follow-up care at the same visit; usually based on diagnosis			x	

Note. From "The Embedded Nurse Navigator Model: A Novel Approach to Providing Survivorship Care in a Community Cancer Center," by D. Burbage and S. Siegel, 2015, *Oncology Issues*, 30(5), p. 38. Table reprinted with permission from the Association of Community Cancer Centers. All rights reserved.

such as endocrinologists for immunotherapy-induced endocrinopathies (Sheikh-Wu et al., 2023). Primary care providers are caring for survivors across all survivorship stages. For care to be successful, primary care providers, specialists, oncologists, and survivors must have the necessary information regarding the treatment course, long-term and late effects, and ongoing surveillance recommendations (Geramita et al., 2020; ONS & ONCC, 2024; Sheikh-Wu et al., 2023).

ONNs can use tools such as survivorship care plans (SCPs) to provide education and facilitate care coordination between the patient, family, and care teams. Often delivered to survivors and care teams in the extended stage of survivorship, SCPs are a comprehensive written resource outlining the treatment summary to date, an expected course for follow-up care, surveillance recommendations, potential long-term and late effects from treatment, common concerns, general screening recommendations, and local resources for cancer survivors. Several SCP templates are available to download at no cost, such as those from the American Society of Clinical Oncology (www.cancer.net/survivorship/follow-care-after-cancer-treatment/asco-cancer-treatment-and-survivorship-care-plans) and OncoLink (www.oncolink.org/support/survivorship).

Evidence-based resource tools are available for ONNs to educate and empower survivors in their care (see Table 14-1). Survivorship resources that can provide aid across the continuum of care include education, targeted assessment tools, clinical practice guidelines on survivorship, SCP templates, patient and caregiver checklists to support survivorship journeys, and advocacy information.

Program Development

Survivorship programs evaluate and address the essential components of survivorship care and aim to deliver quality, coordinated care to survivors. In 2020, the American College of Surgeons Commission on Cancer (ACoS CoC) adjusted its survivorship care standard for accredited programs from a focus on delivering SCPs to survivors treated with curative intent to a more inclusive survivorship care approach. The new *Standard 4.8: Survivorship Program* requires a survivorship program team to assess comprehensive survivorship services, evaluate survivor needs, and focus on enhancing services. SCPs are still recommended to aid in care (ACoS CoC, 2024; Blaes et al., 2020). Services might include screening programs, seminars for survivors, support groups, rehabilitation services, and mental health services. The 2024 ACoS CoC National Accreditation Program for Breast Centers Optimal Resources for Breast Care Standards changed compliance criteria from delivery of SCPs to an expanded survivorship scope. Programs must implement evidence-based guidelines to address the physical and psychosocial effects of breast care and maximize wellness across the continuum of care.

A variety of survivorship models are used across community, rural, and academic institutions to support survivors (see Table 14-2). In a systematic review, Monterosso et al. (2019) found benefits in quality of life for survivors who participated in nurse-led survivorship care, including tumor-specific models that provided patient assessment, management of concerns, and education, as well as encouraged self-management. Survivorship program development can be challenging because of the growing survivor population, the changing landscape of cancer treatments, technological advances, and limited healthcare resources (Blaes et al., 2020; Vaz-Luis et al., 2022). ONNs navigate across all stages of survivorship while collaborating with patients, caregivers, and interprofessional teams to ensure safe, timely, equitable, and effective patient-centered care. They can contribute their knowledge and participate in improvement initiatives when gaps in survivorship services are identified (Franklin et al., 2022). For example, during the first four months of the COVID-19 pandemic, ONNs at Main Line Health in Paoli, Pennsylvania, were receiving a higher volume of calls from caregivers sharing fears of disease progression, concerns about symptoms, and various stressors, including COVID-19 isolation. ONNs collaborated with the interprofessional team, and the decision was made to start a monthly virtual caregiver support group facilitated by ONNs and oncology social workers to support cancer-related treatment questions and psychosocial components of care.

ONNs can advocate for a patient-centered approach to program development and lead efforts within their organizations or communities to develop, implement, and enhance services and resources for survivors (Franklin et al., 2022). Several resources incorporating guidelines, toolkits, and educational opportunities are available to assist in selecting care models and discovering ways to develop and monitor quality, equitable survivorship programs for unique survivors, such as the American Society of Clinical Oncology Survivorship Compendium (www.asco.org/news-initiatives/current-initiatives/cancer-care-initiatives/prevention-survivorship/survivorship-compendium) and George Washington University's National Cancer Survivorship Resource Center (https://cancercontroltap.org/news/national-cancer-survivorship-resource-center).

Future Opportunities in Survivorship Navigation

As survivorship encompasses the individual, family, and community, standardizing quality care models to address unique concerns across the continuum of care can be challenging. Acute management of a cancer diagnosis is often combined with management of comorbidities and concurrent conditions, long-term and late physical and psychosocial effects, screening, and health promotion (Ross et al., 2022). Health disparities, personal risk factors, or other vulnerabilities can intensify across survivorship for adolescent, young adult, or older adult survivors. With increasing numbers of survivors who are living longer after a cancer diagnosis, research is needed to explore the impact and identify evidence-based strategies to assess and manage ongoing challenges, minimize disparities, and improve coordination of care (Avery et al., 2023; Chan et al., 2023; Miller et al., 2022; Soldato et al., 2023). ONNs can explore future opportunities in survivorship delivery to improve outcomes and engage survivors in self-management, including leveraging technology to tailor care with electronic patient-reported outcomes to assess symptoms or needs, providing telehealth to expand access, and offering virtual survivorship seminars (Mollica et al., 2024; Sheikh-Wu et al., 2023; Vaz-Luis et al., 2022).

Summary

As the number of cancer survivors continues to increase, the ONN role is critical in psychosocial, symptom management, and education regarding survivorship. As key interprofessional team members, ONNs can collaborate to support coordinated care and reduce barriers or disparities. Their holistic approach to providing patient-centered care empowers survivors to develop health-related quality-of-life goals, which are essential to improving overall health and well-being and may help reduce the risk of recurrence (Chan et al., 2023; Reb et al., 2023). ONNs are integral to individuals with cancer, embracing survivorship from the time of diagnosis throughout a survivor's lifetime and supporting their unique experience.

The authors would like to acknowledge Susan M. Schneider, PhD, RN, AOCNS®, FAAN, for her contribution to this chapter that remains unchanged from the previous edition of this book.

References

Abrams, H.R., Durbin, S., Huang, C.X., Johnson, S.F., Nayak, R.K., Zahner, G.J., & Peppercorn, J. (2021). Financial toxicity in cancer care: Origins, impact, and solutions. *Translational Behavioral Medicine, 11*(11), 2043–2054. https://doi.org/10.1093/tbm/ibab091

Aman, M.M., Mahmoud, A., Deer, T., Sayed, D., Hagedorn, J.M., Brogan, S.E., ... Narang, S. (2021). The American Society of Pain and Neuroscience (ASPN) Best Practices and Guidelines for the interventional management of cancer-associated pain. *Journal of Pain Research, 14*, 2139–2164. https://doi.org/10.2147/JPR.S315585

American College of Surgeons Commission on Cancer. (2020). *Optimal resources for cancer care: 2020 standards.* https://accreditation.facs.org/accreditationdocuments/CoC/Standards/Optimal_Resources_for_Cancer_Care_Feb_2023.pdf

American College of Surgeons Commission on Cancer. (2024). *Optimal resources for breast care: 2024 standards.* https://accreditation.facs.org/accreditationdocuments/NAPBC/Standards/Optimal_Resources_for_Breast_Care_2024.pdf

Avery, J., Thomas, R., Howell, D., & Dubouloz-Wilner, C.J. (2023). Empowering cancer survivors in managing their own health: A paradoxical dynamic process of taking and letting go of control. *Qualitative Health Research, 33*(5), 412–425. https://doi.org/10.1177/10497323231158629

Bisceglia, I., Canale, M.L., Silvestris, N., Gallucci, G., Camerini, A., Inno, A., ... Colivicchi, F. (2023). Cancer survivorship at heart: A multidisciplinary cardio-oncology roadmap for healthcare professionals. *Frontiers in Cardiovascular Medicine, 10.* https://doi.org/10.3389/fcvm.2023.1223660

Blaes, A.H., Adamson, P.C., Foxhall, L., & Bhatia, S. (2020). Survivorship care plans and the Commission on Cancer Standards: The increasing need for better strategies to improve the outcome for survivors of cancer. *Journal of Clinical Oncology Practice, 16*(8), 447–450. https://doi.org/10.1200/JOP.19.00801

Chan, R.J., Milch, V.E., Crawford-Williams, F., Agbejule, O.A., Joseph, R., Johal, J., ... Hart, N.H. (2023). Patient navigation across the cancer care continuum: An overview of systematic reviews and emerging literature. *CA: A Cancer Journal for Clinicians, 73*(6), 565–589. https://doi.org/10.3322/caac.21788

Fardell, J.E., Tan, S.Y.C., Kerin-Ayres, K., Dhillon, H.M., & Vardy, J.L. (2023). Symptom clusters in survivorship and their impact on ability to work among cancer survivors. *Cancer, 15*(21), 5119. https://doi.org/10.3390/cancers15215119

Franklin, E., Burke, S., Dean, M., Johnston, D., Nevidjon, B., & Booth, L.S. (2022). Oncology navigation standards of professional practice. *Clinical Journal of Oncology Nursing, 26*(3), E14–E25. https://doi.org/10.1188/22.CJON.E14-E25

Geramita, E.M., Parker, I.R., Brufsky, J.W., Diergaarde, B., & van Londen, G.J. (2020). Primary care providers' knowledge, attitudes, beliefs, and practices regarding their preparedness to provide cancer survivorship care. *Journal of Cancer Education, 35*(6), 1219–1226. https://doi.org/10.1007/s13187-019-01585-4

Gulliver, A., Morse, A.R., & Banfield, M. (2023). Cancer survivors' experiences of navigating the Australian health care system for physical and mental health care needs. *International Journal of Environmental Research and Public Health, 20*(5), 3988. https://doi.org/10.3390/ijerph20053988

Gupta, A., Eisenhauer, E., & Booth, C. (2022). The time toxicity of cancer treatment. *Journal of Clinical Oncology, 40*(15), 1611–1619. https://doi.org/10.1200/JCO.21.02810

Han, X., Zhao, J., Zheng, Z., de Moor, J.S., Virgo, K.S., & Yabroff, K.R. (2020). Medical financial hardship intensity and financial sacrifice associated with cancer in the United States. *Cancer Epidemiology, Biomarkers and Prevention, 29*(2), 308–317. https://doi.org/10.1158/1055-9965.EPI-19-0460

Jacobs, J.M., Walsh, E.A., Park, E.R., Berger, J., Peppercorn, J., Partridge, A., ... Greer, J.A. (2020). The patient's voice: Adherence, symptoms, and distress related to adjuvant endocrine therapy after breast cancer. *International Journal of Behavioral Medicine, 27*(6), 687–697. https://doi.org/10.1007/s12529-020-09908-2

Kaplan, M. (2021). Sexual dysfunction: Common side effect. *Clinical Journal of Oncology Nursing, 25*(6), 16–20. https://doi.org/10.1188/21.CJON.S2.16-20

Koczwara, B., Chan, A., Jefford, M., Lam, W.W.T., Taylor, C., Wakefield, C.E., ... Chan, R.J. (2023). Cancer survivorship in the Indo-Pacific: Priorities for progress. *Journal of Clinical Oncology Global Oncology, 9*, e2200305. https://doi.org/10.1200/GO.22.00305

Kozul, C., Stafford, L., Little, R., Bousman, C., Park, A., Shanahan, K., & Mann, G.B. (2020). Breast cancer survivor symptoms: A comparison of physicians' consultation records and nurse-led survivorship care plans. *Clinical Journal of Oncology Nursing, 24*(3), E34–E42. https://doi.org/10.1188/20.CJON.E34-E42

Lai-Kwon, J., Heynemann, S., Hart, N.H., Chan, R.J., Smith, T.J., Nekhlyudov, L., & Jefford, M. (2023). Evolving landscape of metastatic cancer survivorship: Reconsidering clinical care, policy, and research priorities for the modern era. *Journal of Clinical Oncology, 41*(18), 3304–3310. https://doi.org/10.1200/JCO.22.02212

Lambertini, M., Arecco, L., Woodard, T.L., Messelt, A., & Rojas, K.E. (2023). Advances in the management of menopausal symptoms, fertility preservation, and bone health for women with breast cancer on endocrine therapy. *American Society of Clinical Oncology Educational Book, 43*, e390442. https://doi.org/10.1200/EDBK_390442

Lee, L., Ross, A., Griffith, K., Jensen, R.E., & Wallen, G.R. (2020). Symptom clusters in breast cancer survivors: A latent class profile analysis. *Oncology Nursing Forum, 47*(1), 89–100. https://doi.org/10.1188/20.ONF.89-100

Loprinzi, C.L., Lacchetti, C., Bleeker, J., Cavaletti, G., Chauhan, C., Hertz, D.L., ... Hershman, D.L. (2020). Prevention and management of chemotherapy-induced peripheral neuropathy in survivors of adult cancers: ASCO Guideline Update. *Journal of Clinical Oncology, 38*(28), 3325–3348. https://doi.org/10.1200/JCO.20.01399

Miller, K.D., Nogueira, L., Devasia, T., Mariotto, A.B., Yabroff, K.R., Jemal, A., ... Siegel, R.L. (2022). Cancer treatment and survivorship statistics, 2022. *CA: A Cancer Journal for Clinicians, 72*(5), 409–436. https://doi.org/10.3322/caac.21731

Mollica, M.A., McWhirter, G., Tonorezos, E., Fenderson, J., Freyer, D.R., Jefford, M., ... Passero, V.A. (2024). Developing national cancer survivorship standards to inform quality of care in the United States using a consensus approach. *Journal of Cancer Survivorship: Research and Practice, 18*(4), 1190–1199. https://doi.org/10.1007/s11764-024-01602-6

Monterosso, L., Platt, V., Bulsara, M., & Berg, M. (2019). Systematic review and meta-analysis of patient reported outcomes for nurse-led models of survivorship care for adult cancer patients. *Cancer Treatment Reviews, 73*, 62–72. https://doi.org/10.1016/j.ctrv.2018.12.007

Mullan, F. (1985). Seasons of survival: Reflections of a physician with cancer. *New England Journal of Medicine, 313*(4), 270–273. https://doi.org/10.1056/NEJM198507253130421

National Coalition for Cancer Survivorship. (2014). *Defining cancer survivorship.* https://www.canceradvocacy.org/news/defining-cancer-survivorship

National Comprehensive Cancer Network. (2025a). *NCCN Clinical Practice Guidelines in Oncology (NCCN Guidelines®): Adult cancer pain* [v.1.2025]. https://www.nccn.org

National Comprehensive Cancer Network. (2025b). *NCCN Clinical Practice Guidelines in Oncology (NCCN Guidelines®): Cancer-related fatigue* [v.2.2025]. https://www.nccn.org

National Comprehensive Cancer Network. (2025c). *NCCN Clinical Practice Guidelines in Oncology (NCCN Guidelines®): Management of immune checkpoint inhibitor-related toxicities* [v.1.2025]. https://www.nccn.org

National Comprehensive Cancer Network. (2025d). *NCCN Clinical Practice Guidelines in Oncology (NCCN Guidelines®): Survivorship* [v.1.2025]. https://www.nccn.org

Oncology Nursing Society & Oncology Nursing Certification Corporation. (2024). *Oncology nurse navigator competencies.* https://www.ons.org/oncology-nurse-navigator-competencies

Patel, R.P., Parikh, R., Gunturu, K.S., Tariq, R.Z., Dani, S.S., Ganatra, S., & Nohria, A. (2021). Cardiotoxicity of immune checkpoint inhibitors. *Current Oncology Reports, 23*(7), 79. https://doi.org/10.1007/s11912-021-01070-6

Peerenboom, R., Ackroyd, S.A., Chang, C., Moore, E.D., Vogel, T.J., Lippitt, M.H., ... Kirschner, C.V. (2022). Surviving and thriving: What do survivors of gynecologic cancer want? *Gynecologic Oncology Reports, 41*, 101011. https://doi.org/10.1016/j.gore.2022.101011

Reb, A.M., Economou, D., Cope, D.G., Borneman, T., Tejada, M.S., Han, E.S., ... Ferrell, B.R. (2023). Care processes and quality-of-life outcomes affecting the gynecologic cancer survivorship experience. *Oncology Nursing Forum, 50*(2), 185–200. https://doi.org/10.1188/23.ONF.185-200

Rock, C.L., Thomson, C.A., Sullivan, K.R., Howe, C.L., Kushi, L.H., Caan, B.J., ... McCullough, M.L. (2022). American Cancer Society nutrition and physical activity guideline for cancer survivors. *CA: A Cancer Journal for Clinicians, 72*(3), 230–262. https://doi.org/10.3322/caac.21719

Ross, L.W., Townsend, J.S., & Rohan, E.A. (2022). Still lost in transition? Perspectives of ongoing cancer survivorship care needs from comprehensive cancer control programs, survivors, and health care providers. *International Journal of Environmental Research and Public Health, 19*(5), 3037. https://doi.org/10.3390/ijerph19053037

Schagen, S.B., Tsvetkov, A.S., Compter, A., & Wefel, J.S. (2022). Cognitive adverse effects of chemotherapy and immunotherapy: Are interventions within reach? *Neurology, 18*(3), 173–185. https://doi.org/10.1038/s41582-021-00617-2

Sheikh-Wu, S.F., Anglade, D., & Downs, C.A. (2023). A cancer survivorship model for holistic cancer care and research. *Canadian Oncology Nursing Journal, 33*(1), 4–16. https://doi.org/10.5737/236880763314

Sheikh-Wu, S.F., Downs, C.A., & Anglade, D. (2020). Interventions for managing a symptom cluster of pain, fatigue, and sleep disturbances during cancer survivorship: A systematic review. *Oncology Nursing Forum, 47*(4), E107–E119. https://doi.org/10.1188/20.ONF.E107-E119

Smith, A., Wu, V.S., Lambert, S., Lamarche, J., Lebel, S., Leske, S., & Girgis, A. (2022). A systematic mixed studies review of fear of cancer recurrence in families and caregivers of adults diagnosed with cancer. *Journal of Cancer Survivorship: Research and Practice, 16*(6), 1184–1219. https://doi.org/10.1007/s11764-021-01109-4

Soldato, D., Arecco, L., Agostinetto, E., Franzoi, M.A., Mariamidze, E., Begijanashvili, S., ... Lambertini, M. (2023). The future of breast cancer research in the survivorship field. *Oncology and Therapy, 11*(2), 199–229. https://doi.org/10.1007/s40487-023-00225-8

Tonorezos, E., Devasia, T., Mariotto, A.B., Mollica, M.A., Gallicchio, L., Green, P., ... de Moor, J.S. (2024). Prevalence of cancer survivors in the United States. *Journal of the National Cancer Institute, 116*(11), 1784–1790. https://doi.org/10.1093/jnci/djae135

Vaz-Luis, I., Masiero, M., Cavaletti, G., Cervantes, A., Chlebowski, R.T., Curigliano, G., ... Pravettoni, G. (2022). ESMO expert consensus statements on cancer survivorship: Promoting high-quality survivorship care and research in Europe. *Annals of Oncology, 33*(11), 1119–1133. https://doi.org/10.1016/j.annonc.2022.07.1941

Worrell, S.L., Kirschner, M.L., Shatz, R.S., Sengupta, S., & Erickson, M.G. (2021). Interdisciplinary approaches to survivorship with a focus on the low-grade and benign brain tumor populations. *Current Oncology Reports, 23*(2), 19. https://doi.org/10.1007/s11912-020-01004-8

Wu, C.J., Bai, L.Y., Chen, Y.C., Wu, C.F., Lin, K.C., & Wang, Y.J. (2023). Symptom clusters in lymphoma survivors before, during, and after chemotherapy: A prospective study. *Oncology Nursing Forum, 50*(3), 361–371. https://doi.org/10.1188/23.ONF.361-371

CHAPTER 15

Mental Health Issues

Helen Meldrum, EdD

> **KEY TOPICS**
> mental health symptoms, psychiatric conditions, responding to challenging and impaired patients, supporting colleagues who are languishing

Overview

More than one in five adults in the United States live with a mental illness (National Institute of Mental Health, 2024). These conditions include a multitude of challenges that vary in degree and range from mild to severe mental illness and impairment (SMII). The National Institute of Mental Health (2024, para. 4) described SMII as a "mental, behavioral, or emotional disorder resulting in serious functional impairment, which substantially interferes with or limits one or more major life activities" over a long duration. Examples include schizophrenia, major depression, and panic disorder.

Poor mental health is elevated among those with cancer and was further exacerbated by the COVID-19 pandemic as a public health crisis (Kim et al., 2023). Patients with SMII also suffer from increased stigma, which may cause them to avoid the medical system, often to their detriment. A large cohort study indicated that people with schizophrenia had a 64% higher all-cause mortality following a cancer diagnosis (Launders et al., 2022). In addition to patients coping with psychiatric conditions, more than 21% of those aged 12 years or older in the United States reported misuse of prescription drugs in 2023 (National Institute on Drug Abuse, 2023).

Many oncology nurse navigators (ONNs) report they often feel helpless, confused, fearful, and uncertain about what to do when they encounter patients with SMII. These patients often have chronic diseases and poor physical health. Efforts to teach healthcare students communication skills specifically addressing patients with SMII have been limited. Literature on this topic is also decades old, predating significant scientific advances in cognitive neuroscience and psychiatric therapeutics as well as changes in social policies.

This chapter will focus on how ONNs can effectively communicate with patients with cancer and SMII. It will also address chemical coping in patients at all phases of the cancer journey. Finally, it will provide an overview of the causes of psychological adversity for oncology professionals, including common sources of stress found in healthcare settings.

Addressing Mental Health and Cancer

Patients with SMII often have comorbid conditions, such as cardiovascular disease, and risky health behaviors, such as physical inactivity or substance misuse (National Institute of Mental Health, 2024). They may not access care because they do not recognize medical needs, lack health insurance, or fear coercive treatments. Their cancer may be undiagnosed until later stages, and they may have obstacles to receiving adequate treatment, such as their understanding of the disease and commitment to treatment, psychoactive drug interactions, and the ability of staff to deliver care (Decker et al., 2022).

Poorly controlled symptoms of SMII may alter cancer treatment outcomes, as patients can be classified as *difficult* by clinicians. Patients with SMII have reported feeling devalued and dismissed by many healthcare providers (Decker et al., 2022). For example, oncology professionals may be hesitant to recommend a clinical trial for patients with psychosis because they may have overt symptoms and be perceived as disagreeable and nonadherent. Similarly, ONNs may experience frustration with patients with SMII because of their lack of follow-through, self-neglect, or specific behavioral issues. Innovative approaches, including extra training for clinicians, are needed to decrease mental health stigma and facilitate cancer treatment initiation for patients with SMII (Leahy et al., 2023).

The distress associated with the diagnosis and treatment of cancer is complex and can amplify preexisting mental health and substance misuse issues. Studies have reported that high levels of cancer-related distress affect 35%–45% of patients (Bultz, 2016). An Australian study recorded even higher numbers, with 91% indicating clinically significant distress and 56% reporting severe distress (Kirk et al., 2021). Patients with cancer experienced worse psychosocial and financial challenges during the COVID-19 pandemic compared with other chronic disease populations (Baydoun et al., 2023).

Psychosocial distress screening is now a quality care standard. Several national groups require or recommend screening, including the American College of Surgeons Commission on Cancer, the National Comprehensive Cancer Network, the National Academy of Medicine, and the American Psychosocial Oncology Society (Brauer et al., 2022). Screening helps to identify patients whose distress results from or is exacerbated by a preexisting or co-occurring SMII. With an increased focus on survivorship, patient care objectives are expanding beyond medical treatments toward holistic psychosocial care.

ONNs have described feeling uncomfortable caring for patients with SMII and often state that they have not had enough training to build their confidence in this practice. Most ONNs receive little to no education about patients with SMII and feel ineffective in communicating with them (Grudniewicz et al., 2022). Acquiring specific skills for interacting with patients with SMII will improve the patient-centered care of this population. ONNs need to get beyond a quick "call a psych consult" reaction. All oncology professionals involved in direct patient care need guidance on how to consult effectively with patients with SMII because it is impossible to predict when or where they will encounter affected patients.

Research has shown that ONNs can have a positive effect on patient mental health. A study by Yu et al. (2024) found that patients with cancer receiving care from navigators exhibited significantly lower levels of anxiety, demoralization, and emotional distress. This capacity for outreach may be increased in the era of telecommunications. Remote care was prominent before the COVID-19 pandemic, but it was used even more during the pandemic because the need for social distancing was recognized. Singh et al. (2021) noted that patient satisfaction does not decrease with telehealth practices compared to in-person care.

Another development in supporting patients with cancer and SMII has been the innovation of artificial intelligence applications. ONNs may assess these tools for use as an adjunct to professional services. For example, Mika Health provides patients with mobile access to psychological support, reducing patient anxiety and depression in the process (Springer et al., 2024). Although there is a scarcity of new research on remote mental health interventions for patients with cancer, Koc et al. (2022) documented psychoeducational telehealth programs that reduced depressive symptoms and positively affected coping strategies. Telehealth programs can save time and money when used effectively and are a promising format for the management of psychological problems and cognitive functioning issues (Giustiniani et al., 2023).

Patients With Severe Mental Illness and Impairment

The first step when encountering a patient in distress, whether in-person or remote, is to incorporate concepts from psychological first aid (PFA). This method is increasingly recommended for responding to patients who are emotionally charged. Overlapping definitions of PFA exist, but all include a nonintrusive focus on compassionate listening, ensuring that basic needs are met, encouraging support from significant others, and protecting patients from further harm. PFA builds on the concept of human resilience. Numerous organizations, including the American Psychiatric Association (APA), recommend training in this type of assistance. PFA was developed to provide support following traumatic events, such as a cancer diagnosis. This training can equip ONNs with the knowledge they need to better manage stress in their own lives, as well as the lives of patients and coworkers (Hermosilla et al., 2023).

In addition to providing basic PFA, ONNs need to use a Mental Status Examination (MSE). The psychological equivalent of a physical examination, the MSE allows ONNs to gather information to communicate with the healthcare team. When patients exhibit bizarre or unruly behavior in clinical settings, clinicians are often too quick to call for reinforcements from transport emergency medical technicians or law enforcement. Alternatively, use of the MSE may allow navigators to determine the nature of the problem and give patients the opportunity to receive consultation or treatment in the cancer care setting. Although most people subconsciously judge mental status when meeting a new person, navigators need to use a specific list to identify and document symptoms. The MSE includes objective observations by the clinician and subjective descriptions given by the patient. It can help distinguish between mood and thought disorders and cognitive impairments as well as guide appropriate referrals (see Figure 15-1). MSE observations are helpful recordings of patients at that moment in time, which can then be conveyed to other providers on the healthcare team.

Patients With Anxiety and Panic Disorders

Anxiety disorders are the most common challenge to mental health, affecting almost a fifth of the U.S. population (Anxiety and Depression Association of America, 2022). Goerling et al. (2023) observed a high prevalence of anxiety in patients with cancer and at a three times higher rate compared to the general population. A third of patients with cancer who report symptoms of anxiety have no history of precancer anxiety (Grassi et al., 2023).

For some patients with cancer, the diagnosis itself may appear as a significant threat to their well-being, prompting persistent worrying. Anxiety may rise at the time of diagnosis, during treatment transitions, at the end of treatment, or during survivorship. Navigators have said that helping patients with ongoing fears and concerns is a significant part of their mission but that they feel ill-equipped to care for patients who have active anxiety attacks in their practice settings.

Panic disorder (PD) is diagnosed in about 11% of U.S. patients. These individuals experience sudden, unexpected anxiety attacks and are worried about chronic recurrence (Cleveland Clinic, 2023). PD can prompt agoraphobia, which causes people to avoid places or situations that they associate with experiencing panic and feeling trapped, helpless, or embarrassed (Anxiety and Depression Association of America, 2022). PD is often not well recognized by healthcare professionals, yet it is more prevalent in the oncology setting, with one study finding that almost 9% of patients with cancer were afflicted (Goerling et al., 2023).

Patients with PD are also prone to panic attacks, which elicit a rapid, often short-lived, onset of intense fear, usually making medications unhelpful as a resolution. However, if patients report frequent panic attacks, they should be referred for evaluation for management with medication.

Symptoms of Panic Attacks

The *Diagnostic and Statistical Manual of Mental Disorders, Fifth Edition, Text Revision* (*DSM-5-TR*) notes that a panic attack has a rapid onset and short duration.

FIGURE 15-1. Mental Status Examination

Appearance

How does the patient look?	Neat and clean, or dirty and unkempt, bizarre, or inappropriate? Are pupils round, regular and equal, alert, or sleepy looking?

Behavior

How does the patient act?	Strange, threatening, or violent? Unusual motor activity such as grimacing or tremors? Impaired gait, psychomotor retardation, agitation?

Speech

How does the patient talk?	Rate, tone, quantity, quality?

Thought Content

What is on the patient's mind?	Delusions, suicide, bodily preoccupations?
How are thoughts connected?	Randomly, logically?

Mood

How does the patient say he or she feels?	Sad, glad?
What emotions appear to be expressed?	Anger, fear, grief?

Perceptions

What does the patient see, hear, etc.?	Illusions, hallucinations?

Cognitive Capacity

What does the patient know?	Orientation, attention span, intellectual functioning, insight, and judgment?

Memory

Assess recent: "What time was your appointment with me for today?" Assess remote: "What is your Social Security number?"	Note if there is general or selective amnesia.

Insight and Judgment

How is the patient's conduct?	Is the patient cooperative, hostile, seductive, indifferent, or evasive? Assess impulse control. Does the patient seem to understand the cancer diagnosis or deny it?

Note. Based on information from Voss & Das, 2024.

It is not caused by medications, substance misuse, medical conditions, or mental health conditions. Panic attacks are characterized by four or more of the following symptoms (APA, 2022):
- Accelerated heart rate
- Sweating
- Shaking
- Shortness of breath
- Feeling of choking
- Chest pain
- Nausea or abdominal distress
- Feeling dizzy or faint
- Feelings of unreality or being detached from oneself
- Fear of losing control or going crazy
- Fear of dying
- Numbness or tingling sensations
- Chills or hot flushes

During the attack, evidence of reactive phobia may exist, such as a very harsh response triggered by a suggestion that seems noncontroversial (e.g., speaking to an additional doctor) (APA, 2022).

Patients usually feel an abrupt surge of intense fear or discomfort that reaches a peak within a few minutes. Sometimes, the panic attack is sparked by a particular fear or an overall general dread with no apparent trigger. Loss of sanity is often rooted in an underlying major fear, and a fear of panic attacks can actually cause panic attacks.

Communicating With Patients Who Have Panic Attacks

ONNs can develop a repertoire of effective skills to care for patients with PD. Compassionate listening and education are essential in the treatment of panic and anxiety. The main goal should be to help reduce the stigma of the patient's experience because most people are embarrassed by their symptoms. ONNs should think about their own behaviors when managing patients with panic attacks.
- Anxious behavior escalates when there is a lot of noise and visual stimuli. Shifting patients to a quieter, more secluded area might be helpful and reduce the worry that their symptoms are visible to others.
- Determining the attack's origin might be helpful long term but is not to be discussed while the episode is in progress.
- Never say, "Calm down; you are okay." Instead, take what patients are feeling seriously. Confirm reality and say, "It looks like you are very fearful right now."
- Explain everything you do. For example, say, "I am just going to pull this chair over to sit beside you now." For hyperventilators, ask patients to sit down nearby and guide them through slow breathing patterns.
- Avoid sudden movements and be careful with touch, if at all. If patients reach out, offer your hand to hold or a shoulder or arm to rest on. Reassure patients that you will not leave them alone.

- Do not ask open-ended questions that require a thoughtful answer, such as, "Why do you think the attack came on now?" Instead, help patients make simple decisions to regain a sense of control. For example, ask, "Would you like a glass of water?" If they can nod yes or no, it helps them to notice they still have some capacity.
- Determine if calling friends and family will hurt or help. Sometimes, the thought of a loved one witnessing the attack worsens the panic.
- As anxiety subsides, give reassurance by saying, "I can see you are starting to breathe slower now." Communicate that you do not see their anxiety as a weakness or character flaw.
- Model calm behavior, not only for patients but also the nearby staff, who may see their anxiety rising in response to patient behavior.
- If appropriate, at a separate time, discuss common lifestyle recommendations, including reducing possible triggers (e.g., caffeine, stimulants, nicotine, dietary items, stress), improving sleep quality, and increasing physical activity.

To prevent future panic attacks, many patients find success with cognitive behavioral therapy, which teaches them to think in ways that minimize anxiety.

Patients With Suicidal Depression

Among U.S. adults, depression was up by more than 60% from pre-pandemic levels, rising from less than 9% in 2017–2018 to more than 14% in April 2020 (Daly et al., 2021). Another study concluded that the prevalence of depressive symptoms in the United States was more than three-fold higher during the COVID-19 pandemic. People with fewer social and economic resources and greater exposure to stressors (e.g., job loss) reported a more significant burden of depression symptoms (Ettman et al., 2020). A 2023 Gallup poll found that the percentage of U.S. adults who reported a diagnosis of depression at some point in their lifetime had reached 29%, nearly 10% higher than in 2015 (Witter, 2023). As depression is the most substantial risk factor for suicidal behavior, immediate and intensified attention is warranted.

One of the most common disorders among patients with cancer is major depression (Andersen et al., 2023). Despite the widespread effect of depression on patients with cancer, it can be challenging to recognize because it can be hard to distinguish depressive symptoms from treatment- and disease-related effects, such as fatigue (Ha et al., 2019). The co-occurrence of pain, physical impairment, and a loss of autonomy can intensify the emotional burden (Grassi et al., 2023). Depression can also affect outcomes. A robust study of a large cohort of patients with cancer found that the survival of those with major depression was worse than that of those who did not have major depression (Walker et al., 2021).

The risk of suicide among patients with cancer is 11 times that of the general population (Grobman et al., 2023). Research has shown that the desire for death is common among patients with advanced, life-threatening illnesses (Rodríguez-Prat et al., 2024). Further, up to two-thirds of patients who died by suicide gave verbal clues of their intent (Schuler et al., 2021). Specific risk factors for suicide among patients with cancer are cancer prognosis, stage, and time since diagnosis (Heinrich et al., 2022). These findings stress the need for close observation and follow-up.

Despite this research, little has been done to ensure that oncology healthcare providers learn how to identify and potentially prevent suicidal acts in their patients (Granek & Nakash, 2022). Although challenging, these providers need to learn how to listen and respond more effectively when patients are in deep despair.

Symptoms of Depression

Depression can include a wide range of symptoms, and not every person experiences each. *DSM-5-TR* lists the following criteria, denoting depression when five or more symptoms are noted over a two-week span (APA, 2022):
- Depressed mood
- Markedly diminished interest in activities
- Significant weight loss or decrease or increase in appetite
- Insomnia or hypersomnia
- Psychomotor agitation or retardation
- Fatigue
- Feelings of worthlessness or excessive guilt
- Diminished ability to concentrate or indecisiveness
- Recurrent thoughts of death, suicide, or attempt or a specific plan for committing suicide

Communicating With Patients Who Are Suicidal

The World Health Organization has noted that a prior suicide attempt is considered the most critical risk factor for suicide. Pathirathna et al. (2022) reported that domestic conflicts and violence, financial downturns and job loss, anxiety, and preexisting mental health conditions were among the identified risk factors for suicidal attempts and deaths during the COVID-19 pandemic.

Preexisting depression may influence how patients cope with the cancer experience. Using prior coping experiences and skills to manage psychological distress may be beneficial. It is essential to initiate and maintain strong therapeutic relationships with patients who have suicidal depression (Fartacek et al., 2023).

Empathy can help validate the depths of psychological pain. A helpful tool is the BATHE mnemonic (see Figure 15-2). The following points should be considered when addressing these patients:
- Remember not to judge, advise, quiz, or placate. Stick with these types of phrases:
  – "This has got to be a terrifying situation for you."
  – "It is so terribly sad."
  – "Your anger seems understandable."
- Do not try to talk patients out of their feelings.
- Never suggest that patients "take a break" from ruminating.

FIGURE 15-2	BATHE Mnemonic
Background	"What is going on in your life in addition to your cancer treatments?"
Affect	"How do you feel about it?"
Trouble	"What troubles you the most?"
Handle	"What helps you handle the situation?"
Empathy	"I can certainly understand your [anger, sadness, fear]."

Note. Based on information from Thomas et al., 2019.

- Telling depressed patients to "think positively" or "count their blessings" can be felt as dismissive.
- Comparisons to other people fighting emotional battles are rarely helpful.
- Avoid saying anything such as, "I was really sad once, too." Keep the focus on the patients.
- Asking, "Have you tried such and such treatment?" is usually not helpful.
- Find out if patients have a social support system.
- If patients express a wish to die, acknowledge their wish but also support any articulated wish to live.
- Ease into asking about intent with empathy: "Has it gotten so bad or so painful that you have been thinking about ending your life?"
- Determine if patients have thought of a method. Consider whether they have a definite plan and access to lethal means.
- Distinguish between bereavement and suicidal thoughts. Depending on spiritual beliefs, it is common after the loss of a loved one to have thoughts of dying to reunite with the departed.
- Experts in suicide prevention urge counselors to lean in—all the way—and say things that may seem counter-intuitive based on active listening theory, such as the following (Lester, 2005):
  - "I can see that you are at your limit of human capacity for pain and endurance."
  - "I can hear that your suffering is extreme and that the situation feels absolutely unbearable."
  - "I know you feel weakened from the fight, and you do not see any good solutions."
- Be more concerned if patients have someone who has committed suicide in their life or if they have recently experienced a trigger, such as a relationship breakup, job loss, or family conflict.
- Keep listening for excessively negative references and statements indicating guilt and low self-esteem, such as the following:
  - "Things never work out for me."
  - "People should have cared before this."
  - "The people at my work will not even miss me."
- Watch for signs that patients are disheveled and overtired from sleep disturbance (asking for sleep aids), have agitated behavior, or are easily tearful.

- Do not leave patients alone. Have someone else call a referral source or family member and ask, "Would it be okay if I spent more time talking with you today?"
- Realize that some patients who are suicidal must be hospitalized until they are stabilized.

By giving voice to patient anguish, ONNs can initiate a truly empathic relationship. This school of thought says that patients will feel relieved that somebody "gets it" and understands exactly how horrible it feels. Feeling this connection can help patients consider accepting further support (Centers for Disease Control and Prevention, 2024). Recommendations for additional help should be made in a very matter-of-fact manner. If patients resist the suggestion, it should be accepted and deferred to a follow-up talk. It is important to show them that someone is willing to make an immediate phone call to get additional help. This is a complicated process as patients can sometimes feel as if an ONN is trying to "get rid of them" and will feel rejected and passed off by the referral process.

In the past, therapists and healthcare professionals were advised to use no-suicide contracts with patients, but the practice has been proven ineffective. Instead, a safety plan, created in collaboration with patients, provides actions to take to stay safe. This type of planning involves working through several steps (Rogers et al., 2022):
- Recognize warning signs (shifts in thoughts, moods, or behaviors).
- Ask directly, "What can you do if you become suicidal to help yourself not to act on your urges?"
- Collaboratively address potential obstacles and identify coping strategies.
- Help patients make a list of people who they think may help with providing distractions from the crisis.
- Discuss what social settings will help take their minds off their problems, at least for a while.
- Review safe places they can go to be around people (e.g., public library).
- Request that patients have a list handy of several family members or friends who can offer help.
- Prompt patients to think about who is supportive and who they can talk to when stressed.
- Ask patients to consider which professionals and agencies to contact for help (e.g., "Who are the mental health professionals that we should identify to be on your safety plan? Are there other healthcare providers?").
- Have a conversation about making the environment safe.
- Ask patients what means they have access to and could use to attempt suicide and be direct (e.g., "How can we develop a plan to limit access to pills and firearms?").
- Brodsky et al. (2018) provided additional techniques to use in these scenarios.

Patients With Psychosis

When patients are referred to as *psychotic*, it indicates that they have a loss of contact with reality. Several mental illnesses prompt psychotic symptoms, and *psychosis* is used as an overarching term indicating that an individual has sensory experiences of people, places, and things that do not actually exist. The lifetime prevalence of all psychotic disorders in the general population has been estimated at 3%. Schizophrenia, delusional disorder, some bipolar disorders, major depressive disorder with psychotic features, substance-induced psychosis, and other similar disorders fall into this grouping (Sullivan et al., 2020). *Psychosis* is broadly defined by the presence of delusions and hallucinations. Such a condition can also be organic, such as delirium. The risk of violence in patients with these disorders is higher than in the general population but is not actually common, and self-injury is much more likely.

A consensus does not exist regarding the prevalence of schizophrenia among patients with a cancer diagnosis. However, this population has an approximately 50% increased risk of death by cancer compared to age- and sex-matched individuals in the general population (Nordentoft et al., 2021). Studies have confirmed an increased mortality from breast, lung, and colon cancer in patients with schizophrenia. These patients also have lower chances of getting optimal treatment and an increased risk of not being diagnosed or treated before dying from cancer. Screening programs and earlier access to diagnostics and effective treatment can improve outcomes for this highly vulnerable group (Nordentoft et al., 2021).

Collectively, SMII is a factor leading to later cancer diagnosis. This has been described in studies of cancer-related mortality statistics; however, it has not been researched extensively in the literature. This may be the result of diagnostic overshadowing, which can occur when clinicians make assumptions about the medical symptoms patients report (i.e., when descriptions of physical symptoms are attributed to mental illness and not explored further). In addition, medical care received by patients with SMII is often substandard (Charlesworth et al., 2023). Clinicians also spend less time with these patients, as they are often late for appointments, forgetful, disruptive, noisy, poorly groomed, uninsured, and mistrustful. Patients with psychosis often show poor self-management skills and may harbor delusions (e.g., a belief that God will cure them instead of medical interventions). With basic needs (e.g., housing) often in question, disruptions in treatment are common (Tucker-Seeley et al., 2021). In summation, patients with SMII are often treated as "less than" compared to people around them. Maintaining meaning and purpose in life is key to preserving dignity. Unfortunately, the stigma of mental illness creates barriers to managing the cancer itself (Grassi & Riba, 2020).

It is important to remember that a diagnosis of psychosis does not mean patients are unable to have input on decisions about their care. Schizophrenia is a heterogeneous disorder, and any two individuals with the diagnosis may display vastly different symptoms. Disparities in care may become more pronounced when patients have a bizarre effect because the stigma of SMII can also impair interactions with healthcare providers. Agitated patients can be provocative and may challenge the authority, competence, or credentials of the clinician. Providers are less likely to refer these patients to specialized cancer treatment. However, many patients with schizophrenia and cancer can cope well with their disease. When available, family members may also provide important information, serve as advocates, or act as surrogate decision-makers. All professionals must work together to overcome significant problems in communicating with patients with psychosis (Leahy et al., 2023).

Symptoms of Schizophrenia

DSM-5-TR delineates five main criteria for schizophrenia, the most common type of psychotic disorder. Schizophrenia is a disorder in which patients experience gross deficits in reality testing, manifested with at least two or more of the following symptoms, which must be present for at least one month (unless treatment produces symptom remission) (APA, 2022):

1. Delusions: strange beliefs and ideas that are resistant to rational or logical dispute or contradiction from others
2. Hallucinations: typically auditory or, less frequently, visual
3. Disorganized speech: incoherence or irrational content
4. Disorganized or catatonic behavior: repetitive, senseless movements or adopting a pose that may be maintained for hours. Patients may be resistant to efforts to be moved into a different posture or may assume a new posture after they are placed.
5. Negative symptoms: flat affect, lack of motivation, or failure to maintain hygiene

At least one of the symptoms, collectively referred to as *positive symptoms*, must be found in categories 1, 2, or 3. Symptoms must persist for at least six months, during which at least one month of symptoms meets the criteria for positive symptoms and may include periods of residual symptoms. During residual periods, the signs of the disturbance may be manifested by negative symptoms or by two or more positive symptoms present in a less prominent form (e.g., unusual beliefs or perceptions). Schizoaffective disorder, substance misuse, and bipolar disorder with psychotic features must have been ruled out. Associated features may include the following (APA, 2022):

- Inappropriate affect: laughing at sad times
- Depersonalization: detachment or feeling of disconnection from the self
- Derealization: a feeling that surroundings are not real
- Lack of insight into the disorder
- Monotone voice and expressionless face
- Bizarre appearance, odd clothing
- Thought broadcasting: thinking others can hear their unspoken thoughts
- Thought insertion: thinking others have placed voices in their head
- Thought withdrawal: thinking someone has extracted their inner voice
- Appear preoccupied by inner voices and visions, leading to the inability to perceive and follow conversations
- Loudly disturb or "bully" people; may be grandiose or hypercritical
- If potentially violent, there is usually constant body motion (e.g., pacing, fidgeting).
- Paranoid or highly irritated; have more potential for violence

- Patients who are potentially violent often hear command hallucinations (Correll & Schooler, 2020; Onitsuka et al., 2022; Saunders et al., 2011).

Communicating With Patients With Psychosis

Answers to basic questions, such as "Who am I?", "Who are you?", and "Where am I?", are not always clearly defined for patients with psychosis, and they present behavior that is far from accepted norms. It is important for ONNs to keep an even demeanor and not to become reactive.

- Some helpful comments might include stating your name and why you are with them. Say things such as, "I am here to help you as much as I can," or "I am here to see how we can help you feel better." Mention that your practice setting is always a safe place to visit.
- Work on one issue at a time. For example, figure out who accompanies patients on their visits. Determine whom patients trust (e.g., emergency contact, group home staff).
- Reinforce desired behaviors, such as by saying, "Thanks, it really helps me to pay attention to you when you sit quietly instead of pacing."
- Be as agreeable as possible. If agitated patients complain about being disrespected by a doctor, say something vague, such as, "Everyone certainly deserves to be treated respectfully."
- Do not ask loaded questions, such as, "Why are you doing that?"
- Even if you are interested, do not talk with them about their fantasies.
- If patients are seated, do not stand. Seat yourself and avoid using continuous eye contact, touching, or crowding personal space.
- Realize that patients can feel quite vexing. To deflect their sense of vulnerability, many are exquisitely sensitive in detecting clinicians' emotional vulnerabilities and will focus on points of contention. Do not personalize this prodding.
- Warn paranoid patients about any changes in the size, shape, or color of medications or durable equipment. Say things such as, "Other patients were also worried when they noticed that the pill is now pink instead of white."
- Try to maintain a familiar nurse and care team to build trust and comfort over time. Think about combining future oncology appointments with social work or psychiatry visits to provide opportunities for patients to ask questions.
- Keep yourself between patients and the exit; however, do not block the door. Moveable furniture allows for flexible access to exits for both patients and staff.
- Work out an action plan with agreed-upon signals in advance to alert all staff regarding potentially violent behavior.

Trying to subdue an unarmed patient physically is not safe unless accompanied by at least five individuals with advanced training in this area. Modern clinical thinking endorses less coercive interventions. It is important to triage this intervention by determining if there is a history of hostility or if patients have had a criminal arrest in the past. Calls to law enforcement or emergency medical technicians should not supersede trying to help patients connect with medical care. All forms of coercive practices are inconsistent with human rights–based mental health care (Sashidharan et al., 2019).

It is important to consult colleagues to determine if better control of symptoms is needed before the start of cancer treatment. For example, ask if patients report taking medications (particularly antipsychotics) as prescribed. Alternatively, consider having patients visit the radiation therapy area prior to treatment to make it less frightening. It also might make sense for patients to have a brief hospitalization before the first round of chemotherapy or a prolonged rehabilitation stay after surgery.

Patients Using Chemical Coping

More than half of U.S. adults in active cancer treatment and almost 40% of survivors report experiencing pain (Glare et al., 2022). As cancer survivors are projected to grow as a group by 24.4% (to 22.5 million) by 2032, the number of people living with associated ongoing physical pain will increase (National Cancer Institute, 2024). At the same time, concern is rising about the misuse of medications intended to treat pain. In 2021, 46.3 million people aged 12 years or older (16.5% of the population) had a substance misuse disorder, including 29.5 million with an alcohol misuse disorder, 24 million with a drug misuse disorder, and 7.3 million with both (Substance Abuse and Mental Health Services Administration, 2021).

A study of almost 170,000 adult cancer survivors showed a nearly two-fold higher likelihood of prescription opioid use compared with respondents without cancer. Although this does not necessarily translate to a higher risk of misuse, experienced clinicians warn that patients may develop an opioid usage disorder during or after their treatment. Therefore, screening and discussions about potential substance misuse should be routine (Ganguly et al., 2022). Assessing drug-seeking behaviors in patients with cancer can be challenging because many red flags may have valid explanations (Pergolizzi et al., 2021). Nevertheless, cancer likely puts patients at higher risk for substance misuse disorders than the general population because of the increased chance of psychological distress (Paice, 2018). Among patients treated with opioids for cancer pain, approximately 20% developed behaviors consistent with non-medical opioid use (Arthur & Bruera, 2022).

Opioids affect the brain, leading to feelings of pleasure and reducing anxiety. Addictive use taxes the brain and body and reduces the capacity to heal, adding another barrier to successful cancer care. Some substances have adverse interactions or worsen treatment side effects. Indirect effects can include dehydration and nutritional deficits. Persistent opioid use is a common complication in patients after curative intent surgery. This problem requires changes to prescribing guidelines as well as ONNs who can assist with effective patient counseling during the surveillance and survivorship phases (Lee et al., 2017). Screening and additional counseling are necessary to identify individuals who are likely to cope chemically to reduce their suffering or despair. Navigators and their teams need to be proactive in addressing emotional needs, providing targeted education, and monitoring patients and survivors.

Chemical coping occurs when patients use medications, mainly opioids, in a nonprescribed way to cope with the stressful events associated with cancer. There is a proven association between chemical coping and opioid dose escalation, pain complaints, and the inability to discontinue opioids after the resolution of pain (Dalal & Bruera, 2019). Research consistently indicates that seeking out mind-altering products and using multiple sources to obtain them are linked with greater odds of concurrent substance misuse, such as binge alcohol misuse, marijuana misuse, prescription opioid use disorder, or any other substance misuse (Schepis et al., 2020).

A portion of studies support the self-medication hypothesis, and others support the shared vulnerability hypothesis (Garey et al., 2020). Patients who have the assistance of an ONN who understands the complexities of both cancer care and addictive behaviors may feel more comfortable confiding about their realities of substance misuse. ONNs have the opportunity to improve outcomes by incorporating harm-reduction strategies and educational interventions (McNally & Sica, 2021).

Symptoms

DSM-5-TR states that for people to be diagnosed with a disorder related to a substance, they must display 2 of the following 11 symptoms (APA, 2022):
- Consuming more of the substance than initially planned
- Worrying about stopping or consistently failing efforts to control use of the substance
- Spending a significant amount of time using the substance or doing whatever is needed to obtain it
- Using the substance results in the failure to fulfill major role obligations, such as at home, work, or school
- Craving the substance
- Continuing use of the substance despite medical or mental health problems caused or worsened by it
- Continuing use of the substance despite it having negative effects on relationships with others
- Repeatedly using the substance in a dangerous situation (e.g., driving a car)
- Giving up or reducing activities because of substance use
- Building up a tolerance to the substance
- Experiencing withdrawal symptoms after stopping substance use

Behaviors that should raise a red flag for ONNs include dose-escalating, which leads to phone calls for refills; requesting pills for insomnia; finding discrepancies in supply counts; and doctor shopping or hopping.

Navigators need to communicate with other departments about writing prescriptions for opioids (e.g., pharmacy, psychiatry, emergency department) so that patients' medication misuse does not go undetected (Bruera & Del Fabbro, 2018; Merlin et al., 2020). Some patients demand a particular type and dose of opioids. Patients with chemical coping may act up dramatically, including threats and expressions of excessive pain, have concurrent abuse of additional illicit drugs, alter the route of drug delivery, sell prescription drugs, forge prescriptions, report prescription losses, or take another person's drugs (Merlin et al., 2020). The term *drug-seeking* is used by nurses from a variety of practice environments. The use of the term has shifted from objective counts of patient requests for pain medication to a confusing mixture of observable patient behaviors and subjective interpretations of patient motivation (Copeland, 2019).

Trying to help someone with an addiction can be a long, challenging process. Addiction breaks down self-esteem and can leave patients feeling hopeless. Showing unconditional support provides the opportunity for people with a substance misuse disorder to speak honestly. These individuals fear disclosing the truth about their addiction and the idea of living a life without drugs.

The widely used CAGE questions, initially developed for alcohol screening, have been adapted for use in evaluating substance misuse (see Figure 15-3). Researchers have shown that the CAGE-AID questionnaire has had positive results on patients with cancer who need to be screened for substance misuse (Edwards et al., 2023). Item responses on the CAGE-AID are scored 0 for "no" and 1 for "yes" answers. A higher score indicates alcohol or drug problems. A total score of 2 or greater is considered clinically significant.

The standard approach for detox is to replace the problematic opioids with safely prescribed medications, such as methadone. Patients are sustained on these medications for extended periods to stabilize (Holbein et al., 2023). The use of 12-step programs as an adjunct to detox treatment has been demonstrated (Galanter, 2018). Narcotics Anonymous (www.na.org) is a global, community-based organization with a multilingual and multicultural membership. This group support model offers recovery from the effects of addiction through help from peers. Membership is free, making it helpful for patient accessibility.

Communicating With Patients Using Chemical Coping

In the past, confrontational strategies had been designed to make patients using chemical coping to feel scared or humiliated, with the underlying belief that this

FIGURE 15-3 CAGE-AID Questionnaire

C	Have you ever felt you ought to **cut down** on your drinking or drug use?
A	Have people **annoyed** you by criticizing your drinking or drug use?
G	Have you felt bad or **guilty** about your drinking or drug use?
E	Have you **ever** had a drink or used drugs first thing in the morning to steady your nerves or to get rid of a hangover (i.e., an "eye opener")?

Note. Based on information from Aertgeerts et al., 2004.

was helpful. Decades of research have failed to yield evidence that these methods are effective. Furthermore, several studies have shown harmful effects, particularly for more vulnerable populations. A newer school of thought has been developed called motivational interviewing (MI), which has proven effective for patients capable of engaging with clinicians who operate from a strengths-based perspective, tapping into internal wisdom and resources.

MI is based on the idea that people tend to rebel and resist when they feel that they are being forced to choose a specific course of action. Navigators should not attempt to challenge patients who are chemically coping, as arguing can lead them into an ineffective cycle of fighting back. MI encourages collaboration instead of persuasion. Navigators encourage patients to take the lead in brainstorming ideas about how to achieve change. This approach also provides an opportunity for engaging patients who are not ready for complete abstinence from substances and allows for steps toward harm reduction as an option (Rollnick & Miller, 1995). Research has also suggested that MI is a feasible therapeutic tool to help patients with substance misuse disorders with the integrated support of concerned significant others working to achieve mutually agreed-upon goals with the medical team (Tse et al., 2022).

The basic principles of MI, represented by the acronym OARS, are **O**pen-ended questions, **A**ffirmations, **R**eflection, and **S**ummarizing. Phrases might include the following (Adams & Hamera, 2022):

- Reflect: "This is really hard because, on the one hand, it sounds like this, and, yet, on the other hand... ."
- Ask permission: "I have noticed that you have received higher doses and more frequent refills of your pain medications over the past few months. How do you feel about talking about your pain pill use?"
- Explore the reasons for the change: "People usually use extra pain pills because it benefits them in some way. What do you like about having the option to take extra? What are some downsides? What are some aspects of using more pills that you are not happy about?"
- Ask about a time before the opioid addiction: "How were things different then? What may happen if things continue as they are?"
- Explore extremes: "What are the worst things that may happen if you keep using _____? What are the best things that might happen if you stop using _____?"
- Bring out discrepancies: "It sounds like when you started using extra pain meds there were many positives, but now using them is causing tension in your family."
- Explore confidence: "How confident are you that you could cut back on your dose if you decided to? What could you do to reduce some of these problems while you are deciding what to do long term?"

ONNs must not be afraid to set limits and understand that losing a patient to another oncology health center is okay. If the patient is in grave danger or does not respond to concerns, it may be helpful to talk to the medical team and family about staging an intervention led by a specialist.

When Patients Are Peers

This chapter primarily looks at patients with mental health issues, but what if the person who misuses substances is a coworker or peer? Some nurses may have experienced the COVID-19 pandemic as an extended period of intense, traumatic, emotional pain complicated by direct or indirect traumatic events. Many nurses may be suffering from residual symptoms of either trauma or anxiety, which, as data indicate, could function as part of an ongoing cycle of substance misuse and cognitive failure. This negatively affects not only nurses' health but also their ability to provide quality care for their patients (Arble et al., 2023). Organizational leaders may need to think about the environments that might leave healthcare workers susceptible to poor coping choices to offset stress. Identification of impaired nurses and ONNs requires policies that support rapid intervention, including removing or limiting the practice of those affected. Debriefing of peers and colleagues and open discussions with supportive leadership are also essential (Foli et al., 2020).

Whether a peer or a patient, it is important for the ONN to listen to the person who is struggling much more than it is to talk to them. An ONN should ask if the person would be willing to seek professional help. They may become defensive. If this happens, it is best for the ONN to let it go for some time. They should not shame their peer, and they should let the person know they have their best interests at heart; whether the person gets help immediately or later, the ONN should let them know they are not being psychologically punished for their addictive behavior. Change may not come quickly, so a rapport is key. The ONN should remember the old saying: "It is better to keep your foot in the door than get a door slammed in your face."

The Navigator's Wellness in the Post-Pandemic Years

Humankind faced an unprecedented crisis in the COVID-19 era. The decisions made will shape the medical world for decades to come. The pandemic affected all sectors of society, but the crisis hit already overburdened healthcare systems the hardest. Evidence indicates that the pandemic created significant disruptions in service delivery. In its wake, plenty of mental health challenges are ahead, including for ONNs (Cancino et al., 2020).

In a particularly dramatic example of how an entire oncology staff had to be redeployed, a busy inpatient cancer service in Boston that typically treated more than 5,000 patients a year transformed itself into units caring for patients with COVID-19.

"When the moment came, our oncology ward transitioned to a COVID-19 unit in three frenzied hours. The pace was staggering. We became responding clinicians across the general units and [intensive care units]. At the peak, we staffed three COVID-19 units, day and night" (Reynolds et al., 2020, p. 998).

In total, 94 highly specialized oncology staff served over 750 surge shifts and over 130 shifts in the COVID-19 intensive care unit. These 12-hour shifts were stacked on top of keeping up with outpatient cancer care virtual appointments. One of the staff captured the emotional tone.

"COVID-19 is marked by relentless loneliness and fear. These emotions are experienced by individuals, families, and communities. In the face of this, we mobilized our best skills as oncologists to provide individualized and compassionate care while supporting each other as colleagues and friends" (Reynolds et al., 2020, p. 999).

As the pandemic ebbs, a new era of health care begins. In the coming years, the emotional well-being of ONNs should be a topic of interest for researchers and administrators. In addition to a focus on substance misuse and burnout, attending to symptoms of anxiety and trauma may be needed. Healthcare systems should dedicate resources to supporting the psychological and emotional welfare of healthcare professionals. In part, this may mean dedicating education and development activities to promote a culture of self-care and support for implementing strategies to assist ONNs while also deterring substance misuse and negative behaviors (Arble et al., 2023). Many words are used to describe the emotional downside of oncology work, such as *languishing, compassion fatigue, burnout, moral distress, moral injury*, and *loneliness*.

Many ONNs who are not experiencing any diagnosable depression in these post-pandemic years may be languishing. Languishing is a mental state between depression and thriving, characterized by a lack of motivation (Melnyk, 2022). Positive psychologists have defined it as a state that is not a mental disorder, and it does not appear in any diagnostic manuals (e.g., *DSM*). Languishing is a concept used to describe people at the population level as typified by an absence of good mental health. It is associated with a group of affective sensations, including feelings of emptiness, stagnation, and hollowness (Willen, 2022).

Compassion fatigue is often mentioned in the oncology research literature. Signs of compassion fatigue include recurring thoughts of a sad patient scenario, apathy toward work, increased substance misuse, and hypervigilance. Burnout, in contrast, tends to be expressed by sheer exhaustion and typically develops over time as work stress accumulates. Compassion fatigue is more emotional. Compassion is a finite resource that can be depleted. Repeated exposure to trauma can lead to compassion fatigue (Cavanagh et al., 2020; Hegel et al., 2021).

Moral distress is the emotional reaction that comes from an inability to do the right thing. It can be a powerful driver for action (e.g., speaking up when continuing life support is futile). Moral distress is often prompted by close contact with patients in extreme suffering. Moral injury, in contrast, has an existential component leading to a change in worldview. It can develop from perpetrating, failing to prevent, or bearing witness to acts that violate deeply held beliefs. Moral distress and moral injury can lead to impaired resilience and worsening mental health and can prompt the intention to leave the medical profession (Stephenson & Warner-Stidham, 2024; Vig, 2022).

Loneliness in healthcare professionals is a genuine concern, with over one-third of workers reporting that it negatively impacted their well-being during the first wave of the COVID-19 pandemic. Boosting health professionals' mental wellness is beneficial for them, their healthcare systems, and their patients (Stubbs & Achat, 2022).

Loneliness, social isolation, and social support are interrelated but distinct concepts. Although the term *loneliness* often refers to the subjective feeling of being alone, *social isolation* refers to the absence of interpersonal interactions (Clifton et al., 2022). Grief can be isolating and has a significant association with loneliness. Because of exposure to patient suffering and death during the pandemic, healthcare providers are at increased risk of complicated grief, which can result in significant health problems (Hong et al., 2023; Rahmani et al., 2023).

Oncology nurses also suffer from more work-related stressors than other clinicians. An analysis of research studies looked at "feeling lonely" and "being alone," as reported by cancer care nurses. The experience of being alone may relate to the absence of administrative support and organizational issues, whereas the feeling of loneliness derives from an individual's beliefs. Loneliness in the workplace could have a negative effect on both patient care and the nurses' mental health. Research suggests that oncology nurses cope with work-related emotions in isolation, which can lead to loneliness (Phillips & Volker, 2020). Loneliness affects psychological and physical health, and in the context of the workplace, emotional loneliness also contributes to burnout (Melnyk, 2022).

A meta-analysis of oncology nurses' lived experiences found that loneliness was the predominant theme in problematic work issues. Nurses have described an absence of conversation and support between themselves and administrators as leading to high job turnover. Having dedicated time for organized discussion was seen as a sign of support by their supervisors, allowed them to cope with their workplace solitude, and significantly helped them to bear the burden of painful moments by sharing them (Diaw et al., 2020).

Nurses' experiences with loneliness are heterogeneous, highlighting the importance of developing interventions that use various direct and indirect strategies. Thus, a one-size-fits-all approach is insufficient to treat loneliness in oncology practice. A better understanding is needed of how different dimensions of loneliness can be managed on the individual and group levels (Akhter-Khan & Au, 2020). A key component of loneliness interventions is incorporating strategies for addressing underlying negative self-perceptions that stem from and contribute to loneliness. Preliminary evidence indicates that digital platforms may be an effective tool for loneliness interventions and provide the added benefit of offering a productive distraction when feeling lonely (Boucher et al., 2021).

A large survey of healthcare workers during the early phases of the COVID-19 pandemic found that all employees were under high stress, including administrative and non-clinical employees as well as clinical support staff. The stressors included heavy workloads, long hours, lack of organizational support, and the perceived inequity of pay cuts. Greater individual resilience was associated with decreased distress (Meese et al., 2021). Medical professionals are often expected to "absorb" the emotions intrinsic to healthcare work (i.e., emotional labor). In response, clinicians often suppress their responses to stressful scenarios so that patients will feel safe. This means that their psychological needs are not prioritized.

A stigma exists with healthcare professionals admitting to having mental challenges. Researchers have found that nurses are hesitant to discuss problems with

managers because of worries about being misjudged (Bamforth et al., 2023). Fortunately, the following interventions are being brought into the oncology workplace to help on both the individual and organizational levels (Cohen et al., 2023; Davis & Batcheller, 2020; Emami Zeydi et al., 2022):
- Meditation
- Yoga
- Gratitude journaling
- Narrative writing
- Self-help exercises in print and electronic modes
- Massage or acupuncture at work
- Combination of in-person education sessions followed by practice at home
- Resilience training via online delivery methods, either by a smartphone or web-based application
- Altering daily practices and protocols to enhance well-being
- Job crafting strategies based on weekly goals to promote teamwork
- Training and setting personal goals
- Educational workshops
- Relaxation training or promoting a positive mindset
- Communication training

Research with oncology nurses has shown the value of better communication practices. Specific strategies have been used, such as support groups and additional training. Success requires facilitators willing to prepare their learners to endure these emotional experiences without losing their valuable professional skills (Diaw et al., 2020). Organizational interventions are critical mechanisms for addressing ONNs' well-being and fostering resilience. Virtual digital health or social media interventions support and bolster existing, ongoing well-being programming. Tailored interventions should address underlying contributors of burnout and moral distress.

Peer support is an effective and meaningful resource designed to promote institutional resilience. It enhances oncology professionals' mastery of clinical interactions. The value of peer support lies within camaraderie, acceptance, and mutual understanding. A deeper connection to self, patients, and colleagues develops from shared experiences explored through various perspectives, centering on issues such as suffering or grief. Organizations can foster peer relationships through community building, prioritizing workplace factors (i.e., enhancing workflow), scheduling virtual peer meetings, and providing telephone support. Peer support is beneficial for addressing moral distress for significant systemic issues without immediate solutions (e.g., COVID-19 pandemic ramifications). Novel oncology peer support programs (e.g., virtual coffee rounds, nurse meditation groups) are being specifically designed and implemented (Hlubocky et al., 2021).

Systemwide changes that reduce the burdens on healthcare workers are needed. ONNs must be provided with the resources they need to cope. This could involve establishing anonymous feedback forms of communication to speak freely about stressors. Legislative changes that protect the mental health of medical workers also are needed. For example, licensure procedures should focus on a professional's ability to function well instead of their mental health history. Employee counseling should provide support without any sense of stigma, shame, or fear of losing a position (Granek & Nakash, 2022).

Languishing, compassion fatigue, burnout, moral distress, moral injury, and loneliness are significant predictors of quality of life. Increased burnout is also associated with higher anxiety and depression. To address loneliness, healthcare workers are best served by having the opportunity to debrief with each other (Diaw et al., 2020). Importantly, debriefing needs to be conducted in a psychologically safe manner, allowing for authentic communication about work-related emotions. By sharing with colleagues, ONNs can hear each other's experiences and learn that they are not alone with their work-related emotions (Phillips et al., 2021).

Interventions for reducing loneliness are essential. The Schwartz Rounds provide a structured forum where all staff, clinical and non-clinical, come together regularly to discuss the emotional and social aspects of their vocations. Research has shown that Schwartz Rounds work well to reduce feelings of isolation, connect individuals to others, build teams, and strengthen empathy and self-compassion (Jakimowicz & Maben, 2020). ONNs can learn more about how Schwartz Rounds can counterbalance the negative aspects of workplace stress with thoughtful interventions and community efforts by visiting the Schwartz Center for Compassionate Healthcare at www.theschwartzcenter.org/programs/schwartz-rounds.

Summary

ONNs are well placed to coordinate integrated care for people with mental health and substance misuse disorders. They are on the front lines, and the very traits that make them successful—empathy and openness—are also what make navigators vulnerable to their own psychological challenges. Patients and experienced healthcare professionals need help at times, not just with illness but with challenges such as depression, loss, and grief. Stigma still exists inside the medical community regarding patients and peers who are mentally ill; therefore, interventions regarding this matter are crucial to bringing insight about the negative impacts of this bias. Shifting curricula in nursing and allied health schools could reduce the consequences of this type of bias (Oliveira et al., 2020). However, silver linings have emerged from the COVID-19 pandemic. For instance, some oncology professionals have noted that the cancer experience itself may have helped patients to adapt to the stress of COVID-19. Oncology care providers have had to develop innovative strategies to build their resiliency as well (McAndrew et al., 2022).

Much has been written on the pharmacologic approaches to patients with SMII, but relatively little guidance has been given about interpersonal communication methods. Most patients with cancer and SMII do not receive adequate treatment and support. The label of mental illness or impairment can stop patients and their families from seeking help. This often means symptoms will worsen, and the decline can lead to tragic outcomes. Improving cancer care for patients with comorbid SMII requires a holistic understanding of the diagnosis and full collaboration with an interprofessional care team. ONNs need to keep their emotional reactions under control to provide the best care for their patients. By learning more about symptoms, assessments, and response skills, ONNs will know when and how to communicate with mental health teams. This input will also provide ONNs with a better understanding of the need to maintain a safe environment for patients who are vulnerable. In other words, ONNs must learn the specialized language of mental illness and impairment.

The cancer itself, and in many cases, the medications, can further impair patient thinking. Better communication may help patients to seek help earlier and stay in the care system. Navigators should take an active role in the referral process to specialized mental health care and can thereby reassure themselves that they did everything possible to help patients. If ONNs can contribute to positive change in how patients with SMII are treated, then the higher mortality rates from cancer in this population will finally be reduced. It is never easy communicating with patients with SMII, but the process can feel more manageable by following the guidelines and suggestions outlined in this chapter. Also, if a teammate is struggling with mental health, the information in this chapter should help with ideas on how to be supportive. Additional resources are provided in Table 15-1.

TABLE 15-1. Resources for Further Learning

Resource	Website
American Association for the Treatment of Opioid Dependence	www.aatod.org
American Foundation for Suicide Prevention	www.afsp.org
American Hospital Association: Well-Being and Resilience	www.aha.org/topics/well-being-resilience
American Psychiatric Association	www.healthyminds.org
American Psychological Association	www.apa.org/topics
American Psychosocial Oncology Society	www.apos-society.org
Anxiety and Depression Association of America	www.adaa.org
Association for Behavioral and Cognitive Therapies	www.abct.org
Engage	www.engageinitiative.org
National Alliance on Mental Illness	www.nami.org
National Institute of Mental Health	www.nimh.nih.gov
Office of the Surgeon General: Health Worker Burnout	www.hhs.gov/surgeongeneral/priorities/health-worker-burnout/index.html
The Empathy Center	www.theempathycenter.org

ONNs are not expected to transform themselves into experienced psychologists overnight. However, every navigator can be a caring and thoughtful ally to distressed patients with SMII.

Decades ago, I worked briefly with Ellen L. Bassuk, MD, the thoughtful psychiatrist who authored the book Behavioral Emergencies: A Field Guide for EMTs and Paramedics. *The book has had a significant influence on my thinking about communicating with patients with SMII. Everyone in health care should share the knowledge base of a good "first responder." The book is out of print now but still a highly recommended resource if a copy can be obtained.*

References

Adams, S., & Hamera, E. (2022). Motivational interviewing. In K. Wheeler (Ed.), *Psychotherapy for the advanced practice psychiatric nurse: A how-to guide for evidence-based practice* (3rd ed., 401–418). Springer.

Aertgeerts, B., Buntinx, F., & Kester, A. (2004). The value of the CAGE in screening for alcohol abuse and alcohol dependence in general clinical populations: a diagnostic meta-analysis. *Journal of Clinical Epidemiology, 57*(1), 30–39. https://doi.org/10.1016/S0895-4356(03)00254-3

Akhter-Khan, S., & Au, R. (2020). Why loneliness interventions are unsuccessful: A call for precision health. *Advances in Geriatric Medicine and Research, 2*(3), e200016. https://doi.org/10.20900/agmr20200016

American Psychiatric Association. (2022). *Diagnostic and statistical manual of mental disorders* (5th ed., text rev.). https://www.psychiatry.org/psychiatrists/practice/dsm

Andersen, B.L., Lacchetti, C., Ashing, K., Berek, J.S., Berman, B.S., Bolte, S., ... Rowland, J.H. (2023). Management of anxiety and depression in adult survivors of cancer: ASCO guideline update. *Journal of Clinical Oncology, 41*(18), 3426–3453. https://doi.org/10.1200/jco.23.00293

Anxiety and Depression Association of America. (2022). *Anxiety disorders—Facts and statistics.* https://adaa.org/understanding-anxiety/facts-statistics

Arble, E., Manning, D., Arnetz, B.B., & Arnetz, J.E. (2023). Increased substance use among nurses during the COVID-19 pandemic. *International Journal of Environmental Research and Public Health, 20*(3), 2674. https://doi.org/10.3390/ijerph20032674

Arthur, J., & Bruera, E. (2022). Managing cancer pain in patients with opioid use disorder or non-medical opioid use. *JAMA Oncology, 8*(8), 1104–1105. https://doi.org/10.1001/jamaoncol.2022.2150

Bamforth, K., Rae, P., Maben, J., Lloyd, H., & Pearce, S. (2023). Perceptions of healthcare professionals' psychological wellbeing at work and the link to patients' experiences of care: A scoping review. *International Journal of Nursing Studies Advances, 5*, 100148. https://doi.org/10.1016/j.ijnsa.2023.100148

Baydoun, M., McLennan, A.I.G., & Carlson, L.E. (2023). People with cancer experience worse psychosocial and financial consequences of COVID-19 compared with other chronic disease populations: Findings from the International COVID-19 Awareness and Response Evaluation Survey study. *JCO Global Oncology, 9*, e2300085. https://doi.org/10.1200/GO.23.00085

Boucher, E.M., McNaughton, E.C., Harake, N., Stafford, J.L., & Parks, A.C. (2021). The impact of a digital intervention (Happify) on loneliness during COVID-19: Qualitative focus group. *JMIR Mental Health, 8*(2), e26617. https://doi.org/10.2196/26617

Brauer, E.R., Lazaro, S., Williams, C.L., Rapkin, D.A., Madnick, A.B., Dafter, R., ... Wong, D.J. (2022). Implementing a tailored psychosocial distress screening protocol in a head and neck cancer program. *Laryngoscope, 132*(8), 1600–1608. https://doi.org/10.1002/lary.30000

Brodsky, B.S., Spruch-Feiner, A., & Stanley, B. (2018). The Zero Suicide Model: Applying evidence-based suicide prevention practices to clinical care. *Frontiers in Psychiatry, 9*, 33. https://doi.org/10.3389/fpsyt.2018.00033

Bruera, E., & Del Fabbro, E. (2018). Pain management in the era of the opioid crisis. *American Society of Clinical Oncology Educational Book, 38*, 807–812. https://doi.org/10.1200/edbk_208563

Bultz, B.D. (2016). Patient care and outcomes: Why cancer care should screen for distress, the 6th vital sign. *Asia-Pacific Journal of Oncology Nursing, 3*(1), 21–24. https://doi.org/10.4103/2347-5625.178163

Cancino, R.S., Su, Z., Mesa, R., Tomlinson, G.E., & Wang, J. (2020). The impact of COVID-19 on cancer screening: Challenges and opportunities. *JMIR Cancer, 6*(2), e21697. https://doi.org/10.2196/21697

Cavanagh, N., Cockett, G., Heinrich, C., Doig, L., Fiest, K., Guichon, J.R., ... Doig, C.J. (2020). Compassion fatigue in healthcare providers: A systematic review and meta-analysis. *Nursing Ethics, 27*(3), 639–665. https://doi.org/10.1177/0969733019889400

Centers for Disease Control and Prevention. (2024). *Risk and protective factors for suicide.* https://www.cdc.gov/suicide/risk-factors/index.html

Charlesworth, L., Fegan, C., & Ashmore, R. (2023). How does severe mental illness impact on cancer outcomes in individuals with severe mental illness and cancer? A scoping review of the literature. *Journal of Medical Imaging and Radiation Sciences, 54*(2, Suppl.), S104–S114. https://doi.org/10.1016/j.jmir.2023.01.007

Cleveland Clinic. (2023). *Panic attacks and panic disorder.* https://my.clevelandclinic.org/health/diseases/4451-panic-attack-panic-disorder

Clifton, K., Gao, F., Jabbari, J.-A., Van Aman, M., Dulle, P., Hanson, J., & Wildes, T.M. (2022). Loneliness, social isolation, and social support in older adults with active cancer during the COVID-19 pandemic. *Journal of Geriatric Oncology, 13*(8), 1122–1131. https://doi.org/10.1016/j.jgo.2022.08.003

Cohen, C., Pignata, S., Bezak, E., Tie, M., & Childs, J. (2023). Workplace interventions to improve well-being and reduce burnout for nurses, physicians and allied healthcare professionals: A systematic review. *BMJ Open, 13*(6), e071203. https://doi.org/10.1136/bmjopen-2022-071203

Copeland, D. (2019). Drug-seeking: A literature review (and an exemplar of stigmatization in nursing). *Nursing Inquiry, 27*(1), e12329. https://doi.org/https://doi.org/10.1111/nin.12329

Correll, C.U., & Schooler, N.R. (2020). Negative symptoms in schizophrenia: A review and clinical guide for recognition, assessment, and treatment. *Neuropsychiatric Disease and Treatment, 16*, 519–534. https://doi.org/10.2147/NDT.S225643

Dalal, S., & Bruera, E. (2019). Pain management for patients with advanced cancer in the opioid epidemic era. *American Society of Clinical Oncology Educational Book, 39*, 24–35. https://doi.org/10.1200/edbk_100020

Daly, M., Sutin, A.R., & Robinson, E. (2021). Depression reported by US adults in 2017–2018 and March and April 2020. *Journal of Affective Disorders, 278*, 131–135. https://doi.org/10.1016/j.jad.2020.09.065

Davis, M., & Batcheller, J. (2020). Managing moral distress in the workplace: Creating a resiliency bundle. *Nurse Leader, 18*(6), 604–608. https://doi.org/10.1016/j.mnl.2020.06.007

Decker, V.B., Nelson, Z., Corveleyn, A., Gopalan, P.K., & Irwin, K. (2022). Caring for patients with serious mental illness: Guide for the oncology clinician. *Oncology, 36*(7), 450–459. https://doi.org/10.46883/2022.25920966

Diaw, M., Sibeoni, J., Manolios, E., Gouacide, J.-M., Brami, C., Verneuil, L., & Revah-Levy, A. (2020). The lived experience of work-related issues among oncology nurses: A metasynthesis. *Cancer Nursing, 43*(3), 200–221. https://doi.org/10.1097/NCC.0000000000000774

Edwards, T., Arthur, J., Joy, M., Lu, Z., Dibaj, S., Bruera, E., & Zhukovsky, D. (2023). Assessing risk for non-medical opioid use among patients with cancer: Stability of the CAGE-AID questionnaire across clinical care settings. *Palliative and Supportive Care, 22*(6), 1648–1652. https://doi.org/10.1017/S1478951523000871

Emami Zeydi, A., Ghazanfari, M.J., Suhonen, R., Adib-Hajbaghery, M., & Karkhah, S. (2022). Effective interventions for reducing moral distress in critical care nurses. *Nursing Ethics, 29*(4), 1047–1065. https://doi.org/10.1177/09697330211062982

Ettman, C.K., Abdalla, S.M., Cohen, G.H., Sampson, L., Vivier, P.M., & Galea, S. (2020). Prevalence of depression symptoms in US adults before and during the COVID-19 pandemic. *JAMA Network Open, 3*(9), e2019686. https://doi.org/10.1001/jamanetworkopen.2020.19686

Fartacek, C., Kunrath, S., Aichhorn, W., & Plöderl, M. (2023). Therapeutic alliance and change in suicide ideation among psychiatric inpatients at risk for suicide. *Journal of Affective Disorders, 323*, 793–798. https://doi.org/10.1016/j.jad.2022.12.028

Foli, K.J., Reddick, B., Zhang, L., & Krcelich, K. (2020). Substance use in registered nurses: "I heard about a nurse who..." *Journal of the American Psychiatric Nurses Association, 26*(1), 65–76. https://doi.org/10.1177/1078390319886369

Galanter, M. (2018). Combining medically assisted treatment and Twelve-Step programming: A perspective and review. *American Journal of Drug and Alcohol Abuse, 44*(2), 151–159. https://doi.org/10.1080/00952990.2017.1306747

Ganguly, A., Michael, M., Goschin, S., Harris, K., & McFarland, D.C. (2022). Cancer pain and opioid use disorder. *Oncology, 36*(9), 535–541. https://doi.org/10.46883/2022.25920973

Garey, L., Olofsson, H., Garza, T., Rogers, A.H., Kauffman, B.Y., & Zvolensky, M.J. (2020). Directional effects of anxiety and depressive disorders with substance use: A review of recent prospective research. *Current Addiction Reports, 7*(3), 344–345. https://doi.org/10.1007/s40429-020-00321-z

Giustiniani, A., Danesin, L., Pezzetta, R., Masina, F., Oliva, G., Arcara, G., ... Conte, P. (2023). Use of telemedicine to improve cognitive functions and psychological well-being in patients with breast cancer: A systematic review of the current literature. *Cancers, 15*(4), 1353. https://doi.org/10.3390/cancers15041353

Glare, P., Aubrey, K., Gulati, A., Lee, Y.C., Moryl, N., & Overton, S. (2022). Pharmacologic management of persistent pain in cancer survivors. *Drugs, 82*(3), 275–291. https://doi.org/10.1007/s40265-022-01675-6

Goerling, U., Hinz, A., Koch-Gromus, U., Hufeld, J.M., Esser, P., & Mehnert-Theuerkauf, A. (2023). Prevalence and severity of anxiety in cancer patients: Results from a multi-center cohort study in Germany. *Journal of Cancer Research and Clinical Oncology, 149*(9), 6371–6379. https://doi.org/10.1007/s00432-023-04600-w

Granek, L., & Nakash, O. (2022). Oncology healthcare professionals' mental health during the COVID-19 pandemic. *Current Oncology, 29*(6), 4054–4067. https://doi.org/10.3390/curroncol29060323

Grassi, L., Caruso, R., Riba, M.B., Lloyd-Williams, M., Kissane, D., Rodin, G., ... Ripamonti, C.I. (2023). Anxiety and depression in adult cancer patients: ESMO Clinical Practice Guideline. *ESMO Open, 8*(2), 101155. https://doi.org/10.1016/j.esmoop.2023.101155

Grassi, L., & Riba, M. (2020). Cancer and severe mental illness: Bi-directional problems and potential solutions. *Psycho-Oncology, 29*(10), 1445–1451.

Grobman, B., Mansur, A., Babalola, D., Srinivasan, A.P., Antonio, J.M., & Lu, C.Y. (2023). Suicide among cancer patients: Current knowledge and directions for observational research. *Journal of Clinical Medicine, 12*(20), 6563. https://doi.org/10.3390/jcm12206563

Grudniewicz, A., Peckham, A., Rudoler, D., Lavergne, M.R., Ashcroft, R., Corace, K., ... Kurdyak, P. (2022). Primary care for individuals with serious mental illness (PriSMI): Protocol for a convergent mixed methods study. *BMJ Open, 12*(9), e065084. https://doi.org/10.1136/bmjopen-2022-065084

Ha, S.H., Shim, I.H., & Bae, D.S. (2019). Differences in depressive and anxiety symptoms between cancer and noncancer patients with psychological distress. *Indian Journal of Psychiatry, 61*(4), 395–399. https://doi.org/10.4103/psychiatry.IndianJPsychiatry_342_18

Hegel, J., Halkett, G.K.B., Schofield, P., Rees, C.S., Heritage, B., Suleman, S., ... Breen, L.J. (2021). The relationship between present-centered awareness and attention, burnout, and compassion fatigue in oncology health professionals. *Mindfulness, 12*(5), 1224–1233. https://doi.org/10.1007/s12671-020-01591-4

Heinrich, M., Hofmann, L., Baurecht, H., Kreuzer, P.M., Knüttel, H., Leitzmann, M.F., & Seliger, C. (2022). Suicide risk and mortality among patients with cancer. *Nature Medicine, 28*(4), 852–859. https://doi.org/10.1038/s41591-022-01745-y

Hermosilla, S., Forthal, S., Sadowska, K., Magill, E.B., Watson, P., & Pike, K.M. (2023). We need to build the evidence: A systematic review of psychological first aid on mental health and well-being. *Journal of Traumatic Stress, 36*(1), 5–16. https://doi.org/10.1002/jts.22888

Hlubocky, F.J., Symington, B.E., McFarland, D.C., Gallagher, C.M., Dragnev, K.H., Burke, J.M., ... Shanafelt, T.D. (2021). Impact of the COVID-19 pandemic on oncologist burnout, emotional well-being, and moral distress: Considerations for the cancer organization's response for readiness, mitigation, and resilience. *JCO Oncology Practice, 17*(7), 365–374. https://doi.org/10.1200/op.20.00937

Holbein, M.M., Walter, M., Ho, J.J., Tapper, C., Brontman, B., Pailler, M., & Case, A.A. (2023). Empowering oncologists to successfully address non-medical opioid use during cancer treatment: A review of best practices. *Journal on Oncology, 3*(2), 1120. https://doi.org/10.52768/2692-563X/1120

Hong, J., Park, C.H.K., Kim, H., Hong, Y., Ahn, J., Jun, J.Y., ... Chung, S. (2023). Grief response of nursing professionals is associated with their depression, loneliness, insomnia, and work-related stress while working in COVID-19 inpatient wards. *Psychiatry Investigation, 20*(4), 374–381. https://doi.org/10.30773/pi.2022.0375

Jakimowicz, S., & Maben, J. (2020). "I can't stop thinking about it": Schwartz Rounds® an intervention to support students and higher education staff with emotional, social and ethical experiences at work. *Journal of Clinical Nursing, 29*(23–24), 4421–4424. https://doi.org/10.1111/jocn.15354

Kim, J., Linos, E., Dove, M.S., Hoch, J.S., & Keegan, T.H. (2023). Impact of COVID-19, cancer survivorship and patient–provider communication on mental health in the US: Difference-In-Difference. *NPJ Mental Health Research, 2*(1), 14. https://doi.org/10.1038/s44184-023-00034-x

Kirk, D., Kabdebo, I., & Whitehead, L. (2021). Prevalence of distress, its associated factors and referral to support services in people with cancer. *Journal of Clinical Nursing, 30*(19–20), 2873–2885. https://doi.org/10.1111/jocn.15794

Koc, Z., Kaplan, E., & Tanrıverdi, D. (2022). The effectiveness of telehealth programs on the mental health of women with breast cancer: A systematic review. *Journal of Telemedicine and Telecare, 30*(3), 405–419. https://doi.org/10.1177/1357633X211069663

Launders, N., Scolamiero, L., Osborn, D.P.J., & Hayes, J.F. (2022). Cancer rates and mortality in people with severe mental illness: Further evidence of lack of parity. *Schizophrenia Research, 246*, 260–267. https://doi.org/10.1016/j.schres.2022.07.008

Leahy, D., Irwin, K., & Murphy, G. (2023). Cancer care for people with significant mental health difficulties (SMHD)—Patient perspectives. *Journal of Psychosocial Oncology, 42*(4), 506–525. https://doi.org/10.1080/07347332.2023.2291203

Lee, J.S.-J., Hu, H.M., Edelman, A.L., Brummett, C.M., Englesbe, M.J., Waljee, J.F., ... Dossett, L.A. (2017). New persistent opioid use among patients with cancer after curative-intent surgery. *Journal of Clinical Oncology, 35*(36), 4042–4049. https://doi.org/10.1200/jco.2017.74.1363

McAndrew, N.S., Strong, Y., Morris, K.J., Sannes, T.S., Pirl, W.F., Cole, S., ... Knight, J.M. (2022). Impact of the COVID-19 pandemic on cancer patients and psycho-oncology providers: Perspectives, observations, and experiences of the American Psychosocial Oncology Society membership. *Psycho-Oncology, 31*(6), 1031–1040. https://doi.org/https://doi.org/10.1002/pon.5894

McNally, G.A., & Sica, A. (2021). Addiction in patients with cancer: Challenges and opportunities. *Journal of the Advanced Practitioner in Oncology, 12*(7), 740–746. https://doi.org/10.6004/jadpro.2021.12.7.7

Meese, K.A., Colón-López, A., Singh, J.A., Burkholder, G.A., & Rogers, D.A. (2021). Healthcare is a team sport: Stress, resilience, and correlates of well-being among health system employees in a crisis. *Journal of Healthcare Management, 66*(4), 304–322. https://doi.org/10.1097/JHM-D-20-00288

Melnyk, B.M. (2022). Battling burnout and languishing. *American Nurse Journal, 17*(8), 44.

Merlin, J.S., Young, S.R., Arnold, R., Bulls, H.W., Childers, J., Gauthier, L., ... Liebschutz, J.M. (2020). Managing opioids, including misuse and addiction, in patients with serious illness in ambulatory palliative care: A qualitative study. *American Journal of Hospice and Palliative Medicine, 37*(7), 507–513. https://doi.org/10.1177/1049909119890556

National Cancer Institute. (2024, May 9). *Cancer statistics*. https://www.cancer.gov/about-cancer/understanding/statistics

National Institute of Mental Health. (2024). *Mental illness*. https://www.nimh.nih.gov/health/statistics/mental-illness

National Institute on Drug Abuse. (2023). *NIDA IC fact sheet 2024*. https://nida.nih.gov/about-nida/legislative-activities/budget-information/fiscal-year-2024-budget-information-congressional-justification-national-institute-drug-abuse/ic-fact-sheet-2024

Nordentoft, M., Plana-Ripoll, O., & Laursen, T.M. (2021). Cancer and schizophrenia. *Current Opinion in Psychiatry, 34*(3), 260–265. https://doi.org/10.1097/yco.0000000000000697

Oliveira, A.M., Machado, D., Fonseca, J.B., Palha, F., Silva Moreira, P., Sousa, N., ... Morgado, P. (2020). Stigmatizing attitudes toward patients with psychiatric disorders among medical students and professionals. *Frontiers in Psychiatry, 11*, 326. https://doi.org/10.3389/fpsyt.2020.00326

Onitsuka, T., Hirano, Y., Nakazawa, T., Ichihashi, K., Miura, K., Inada, K., ... Hashimoto, R. (2022). Toward recovery in schizophrenia: Current concepts, findings, and future research directions. *Psychiatry and Clinical Neurosciences, 76*(7), 282–291. https://doi.org/10.1111/pcn.13342

Paice, J.A. (2018). Cancer pain management and the opioid crisis in America: How to preserve hard-earned gains in improving the quality of cancer pain management. *Cancer, 124*(12), 2491–2497. https://doi.org/10.1002/cncr.31303

Pathirathna, M.L., Nandasena, H.M.R.K.G., Atapattu, A.M.M.P., & Weerasekara, I. (2022). Impact of the COVID-19 pandemic on suicidal attempts and death rates: A systematic review. *BMC Psychiatry, 22*(1), 506. https://doi.org/10.1186/s12888-022-04158-w

Pergolizzi, J.V., Jr., Magnusson, P., Christo, P.J., LeQuang, J.A., Breve, F., Mitchell, K., & Varrassi, G. (2021). Opioid therapy in cancer patients and survivors at risk of addiction, misuse or complex dependency. *Frontiers in Pain Research, 2*, 691720. https://doi.org/10.3389/fpain.2021.691720

Phillips, C.S., Becker, H., & Gonzalez, E. (2021). Psychosocial well-being: An exploratory cross-sectional evaluation of loneliness, anxiety, depression, self-compassion, and professional quality of life in oncology nurses. *Clinical Journal of Oncology Nursing, 25*(5), 530–538. https://doi.org/10.1188/21.CJON.530-538

Phillips, C.S., & Volker, D.L. (2020). Riding the roller coaster: A qualitative study of oncology nurses' emotional experience in caring for patients and their families. *Cancer Nursing, 43*(5), e283–e290. https://doi.org/10.1097/ncc.0000000000000734

Rahmani, F., Hosseinzadeh, M., & Gholizadeh, L. (2023). Complicated grief and related factors among nursing staff during the Covid-19 pandemic: A cross-sectional study. *BMC Psychiatry, 23*(1), 73. https://doi.org/10.1186/s12888-023-04562-w

Reynolds, K.L., Klempner, S.J., Parikh, A., Hochberg, E.P., Michaelson, M.D., Mooradian, M.J., ... Ryan, D.P. (2020). The art of oncology: COVID-19 era. *Oncologist, 25*(11), 997–1000. https://doi.org/10.1634/theoncologist.2020-0512

Rodríguez-Prat, A., Pergolizzi, D., Crespo, I., Julià-Torras, J., Balaguer, A., Kremeike, K., ... Monforte-Royo, C. (2024). The wish to hasten death in patients with life-limiting conditions: A systematic overview. *Journal of Pain and Symptom Management, 68*(2), e91–e115. https://doi.org/10.1016/j.jpainsymman.2024.04.023

Rogers, M.L., Gai, A.R., Lieberman, A., Musacchio Schafer, K., & Joiner, T.E. (2022). Why does safety planning prevent suicidal behavior? *Professional Psychology: Research and Practice, 53*(1), 33–41. https://doi.org/10.1037/pro0000427

Rollnick, S., & Miller, W.R. (1995). What is motivational interviewing? *Behavioural and Cognitive Psychotherapy, 23*(4), 325–334. https://doi.org/10.1017/S135246580001643X

Sashidharan, S.P., Mezzina, R., & Puras, D. (2019). Reducing coercion in mental healthcare. *Epidemiology and Psychiatric Sciences, 28*(6), 605–612. https://doi.org/10.1017/S2045796019000350

Saunders, K., Brain, S., & Ebmeier, K.P. (2011). Diagnosing and managing psychosis in primary care. *Practitioner, 255*(1740), 17–20.

Schepis, T.S., Klare, D.L., Ford, J.A., & McCabe, S.E. (2020). Prescription drug misuse: Taking a lifespan perspective. *Substance Abuse: Research and Treatment, 14*. https://doi.org/10.1177/1178221820909352

Schuler, K.R., LaCroix, J.M., Perera, K.U., Baer, M.M., Trieu, T.H., Nademin, E., ... Ghahramanlou-Holloway, M. (2021). Interpersonal precipitants are associated with suicide intent communication among United States Air Force suicide decedents. *Journal of Affective Disorders Reports, 5*, 100176. https://doi.org/10.1016/j.jadr.2021.100176

Singh, S., Fletcher, G.G., Yao, X., & Sussman, J. (2021). Virtual care in patients with cancer: A systematic review. *Current Oncology, 28*(5), 3488–3506. https://doi.org/10.3390/curroncol28050301

Springer, F., Maier, A., Friedrich, M., Raue, J.S., Finke, G., Lordick, F., ... Mehnert-Theuerkauf, A. (2024). Digital therapeutic (Mika) targeting distress in patients with cancer: Results from a nationwide waitlist randomized controlled trial. *Journal of Medical Internet Research, 26*, e51949. https://doi.org/10.2196/51949

Stephenson, P., & Warner-Stidham, A. (2024). Nurse reports of moral distress during the COVID-19 pandemic. *SAGE Open Nursing, 10*. https://doi.org/10.1177/23779608231226095

Stubbs, J.M., & Achat, H.M. (2022). Are healthcare workers particularly vulnerable to loneliness? The role of social relationships and mental well-being during the COVID-19 pandemic. *Psychiatry Research Communications, 2*(2). https://doi.org/10.1016/j.psycom.2022.100050

Substance Abuse and Mental Health Services Administration. (2021). *Key substance use and mental health indicators in the United States: Results from the 2020 National Survey on Drug Use and Health*. https://www.samhsa.gov/data/sites/default/files/reports/rpt35319/2020NSDUHFFR1PDFW102121.pdf

Sullivan, S.A., Kounali, D., Cannon, M., David, A.S., Fletcher, P.C., Holmans, P., ... Zammit, S. (2020). A population-based cohort study examining the incidence and impact of psychotic experiences from childhood to adulthood, and prediction of psychotic disorder. *American Journal of Psychiatry, 177*(4), 308-317. https://doi.org/10.1176/appi.ajp.2019.19060654

Thomas, C., Cramer, H., Jackson, S., Kessler, D., Metcalfe, C., Record, C., & Barnes, R.K. (2019). Acceptability of the BATHE technique amongst GPs and frequently attending patients in primary care: A nested qualitative study. *BMC Family Practice, 20*(1), 121. https://doi.org/10.1186/s12875-019-1011-y

Tse, N., Tse, S., & Wong, P.W.C. (2022). Collective motivational interviewing for individuals with drug use problems: A pre-post–follow-up, uncontrolled pilot study. *International Journal of Environmental Research and Public Health, 19*(23), 16344. https://doi.org/10.3390/ijerph192316344

Tucker-Seeley, R.D., Wallington, S.F., Canin, B., Tang, W., & McKoy, J.M. (2021). Health equity for older adults with cancer. *Journal of Clinical Oncology, 39*(19), 2205-2216. https://doi.org/10.1200/jco.21.00027

Vig, E.K. (2022). As the pandemic recedes, will moral distress continue to surge? *American Journal of Hospice and Palliative Medicine, 39*(4), 401-405. https://doi.org/10.1177/10499091211030456

Voss, R.M.M., & Das, J. (2022). Mental Status Examination. In *StatPearls*. StatPearls Publishing. https://www.ncbi.nlm.nih.gov/books/NBK546682/

Walker, J., Mulick, A., Magill, N., Symeonides, S., Gourley, C., Burke, K., ... Sharpe, M. (2021). Major depression and survival in people with cancer. *Psychosomatic Medicine, 83*(5), 410-416. https://doi.org/10.1097/PSY.0000000000000942

Willen, S.S. (2022). "Languishing" in critical perspective: Roots and routes of a traveling concept in COVID-19 times. *SSM Mental Health, 2*, 100128. https://doi.org/10.1016/j.ssmmh.2022.100128

Witter, D. (2023, May 17). *U.S. depression rates reach new highs*. Gallup. https://news.gallup.com/poll/505745/depression-rates-reach-new-highs.aspx

Yu, W.-Z., Wang, H.-F., Lin, Y.-K., Liu, Y.-L., Yen, Y., Whang-Peng, J., ... Chang, H.-J. (2024). The effect of oncology nurse navigation on mental health in patients with cancer in Taiwan: A randomized controlled clinical trial. *Current Oncology, 31*(7), 4105-4122. https://doi.org/10.3390/curroncol31070306

CHAPTER 16

Gero-Oncology Considerations

Sarah H. Kagan, PhD, RN, AOCN®, GCNS-BC, FAAN, FGSA

> **KEY TOPICS**
> gero-oncology, age friendly, frailty, frailty screening, geriatric assessment, multimorbidity, oncology nurse navigation

Overview

Older adults represent a rapidly growing majority of those living as cancer survivors (National Cancer Institute, n.d., 2021; Siegel et al., 2023). The needs and preferences of this population are distinctive in many respects when compared to those experienced by their younger counterparts.

The needs experienced by older adult patients and their care partners result from risks for iatrogenic and other complications when receiving cancer care and other healthcare services (Krasovitsky et al., 2023; Mohile et al., 2020; Nightingale et al., 2021). Older adults and their care partners may also experience distress during cancer care differently than that experienced by younger people. Care partners of older adults with cancer, often referred to as *caregivers*, may be spouses or intimate partners, children, grandchildren, or other family members. They may also be outside of the family circle, such as friends, neighbors, or faith community members. *Care partner* is the more inclusive term for the diverse group of people who support older adults living with cancer and other conditions and will be used throughout this chapter (Bennett et al., 2017).

Clinical phenomena, such as frailty and delirium, differentially and often disproportionately affect older adults living with and surviving cancer (Jung et al., 2021; Ness et al., 2014; Yu et al., 2020). Evidence suggests structural and individual ageism threaten health, as well as the outcomes and experiences of cancer care and health care more broadly (Chang et al., 2020; Haase et al., 2023; Krasovitsky et al., 2023; Levy, 2022; Nakamura et al., 2022). As a result, this population may interact more frequently with many different elements within the continuum of health and social care but may not receive better care or enjoy optimal cancer care experiences (Fulmer et al., 2017; Mohile et al., 2021).

Oncology nurse navigators (ONNs) care for older adult patients across disease and survivorship trajectories in various settings. However, many ONNs often possess limited knowledge and skills specific to care for older adult patients in contrast to their oncology-specific expertise (Chan et al., 2023). Resources to improve clinical knowledge and skill in delivering care to older adults are widely available, offering support to ONNs aiming to improve patient and care partner experiences and clinical outcomes. The age-friendly gero-oncology approach to navigation and related resources typically enhances care for younger patients as well.

Evidence indicates premature expression of frailty among childhood cancer survivors as they age, suggesting the value of ONNs screening their patients for frailty across all age groups (Delaney et al., 2021). Younger individuals living with and after cancer also experience syndromes such as frailty, delirium, polypharmacy, and functional impairments (Johnston & Rosenberg, 2024; Oberoi et al., 2024). These syndromes in both older and younger populations may be exacerbated by alterations in social determinants of health, making assessment and intervention from ONNs even more necessary for patients of all ages (Bhandari & Armenian, 2023; Schwartz et al., 2023).

This chapter will provide essential background, evidence, and resources to achieve foundational competency in age-friendly gero-oncology nursing navigation.

Foundations of Age-Friendly Oncology Care

The Gero-Oncology Perspective and Age Friendliness

Aging populations are often described in negative terms, such as the *silver tsunami* (Boyle, 2023; Calasanti, 2020). The needs of older adults living with and surviving cancer are similarly described in negative ways, often accompanied by the word *burden*. The use of such negative terms and metaphors reinforces prevalent structural and individual ageism across health care and in oncology specifically (Calasanti, 2020; Chang et al., 2020; Haase et al., 2023). The effects of structural ageism and resultant bleak perspectives on older adults and their healthcare needs impinge upon the ability of ONNs and other clinicians to provide effective and satisfying care. Understanding what matters to older adults and knowing their goals serves as a foundation from which to complete specialized assessments and follow-up with targeted interventions, including education and support. Further, understanding what matters helps to scale age-friendly expectations for cancer and other health concerns for patients, care partners, and the cancer care team (Fulmer et al., 2020, 2021; Kwak et al., 2024).

Employing a people-centered approach, inclusive of older adults and their care partners, underscores the need to set personalized health and functional goals collaboratively (Young et al., 2020). Using this approach then enables ONNs to fully integrate evidence-based navigation for older adults living with and after cancer. The term *gero-oncology* captures this people-centeredness better than the more common biomedical term *geriatric oncology*. The prefix *gero-* comes from *gerontology* and represents a focus on aging, emphasizing health and function for the person and care partner instead of accentuating the cancer diagnosis alone. *Geriatric oncology* identifies populations of people diagnosed with and treated for cancer by advanced age and, increasingly, by the presence of frailty (Chapman et al., 2021). Specialists who possess education in the biomedical specialties of geriatrics and oncology play important roles in the assessment and treatment of these older adults. Age-friendly gero-oncology care nurse navigation offers the advantage of people-centered holism, in line with the nursing metaparadigm, to place the older adult and their care partner at the center of care regardless of their chronological age and presence of frailty. Thus, even those who are younger than the age cutoffs for geriatric oncology programs (e.g., over age 70 years or over age 75 years) and who are not yet frail can benefit.

Evidence that supports cancer care navigation specifically for older adults, either within geriatric or general oncology care, is limited (Chan et al., 2023). Nonetheless, careful interpretation of evidence from geriatric and oncology research underscores the value of specific screening, assessment, and interventions for older adult patients and their care partners (Extermann et al., 2021; Hamaker et al., 2022). Framing an age-friendly approach to health care with a gero-oncology perspective enables ONNs to facilitate improved evidence-based oncology care for older adult patients and their care partners while meeting their expectations and creating individualized care experiences (Hudson et al., 2019).

Structural ageism puts both quality of cancer care outcomes and experiences at risk for older adults living with and surviving cancer, suggesting that they may be left behind in the current system. Thus, this population is likely to experience significant inequity as they receive cancer and other healthcare services. Although Louart et al. (2020) focused on a different population, the authors posited that navigation may be the solution to preventing those who have limited access to care from being left behind. Age-friendly ONNs employed within a gero-oncology perspective promote equity, as they provide the necessary care, support, and resources needed in a timely fashion (Kagan et al., 2020).

The Planetary Crisis Is a Health Crisis

Achieving and maintaining age-friendly gero-oncology care coordinated by ONNs and performed by all members of the cancer care team requires consideration of the planetary crisis—comprising the climate crisis, the air pollution crisis, and the biodiversity crisis (Hellweg et al., 2023). These aspects affect health across the life span. All health care is affected, but high-intensity services, such as cancer care, are more likely to be disrupted. Additionally, the healthcare industry actively contributes a sizable proportion of greenhouse gas emissions, worsening conditions for health and generating carcinogenic substances in some cases (Eckelman et al., 2020; Hiatt & Beyeler, 2020; Kagan, 2022; Lenzen et al., 2020; Nogueira et al., 2023).

ONNs can play active roles in both adapting to and mitigating the effects of the planetary crisis with their patients and institutions (Lenzen et al., 2020). Integrating issues into navigation, such as finding a mode of transportation to cancer treatments and provider appointments and encouraging plant-based diets, ensures planet- and age-friendly gero-oncology care. As a result, age-friendly gero-oncology nurse navigation merits deliberate consideration of the planetary crisis and the means to help patients and care partners adapt. It also emphasizes sustainable health care to support the mitigation of the crisis itself.

The M's of Age-Friendly Oncology Nurse Navigation

Age-friendly health care and health systems emphasize domains where the risks of iatrogenic events and poor health outcomes are high, and where opportunities to improve health care result in measurable benefits to the healthcare experiences and outcomes of older adults and their families. The Institute for Healthcare Improvement (2023) Age-Friendly Health Systems initiative outlines four domains: What Matters, Medication, Mentation, and Mobility (Emery-Tiburcio et al., 2021; see Figure 16-1). Modern geriatric medicine outlines five domains that overlap nearly completely—Mind, Mobility, Medication, Multicomplexity, and Matters Most. The outlier, multicomplexity, captures the way in which many high-risk clinical and social phenomena intersect at biologic, psychological, and social levels, especially when an individual is frail and without a combination of robust functional reserves, personal resilience, social capital, and social support.

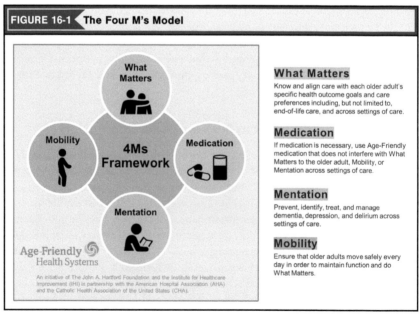

FIGURE 16-1 The Four M's Model

Note. Image courtesy of Age-Friendly Health Systems. For related work, this graphic may be used in its entirety without requesting permission. Graphic files and guidance at https://ihi.org/AgeFriendly.

Frailty is a complex epigenetic phenomenon characterized by weight loss, fatigue, loss of skeletal muscle mass, and slowed mobility (Fried et al., 2001; Pilotto et al., 2020). Physical frailty may also be associated with cognitive decline and psychological changes, such as anxiety and depression (Pilotto et al., 2020). Frailty often mimics or compounds cachexia resulting from cancer treatment and disease progression. Assessing the presence and trajectory of frailty is then key to accurate identification, making screening and intervention at diagnosis essential. However, most cancer centers also lack the resources to conduct an integrated, interprofessional geriatric assessment of multicomplexity, including that for frailty (Williams et al., 2020). Although multicomplexity often proves difficult to fully measure feasibly, validly, and reliably in practice, screening for the presence of frailty makes it easy to incorporate consideration of multicomplexity into ONN practice effectively.

Initiation of Age-Friendly Care

Attaining age-friendly navigation requires patient and care partner education, interprofessional team member and service referrals, and care coordination into the Institute for Healthcare Improvement domains. Improving the cancer experience and outcomes for older adult patients relies on interprofessional geriatric assessment and subsequent intervention to detect frailty and then identify and mitigate high-risk clinical phenomena, such as polypharmacy and repeated falls. These phenomena, classically termed *geriatric syndromes*, incur significant risk for poor outcomes, functional decline, and other complications. Contemporary approaches reframe the understanding of geriatric syndromes into the M's of age-friendly and geriatric health care. Application of these M's begins with detecting underlying frailty, allowing for timely, proactive intervention to limit sequelae, offer prehabilitation where possible, and initiate rehabilitation when functional changes are already present (Kenig et al., 2020; Ness & Wogksch, 2020; O'Donovan & Leech, 2020). Ideally, frailty screening begins at the time a malignancy is diagnosed and continues periodically throughout the cancer care trajectory, primarily when a change in treatment or disease occurs.

ONNs are well-positioned to coordinate a more equitable, alternative approach to the usual understanding of geriatric oncology. Using age-friendly practices within a gero-oncology perspective, ONNs can replicate the benefits of geriatric assessment using a frailty screening tool followed by navigating a process of targeted referral and use of specific resources. This model of ONN care departs from what Chapman et al. (2021) described as the "screen and refer model" by making ONNs the constant in the care experiences of patients and care partners and relying on age-friendly care from a gero-oncology perspective. When guided by the application of the four M's of age-friendly health care, assessment findings help refine goals for prehabilitation, rehabilitation, and supportive care, which guide patient and care partner education and direct subsequent referrals.

Positive screening for frailty also prompts the timely introduction of resources such as homecare services and care partner support. Early introduction of resources may reduce a sense of burden and promote the introduction of prehabilitative and rehabilitative services. Moreover, such referrals, resources, and services may support a future-proofed plan for when climate-related and other events affect access to health care, supportive care, and social services (Espinel et al., 2022). Whether frailty or other concerns are present, all patients should have a disaster plan in place that considers necessary medication, essential services, and potential evacuation plans (Sahar et al., 2020).

Frailty Screening

Frailty screening tools are short instruments designed for use by nurses, social workers, and other healthcare providers to identify people at risk for functional decline who are seeking health care in ways indicative of clinical frailty. Screening tools widely used to improve cancer care for older adults are the Abbreviated Comprehensive Geriatric Assessment, Geriatric 8, Groningen Frailty Indicator, Tilburg Frailty Indicator, Triage Risk Screening Tool (including the Flemish version), and the Vulnerable Elder Survey-13 (Kenig et al., 2020). A newer tool, the Practical Geriatric Assessment, was developed by the Cancer and Aging Research Group and the American Society of Clinical Oncology (Dale et al., 2023; Williams et al., 2023). Table 16-1 lists the most widely used frailty tools and where they can be found. The eFrailty

TABLE 16-1. Frailty Screening Tools

Tool	Access Links and Resources
Abbreviated Comprehensive Geriatric Assessment (aCGA)	The aCGA is presented in the original publication by Overcash et al. (2005) and then further analyzed by Overcash et al. (2006).
Geriatric 8 (G8)	https://efrailty.hsl.harvard.edu/ToolG8.html
Groningen Frailty Indicator (GFI)	https://efrailty.hsl.harvard.edu/ToolGroningenFrailtyIndicator.html
Tilburg Frailty Indicator (TFI)	https://efrailty.hsl.harvard.edu/ToolTilburgFrailtyIndicator.html
Triage Risk Screening Tool (TRST) and Flemish version of the Triage Risk Screening Tool (fTRST): fTRST is easily integrated into ONN assessment.	The fTRST is fully presented in an abstract (Kenis et al., 2006) and is included as a table in an article comparing it with G8 (Kenis et al., 2014).
Vulnerable Elder Survey-13 (VES-13): This tool can direct referrals to physical and occupational therapy and social work for further assessment.	https://efrailty.hsl.harvard.edu/ToolVulnerableElderSurvey-13.html

site (https://efrailty.hsl.harvard.edu/index.html) offers several tools commonly used in cancer care and for relevant oncology practices with specific needs.

A screening result indicative of frailty provides a clinical threshold to trigger referrals for the domains of mental, physical, and social function. Routine application of one of these tools in ONNs' intake or initial assessment quickly identifies aspects of health and function. Kenig et al. (2020) identified the Geriatric 8 and the Abbreviated Comprehensive Geriatric Assessment tools as having desirable measurement characteristics. Garcia et al. (2021) noted that the Vulnerable Elder Survey-13 is well suited in settings where clinicians' availability or time is limited. ONNs should gauge the feasibility of multiple screening tools within their practice, consulting with colleagues both within their cancer program and in gerontologic nursing and geriatric medicine when possible.

Positive results from frailty screening require referral for further assessment and subsequent decision-making and individualized intervention by the cancer team or others, such as the primary care provider (Williams et al., 2020). Close collaboration with the interprofessional team ensures relevant decision-making and care planning rounds, which are essential aspects of geriatric assessment and intervention that outline priorities for clinical follow-up. ONNs' use of frailty screening is a best practice in gero-oncology care.

Multicomplexity and High-Risk Clinical Phenomena

Clinical phenomena associated with elevated risk of functional decline and disability detected in frailty screening and geriatric assessment are classically termed *geriatric syndromes* (Inouye et al., 2007). In an age-friendly context, these clinical events are better labeled as *multimorbidity* and *high-risk clinical phenomena* to avoid the association that only older adults develop these conditions (Hayek et al., 2020). Clinical and scientific evidence suggests that preventing and intervening in effects stemming from the intersection of frailty and multimorbidity in a timely fashion are keys to improving oncology care for older adult patients and their care partners (Extermann et al., 2021; Nightingale et al., 2021).

Common high-risk clinical phenomena include polypharmacy, falls, depression, delirium and other cognitive impairment, and undue burden on care partners. Individuals who are frail and multimorbid are more likely to develop these conditions, though they also occur in people who are younger, prefrail, or without comorbidities. These clinical phenomena are often interrelated and complex, resulting in care planning that quickly becomes overwhelming for patients and care partners. The age-friendly gero-oncology perspective enables ONNs to intervene, reducing the burden and feelings of being overwhelmed for patients and their care partners. Using routine frailty screening as an age-friendly gero-oncology best practice to address high-risk clinical phenomena enables ONNs to leverage principles of care coordination and transitional care central to models of nurse navigation (Franklin et al., 2022). Thus, the combination of age-friendly gero-oncology care initiated with periodic frailty screening and followed by care coordination and transitional care facilitates more clinically effective care and promotes patient and care partner concordance and self-care capacity.

Applying the Four M's

Age-friendly gero-oncology ONN practice uses the four M's to integrate specialty cancer care with other health and social care to achieve person-centered and individualized care to meet patient and care partner needs. ONNs applying the four M's in conjunction with frailty screening can deliver timely patient and care partner education, make targeted referrals to interprofessional team members and ambulatory or homecare services, and coordinate with primary and other specialty care providers to individualize care for patients identified as possibly frail on screening. Care coordination aims to enhance adherence and concordance, bolster patient and care partner satisfaction, avoid overuse and misuse of healthcare resources, and promote optimal outcomes to guide the application of these overarching interventions.

What Matters

Knowing what matters to older adults diagnosed with cancer and their families is critical to all health care (Carbonell et al., 2022). Identification and alignment of values, priorities, and goals for cancer care between patients and providers is frequently challenging, regardless of a patient's age, because of the complexity of the disease and its treatment, as well as the emotional response to the diagnosis and treatment (Fitch et al., 2020). Ageism and poor communication limit clinicians' understanding of older adults' wishes and expectations (Haase et al., 2023; Krasovitsky et al., 2023). Detailed navigation assessments coupled with sensitivity to patient and care partner lifeways provide a platform for ONNs to educate providers, patients, and care partners (Chan et al., 2023; Franklin et al., 2022; Kagan et al., 2020).

Age-friendly care points ONNs toward educating providers and other team members about what matters to older adult patients. This bilateral education helps close the gaps in treatment decision-making and promote access to equitable, effective care that matches patient priorities and goals as closely as possible (Budde et al., 2021; Louart et al., 2020). ONNs can focus on understanding and monitoring evolving preferences and goals and assessing and tracking individual and care partner needs as they develop. Such detailed knowledge of patients and care partners enables ONNs to intervene in a timely manner with referrals to resources, such as social work and chaplaincy services, to achieve tighter coordination with oncology, primary care, and other specialty providers (Extermann et al., 2021). Proactive, timely intervention allows healthcare personnel to avoid reactive responses to crises within the home when patients or care partners cannot compensate for changes in health and functional status and when climate or other related disasters occur.

Medication

Older adults are at risk for complications and sentinel events related to medication use, making optimal use of prescription and over-the-counter medications and dietary supplements critical to safe and effective health care (Zonsius et al., 2022). Shifts in delivery routes for anticancer agents, the high prevalence of potentially inappropriate medications (PIMs), and the possibility of polypharmacy make identifying, preventing, and mitigating medication-related events a high priority for this population (Khezrian et al., 2020; Li et al., 2021; Lu-Yao et al., 2020; Mohamed et al., 2020). Medication overuse and misuse are prime mechanisms for iatrogenic care complications with an attendant risk of worse cancer therapy toxicities, emergency department visits, and inpatient hospitalization (Lu-Yao et al., 2020; Mohamed et al., 2020). Using PIM screening tools, undergoing medication reviews, and deprescribing algorithms are best practices to help avoid toxicity or side effects related to PIMs and polypharmacy (Barlow et al., 2021).

Early referrals to pharmacists for PIMs, polypharmacy education, and deprescribing assistance are fundamental to age-friendly gero-oncology nurse navigation (Turner et al., 2020). Corollary referral to a registered dietitian when food–drug interactions, anorexia, and cachexia occur further supports best practice. Additionally, education for medication safety and coaching to promote engagement with prescribing providers for patients and their care partners is essential. Care coordination warrants the consideration of creating master medication lists, especially for patients who are frail and multimorbid and have many prescribing providers. ONNs and pharmacists should routinely review master medication lists to educate patients and care partners, anticipate medication supply concerns, and alert prescribing providers as needed. These lists also ensure adequate medication supplies and appropriate storage during severe weather events, especially heat waves, and in other climate-related and human-caused disasters.

Mobility

Physical function is critically important for older adults living with and surviving cancer (Ezzatvar et al., 2020; Olson et al., 2022). Mobility influences clinical outcomes and shapes outlook on life in ways that are often underestimated. Changes in mobility and falls frequently result in injury and loss of independence, serious multisystem injury, and may even affect subsequent cancer treatment plans (Gearhart et al., 2020; Montero-Odasso et al., 2022; Sattar et al., 2021). Ambulation and the ability to transit a larger life space are linked to quality of life and mortality (Montero-Odasso et al., 2022; Williams et al., 2021).

Early referral to physical therapy offers optimal opportunities for prehabilitation, rehabilitation, and in-home modifications for safety and mobility (Merchant et al., 2022). Referral to occupational therapy when cognitive function and changes in activities of daily living may affect mobility is similarly crucial. Additionally, referral to a registered dietitian is essential to a complete plan of care for mobility, especially when nutritional states are suboptimal and sarcopenia may underlie weakness and fatigue (Williams et al., 2021). Patients and care partners require education to be able to alert ONNs and other interprofessional team members to increasing fatigue. As the most common cancer symptom and treatment side effect, fatigue negatively affects mobility and puts older patients at risk of rapid deconditioning (Morris & Lewis, 2020).

Barriers to life space mobility outside the home entail referral to an ongoing collaboration with oncology or geriatric social workers. Assistance with transportation is essential to supporting attendance at cancer treatments and other healthcare appointments and to help mitigate social isolation when independent travel is not possible. Efforts to promote low-carbon transportation are valuable and prompt consideration of walkability. Journeys of walkable distances offer potential health benefits that a physical therapist can help patients, care partners, and ONNs evaluate.

Mentation

Changes in mentation in later life include delirium, depression, and dementia, which are sometimes referred to as the 3 D's (Mack et al., 2022). Delirium may be less familiar to ONNs. This acute syndrome is prevalent among older adults living with cancer (Martínez-Arnau et al., 2023). With multifactorial etiology, it is a frequent presenting sign in acute infections, such as those of the urinary tract and lungs, as well as in cases of metabolic derangements, such as electrolyte imbalances. The extent to which phenomena such as "chemobrain" overlap with delirium remains unclear. However, delirium is frequently superimposed on dementia, posing diagnostic and therapeutic challenges. Anxiety is also a common concern for this patient population. Notably, anxiety in the context of cancer may be situational, generalized, or a symptom of depression or dementia.

Mentation and especially cognitive changes in later life elicit worry and, frequently, avoidance on the part of older adult patients and their care partners. Anxiety and avoidance can contribute to depression, which can further alter mentation. Untreated changes in mentation, especially delirium, commonly lead to complications, including increased morbidity and risk of premature mortality (Seiler et al., 2021; Tao et al., 2023). Cancer clinicians, including ONNs, are usually not experts in the assessment of age- and cancer-related changes in mentation. These needs often require adept use of referrals to colleagues outside the cancer care team.

Effective frailty screening always includes consideration of mentation and cognition. Geriatric assessment comprises multifaceted evaluation of cognition and identification of changes in mentation, including delirium, depression, and dementia. ONNs can then pinpoint referrals to achieve a detailed assessment of mentation through the routine use of frailty screening. Further screening for delirium may be necessary, especially for patients who are acutely ill or experiencing new problems with attention. A variety of reliable and valid delirium screening tools are available. Helfand et al. (2021) highlighted the strength of the Confusion Assessment Method, Delirium Observation Screening Scale, Delirium Rating Scale–Revised-98, and Memorial Delirium Assessment Scale. The combination of the Ultra Brief screen and the Confusion Assessment Method (UB-CAM) may offer valuable efficiency in busy ONN practices (Motyl et al., 2020).

Clinicians performing subsequent geriatric assessments include recommendations for specialty follow-up, such as referrals to specialist services similar to those offered by neurology or in an interprofessional memory center. In the absence of easily accessed specialist services, occupational therapists and speech-language pathologists provide valuable expertise because of their focus on cognition and, more broadly, mentation (Habib et al., 2024). Moreover, referrals to audiology often offer clinically significant insight, given the yet-to-be fully-described associations between hearing and cognitive function (Powell et al., 2021).

The role of social isolation and feelings of loneliness cannot be discounted in contributing to changes in mentation (Kuiper et al., 2020). Loneliness may promote and interact with cognitive changes, even to the extent of altering decision-making abilities in older adults (Stewart et al., 2020). Thus, early social work referrals are valuable in addressing mentation. The 3 D's effortlessly intertwine and may occur and co-occur over time for frail, multimorbid older adult patients with cancers. ONNs must lead efforts to ensure that older adults and their care partners access the best possible resources within a given health system to prevent, treat, and mitigate alterations in mentation.

Care partners of older adult patients may be similarly affected by temporary or progressive changes in cognition and mentation (Adashek & Subbiah, 2020). Consequently, ONNs delivering age-friendly navigation must rely on careful ongoing assessment of patient and care partner status, collaboration with social workers, and targeted specialist or therapeutic discipline integration to evaluate cognitive changes (Sun et al., 2021). Supporting, maintaining, or even enhancing mentation requires consistent assessment of care partners by ONNs. However, evidence describing the salience of care partner health and experience underscores treating the older adult patient and care partner as a unit, when possible, to improve navigation and overall care (Kadambi et al., 2020). This understanding is essential when considering events and activities, such as food security and transportation, in this era of planetary crisis.

Summary

ONNs play an essential role in improving cancer care and optimizing the experience of older adult patients and their care partners. Relying on age-friendly gero-oncology nursing navigation enables ONNs to organize assessments and develop a plan of care using a positive approach, understanding what matters most to older adult patients and their care partners. Applying age-friendly gero-oncology nursing navigation begins with frailty screening and focuses on timely intervention and support in the four M's of age-friendly health care. The four M's highlight areas where older adult patients and their care partners are likely to encounter challenges and benefit from early intervention and ongoing collaboration with ONNs. Patients, care partners, and ONNs can make use of various resources available online, including those in age-friendly, planet-friendly, and gero-oncology initiatives (see Table 16-2).

TABLE 16-2. Online Resources for Age-Friendly Gero-Oncology Nurse Navigation	
Resource	Website
AARP Home and Family Caregiving Resource Center: offers information about a variety of resources for care partners of older Americans	www.aarp.org/home-family/caregiving
Age-Friendly Health Systems: details the Age-Friendly Health Systems initiative, offers updates on the status of the initiative, describes age-friendly health care, and includes resources	www.ihi.org/Engage/Initiatives/Age-Friendly-Health-Systems/Pages/default.aspx
Alliance of Nurses for Healthy Environments: offers an extensive array of links to resources and free access to the third edition of *Environmental Health in Nursing*, which offers current knowledge on topics relevant to oncology nursing and navigation practice	www.envirn.org/resources
American Geriatrics Society CoCare: aims at improving health care and integrating geriatric resources into care for older adults	https://agscocare.org
American Geriatrics Society Publications and Tools: provides a resource center for geriatricians, gerontologic nurse practitioners, and other clinicians dedicated to the care of older adults	www.americangeriatrics.org/publications-tools
American Journal of Nursing: offers a series of articles titled *Supporting Family Caregivers in the 4 Ms of an Age-Friendly Health System,* which outline the application of the 4 M's in health and social care for older adults and their care partners	https://journals.lww.com/ajnonline/pages/results.aspx?txtKeywords=Supporting+Family+Caregivers+in+the+4Ms+of+an+Age-Friendly+Health+System
American Red Cross: offers a page on emergency preparedness for older adults that oncology nurse navigators can use to educate themselves and review with patients and care partners	www.redcross.org/get-help/how-to-prepare-for-emergencies/older-adults.html
Cancer and Aging Research Group: includes the Practical Geriatric Assessment and cancer toxicity risk assessment tools that oncology nurse navigators, physicians, and nurse practitioners can incorporate into practices and programs	www.mycarg.org
Columbia University's Mailman School of Public Health Global Consortium on Climate and Health Education: a renowned resource for learning about the effects of the climate crisis on health	www.publichealth.columbia.edu/research/programs/global-consortium-climate-health-education

(Continued on next page)

TABLE 16-2	Online Resources for Age-Friendly Gero-Oncology Nurse Navigation *(Continued)*
Resource	**Website**
GeriatricsCareOnline.org: a searchable database of guidelines and recommendations from the American Geriatrics Society, including the Beers criteria, which lists potentially inappropriate medication use in older adults	https://geriatricscareonline.org/ProductTypeStore/clinical-guidelines-recommendations/8
Gerontological Advanced Practice Nurses Association: offers conferences and other education beneficial to oncology nurse navigators seeking to improve their gerontologic knowledge and skills	www.gapna.org
Hartford Institute for Geriatric Nursing: a robust web-based resource for best practice and evidence-based nursing practice	www.hign.org
National Institute on Aging blog entry *Don't Call Me "Old": Avoiding Ageism When Writing About Aging:* a useful entry about combating ageism in spoken and written communications with patients and care partners and in clinical documents	www.nia.nih.gov/research/blog/2023/12/dont-call-me-old-avoiding-ageism-when-writing-about-aging
Washington University in St. Louis Institute for Public Health blog entry *Age-Inclusive Language: Are You Using It in Your Writing and Everyday Speech?:* offers guidance on using age-inclusive language when communicating with patients, care partners, and colleagues and writing documents in oncology nurse navigation and general oncology practice	https://publichealth.wustl.edu/age-inclusive-language-are-you-using-it-in-your-writing-and-everyday-speech
U.S. Aging: includes an overview of many different resources for older people and their families	www.usaging.org

The author is grateful to Kristen W. Maloney, PhD, RN, AOCNS®, for her careful and helpful review of this chapter.

References

Adashek, J.J., & Subbiah, I.M. (2020). Caring for the caregiver: A systematic review characterising the experience of caregivers of older adults with advanced cancers. *ESMO Open, 5*(5), e000862. https://doi.org/10.1136/esmoopen-2020-000862

Barlow, A., Prusak, E.S., Barlow, B., & Nightingale, G. (2021). Interventions to reduce polypharmacy and optimize medication use in older adults with cancer. *Journal of Geriatric Oncology, 12*(6), 863–871. https://doi.org/10.1016/j.jgo.2020.12.007

Bennett, P.N., Wang, W., Moore, M., & Nagle, C. (2017). Care partner: A concept analysis. *Nursing Outlook, 65*(2), 184–194. https://doi.org/10.1016/j.outlook.2016.11.005

Bhandari, R., & Armenian, S.H. (2023). Risk of frailty in survivors of childhood cancer: The role of socio-environmental factors. *Cancer Epidemiology, Biomarkers and Prevention, 32*(8), 997–998. https://doi.org/10.1158/1055-9965.EPI-23-0642

Boyle, D.A. (2023). The geriatric Asia-Pacific oncology nursing imperative. *Asia-Pacific Journal of Oncology Nursing, 10*(12). https://doi.org/10.1016/j.apjon.2023.100319

Budde, H., Williams, G.A., Winkelmann, J., Pfirter, L., & Maier, C.B. (2021). The role of patient navigators in ambulatory care: Overview of systematic reviews. *BMC Health Services Research, 21*(1), 1166. https://doi.org/10.1186/s12913-021-07140-6

Calasanti, T. (2020). Brown slime, the silver tsunami, and apocalyptic demography: The importance of ageism and age relations. *Social Currents, 7*(3), 195–211. https://doi.org/10.1177/2329496520912736

Carbonell, E., Zonsius, M.C., Rodriguez-Morales, G., Newman, M., & Emery-Tiburcio, E.E. (2022). Addressing what matters. *American Journal of Nursing, 122*(1), 54–58. https://doi.org/10.1097/01.NAJ.0000815440.19544.ed

Chan, R.J., Milch, V.E., Crawford-Williams, F., Agbejule, O.A., Joseph, R., Johal, J., ... Hart, N.H. (2023). Patient navigation across the cancer care continuum: An overview of systematic reviews and emerging literature. *CA: A Cancer Journal for Clinicians, 73*(6), 565–589. https://doi.org/10.3322/caac.21788

Chang, E.-S., Kannoth, S., Levy, S., Wang, S.-Y., Lee, J.E., & Levy, B.R. (2020). Global reach of ageism on older persons' health: A systematic review. *PLOS ONE, 15*(1), e0220857. https://doi.org/10.1371/journal.pone.0220857

Chapman, A.E., Elias, R., Plotkin, E., Lowenstein, L.M., & Swartz, K. (2021). Models of care in geriatric oncology. *Journal of Clinical Oncology, 39*(19), 2195–2204. https://doi.org/10.1200/JCO.21.00118

Dale, W., Klepin, H.D., Williams, G.R., Alibhai, S.M.H., Bergerot, C., Brintzenhofeszoc, K., ... Mohile, S.G. (2023). Practical assessment and management of vulnerabilities in older patients receiving systemic cancer therapy: ASCO guideline update. *Journal of Clinical Oncology, 41*(26), 4293–4312. https://doi.org/10.1200/JCO.23.00933

Delaney, A., Howell, C.R., Krull, K.R., Brinkman, T.M., Armstrong, G.T., Chemaitilly, W., ... Ness, K.K. (2021). Progression of frailty in survivors of childhood cancer: A St. Jude Lifetime Cohort report. *Journal of the National Cancer Institute, 113*(10), 1415–1421. https://doi.org/10.1093/jnci/djab033

Eckelman, M.J., Huang, K., Lagasse, R., Senay, E., Dubrow, R., & Sherman, J.D. (2020). Health care pollution and public health damage in the United States: An update. *Health Affairs, 39*(12), 2071–2079. https://doi.org/10.1377/hlthaff.2020.01247

Emery-Tiburcio, E.E., Mack, L., Zonsius, M.C., Carbonell, E., & Newman, M. (2021). The 4Ms of an age-friendly health system. *American Journal of Nursing, 121*(11), 44–49. https://doi.org/10.1097/01.NAJ.0000799016.07144.0d

Espinel, Z., Nogueira, L.M., Gay, H.A., Bryant, J.M., Hamilton, W., Trapido, E.J., ... Shultz, J.M. (2022). Climate-driven Atlantic hurricanes create complex challenges for cancer care. *Lancet Oncology, 23*(12), 1497–1498. https://doi.org/10.1016/S1470-2045(22)00635-0

Extermann, M., Brain, E., Canin, B., Cherian, M.N., Cheung, K.-L., de Glas, N., ... Karnakis, T. (2021). Priorities for the global advancement of care for older adults with cancer: An update of the International Society of Geriatric Oncology Priorities Initiative. *Lancet Oncology, 22*(1), e29–e36. https://doi.org/10.1016/S1470-2045(20)30473-3

Ezzatvar, Y., Ramírez-Vélez, R., Sáez de Asteasu, M.L., Martínez-Velilla, N., Zambom-Ferraresi, F., Izquierdo, M., & García-Hermoso, A. (2020). Physical function and all-cause mortality in older adults diagnosed with cancer: A systematic review and meta-analysis. *Journals of Gerontology: Series A, 76*(8), 1447–1453. https://doi.org/10.1093/gerona/glaa305

Fitch, M.I., Coronado, A.C., Schippke, J.C., Chadder, J., & Green, E. (2020). Exploring the perspectives of patients about their care experience: Identifying what patients perceive are important qualities in cancer care. *Supportive Care in Cancer, 28*(5), 2299–2309. https://doi.org/10.1007/s00520-019-05057-9

Franklin, E., Burke, S., Dean, M., Johnston, D., Nevidjon, B., & Booth, L.S. (2022). Oncology navigation standards of professional practice. *Journal of Oncology Navigation and Survivorship, 13*(3), 74–85. https://www.jons-online.com/issues/2022/march-2022-vol-13-no-3/oncology-navigation-standards-of-professional-practice

Fried, L.P., Tangen, C.M., Walston, J., Newman, A.B., Hirsch, C., Gottdiener, J., ... McBurnie, M.A. (2001). Frailty in older adults: Evidence for a phenotype. *Journals of Gerontology Series A, 56*(3), M146–M157. https://doi.org/10.1093/gerona/56.3.M146

Fulmer, T., Mate, K.S., & Berman, A. (2017). The Age-Friendly Health System Imperative. *Journal of the American Geriatrics Society, 66*(1), 22–24. https://doi.org/10.1111/jgs.15076

Fulmer, T., Patel, P., Levy, N., Mate, K., Berman, A., Pelton, L., ... Auerbach, J. (2020). Moving toward a global age-friendly ecosystem. *Journal of the American Geriatrics Society, 68*(9), 1936–1940. https://doi.org/10.1111/jgs.16675

Fulmer, T., Reuben, D.B., Auerbach, J., Fick, D.M., Galambos, C., & Johnson, K.S. (2021). Actualizing better health and health care for older adults. *Health Affairs, 40*(2), 219–225. https://doi.org/10.1377/hlthaff.2020.01470

Garcia, M.V., Agar, M.R., Soo, W.-K., To, T., & Phillips, J.L. (2021). Screening tools for identifying older adults with cancer who may benefit from a geriatric assessment: A systematic review. *JAMA Oncology, 7*(4), 616–627. https://doi.org/10.1001/jamaoncol.2020.6736

Gearhart, S.L., Do, E.M., Owodunni, O., Gabre-Kidan, A.A., & Magnuson, T. (2020). Loss of independence in older patients after operation for colorectal cancer. *Journal of the American College of Surgeons, 230*(4), 573–582. https://doi.org/10.1016/j.jamcollsurg.2019.12.021

Haase, K.R., Sattar, S., Pilleron, S., Lambrechts, Y., Hannan, M., Navarrete, E., ... Puts, M. (2023). A scoping review of ageism towards older adults in cancer care. *Journal of Geriatric Oncology, 14*(1), 101385. https://doi.org/10.1016/j.jgo.2022.09.014

Habib, M.H., Zheng, J., Radwan, A., Tolchin, D.W., Smith, S., Inzana, R.S., ... Schlögl, M. (2024). Top ten tips palliative care clinicians should know about physical therapy, occupational therapy, and speech language pathology. *Journal of Palliative Medicine, 27*(5), 681–687. https://doi.org/10.1089/jpm.2023.0545

Hamaker, M., Lund, C., te Molder, M., Soubeyran, P., Wildiers, H., van Huis, L., & Rostoft, S. (2022). Geriatric assessment in the management of older patients with cancer—A systematic review (update). *Journal of Geriatric Oncology, 13*(6), 761–777. https://doi.org/10.1016/j.jgo.2022.04.008

Hayek, S., Gibson, T.M., Leisenring, W.M., Guida, J.L., Gramatges, M.M., Lupo, P.J., ... Ness, K.K. (2020). Prevalence and predictors of frailty in childhood cancer survivors and siblings: A report from the childhood cancer survivor study. *Journal of Clinical Oncology, 38*(3), 232–247. https://doi.org/10.1200/JCO.19.01226

Helfand, B.K., D'Aquila, M.L., Tabloski, P., Erickson, K., Yue, J., Fong, T.G., ... Jones, R.N. (2021). Detecting delirium: A systematic review of identification instruments for non-ICU settings. *Journal of the American Geriatrics Society, 69*(2), 547–555. https://doi.org/10.1111/jgs.16879

Hellweg, S., Benetto, E., Huijbregts, M.A., Verones, F., & Wood, R. (2023). Life-cycle assessment to guide solutions for the triple planetary crisis. *Nature Reviews Earth and Environment, 4*(7), 471–486. https://doi.org/10.1038/s43017-023-00449-2

Hiatt, R.A., & Beyeler, N. (2020). Cancer and climate change. *Lancet Oncology, 21*(11), e519–e527. https://doi.org/10.1016/S1470-2045(20)30448-4

Hudson, A.P., Spooner, A.J., Booth, N., Penny, R.A., Gordon, L.G., Downer, T.-R., ... Chan, R.J. (2019). Qualitative insights of patients and carers under the care of nurse navigators. *Collegian, 26*(1),110–117. https://doi.org/10.1016/j.colegn.2018.05.002

Inouye, S.K., Studenski, S., Tinetti, M.E., & Kuchel, G.A. (2007). Geriatric syndromes: Clinical, research, and policy implications of a core geriatric concept. *Journal of the American Geriatrics Society, 55*(5), 780–791. https://doi.org/10.1111/j.1532-5415.2007.01156.x

Institute for Healthcare Improvement. (2023). *Age-Friendly Health Systems.* https://www.ihi.org/networks/initiatives/age-friendly-health-systems

Johnston, E.E., & Rosenberg, A.R. (2024). Palliative care in adolescents and young adults with cancer. *Journal of Clinical Oncology, 42*(6), 755–763. https://doi.org/10.1200/JCO.23.00709

Jung, P., Puts, M., Frankel, N., Syed, A.T., Alam, Z., Yeung, L., ... Alibhai, S.M.H. (2021). Delirium incidence, risk factors, and treatments in older adults receiving chemotherapy: A systematic review and meta-analysis. *Journal of Geriatric Oncology, 12*(3), 352–360. https://doi.org/10.1016/j.jgo.2020.08.011

Kadambi, S., Loh, K.P., Dunne, R., Magnuson, A., Maggiore, R., Zittel, J., ... Mohile, S. (2020). Older adults with cancer and their caregivers—Current landscape and future directions for clinical care. *Nature Reviews Clinical Oncology, 17*(12), 742–755. https://doi.org/10.1038/s41571-020-0421-z

Kagan, S.H. (2022). Treating our malignant climate: Global heating, healthy climate, and cancer nursing. *Cancer Nursing, 45*(2), 85–86. https://doi.org/10.1097/NCC.0000000000001059

Kagan, S.H., Morgan, B., Smink, T., DeMille, D., Huntzinger, C., Pauly, M., & Lynch, M.P. (2020). The oncology nurse navigator as "gate opener" to interdisciplinary supportive and palliative care for people with head and neck cancer. *Journal of Oncology Navigation and Survivorship, 11*(8), 259–266.

Kenig, J., Szabat, K., Mituś, J., Mituś-Kenig, M., & Krzeszowiak, J. (2020). Usefulness of eight screening tools for predicting frailty and postoperative short-and long-term outcomes among older patients with cancer who qualify for abdominal surgery. *European Journal of Surgical Oncology, 46*(11), 2091–2098. https://doi.org/10.1016/j.ejso.2020.07.040

Kenis, C., Decoster, L., Van Puyvelde, K., De Grève, J., Conings, G., Milisen, K., ... Wildiers, H. (2014). Performance of two geriatric screening tools in older patients with cancer. *Journal of Clinical Oncology, 32*(1), 19–26. https://doi.org/10.1200/JCO.2013.51.1345

Kenis, C., Geeraerts, A., Braes, T., Milisen, K., Flamaing, J., & Wildiers, H. (2006). 19 The Flemish version of the Triage Risk Screening Tool (TRST): A multidimensional short screening tool for the assessment of elderly patients. *Critical Reviews in Oncology/Hematology, 60*, S31. https://doi.org/10.1016/S1040-8428(13)70090-8

Khezrian, M., McNeil, C.J., Murray, A.D., & Myint, P.K. (2020). An overview of prevalence, determinants and health outcomes of polypharmacy. *Therapeutic Advances in Drug Safety, 11*, https://doi.org/10.1177/2042098620933741

Krasovitsky, M., Porter, I., & Tuch, G. (2023). The impact of ageism in the care of older adults with cancer. *Current Opinion in Supportive and Palliative Care, 17*(1), 8–14. https://doi.org/10.1097/SPC.0000000000000629

Kuiper, J.S., Smidt, N., Zuidema, S.U., Comijs, H.C., Oude Voshaar, R.C., & Zuidersma, M. (2020). A longitudinal study of the impact of social network size and loneliness on cognitive performance in depressed older adults. *Aging and Mental Health, 24*(6), 889–897. https://doi.org/10.1080/13607863.2019.1571012

Kwak, M.J., Inouye, S.K., Fick, D.M., Bonner, A., Fulmer, T., Carter, E., ... Oh, E.S. (2024). Optimizing delirium care in the era of Age-Friendly Health System. *Journal of the American Geriatrics Society, 72*(1), 14–23. https://doi.org/10.1111/jgs.18631

Lenzen, M., Malik, A., Li, M., Fry, J., Weisz, H., Pichler, P.-P., ... Pencheon, D. (2020). The environmental footprint of health care: A global assessment. *Lancet Planetary Health, 4*(7), e271–e279. https://doi.org/10.1016/S2542-5196(20)30121-2

Levy, B.R. (2022). The role of structural ageism in age beliefs and health of older persons. *JAMA Network Open, 5*(2), e2147802. https://doi.org/10.1001/jamanetworkopen.2021.47802.

Li, D., Sun, C.-L., Kim, H., Soto-Perez-de-Celis, E., Chung, V., Koczywas, M., ... Dale, W. (2021). Geriatric Assessment–Driven Intervention (GAIN) on chemotherapy-related toxic effects in older adults with cancer: A randomized clinical trial. *JAMA Oncology, 7*(11), e214158. https://doi.org/10.1001/jamaoncol.2021.4158

Louart, S., Bonnet, E., & Ridde, V. (2020). Is patient navigation a solution to the problem of "leaving no one behind"? A scoping review of evidence from low-income countries. *Health Policy and Planning, 36*(1), 101–116. https://doi.org/10.1093/heapol/czaa09

Lu-Yao, G., Nightingale, G., Nikita, N., Keith, S., Gandhi, K., Swartz, K., ... Chapman, A. (2020). Relationship between polypharmacy and inpatient hospitalization among older adults with cancer treated with intravenous chemotherapy. *Journal of Geriatric Oncology, 11*(4), 579–585. https://doi.org/10.1016/j.jgo.2020.03.001

Mack, L., Zonsius, M.C., Newman, M., & Emery-Tiburcio, E.E. (2022). Recognizing and acting on mentation concerns. *American Journal of Nursing, 122*(5), 50–55. https://doi.org/10.1097/01.NAJ.0000830764.74949.fd

Martínez-Arnau, F.M., Buigues, C., & Pérez-Ros, P. (2023). Incidence of delirium in older people with cancer: Systematic review and meta-analysis. *European Journal of Oncology Nursing, 67*, 102457. https://doi.org/10.1016/j.ejon.2023.102457

Merchant, Z., Denchy, L., Santa Mina, D., Alibhai, S., & Moore, J. (2022). Prehabilitation and rehabilitation in older adults with cancer and frailty. In F. Gomes (Ed.), *Frailty in older adults with cancer* (pp. 155–176). Springer.

Mohamed, M.R., Ramsdale, E., Loh, K.P., Arastu, A., Xu, H., Obrecht, S., ... Mohile, S.G. (2020). Associations of polypharmacy and inappropriate medications with adverse outcomes in older adults with cancer: A systematic review and meta-analysis. *Oncologist, 25*(1), e94–e108. https://doi.org/10.1007/978-3-030-89162-6_9

Mohile, S.G., Epstein, R.M., Hurria, A., Heckler, C.E., Canin, B., Culakova, E., ... Dale, W. (2020). Communication with older patients with cancer using geriatric assessment: A cluster-randomized clinical trial from the National Cancer Institute Community Oncology Research Program. *JAMA Oncology, 6*(2), 196–204. https://doi.org/10.1001/jamaoncol.2019.4728

Mohile, S.G., Mohamed, M.R., Xu, H., Culakova, E., Loh, K.P., Magnuson, A., ... Dale, W. (2021). Evaluation of geriatric assessment and management on the toxic effects of cancer treatment (GAP70+): A cluster-randomised study. *Lancet, 398*(10314), 1894–1904. https://doi.org/10.1016/S0140-6736(21)01789-X

Montero-Odasso, M., van der Velde, N., Martin, F.C., Petrovic, M., Tan, M.P., Ryg, J., ... Masud, T. (2022). World guidelines for falls prevention and management for older adults: A global initiative. *Age and Ageing, 51*(9), afac205. https://doi.org/10.1093/ageing/afac205

Morris, R., & Lewis, A. (2020). Falls and cancer. *Clinical Oncology, 32*(9), 569–578. https://doi.org/10.1016/j.clon.2020.03.011

Motyl, C.M., Ngo, L., Zhou, W., Jung, Y., Leslie, D., Boltz, M., ... Marcantonio, E.R. (2020). Comparative accuracy and efficiency of four delirium screening protocols. *Journal of the American Geriatrics Society, 68*(11), 2572–2578. https://doi.org/10.1111/jgs.1671

Nakamura, J.S., Hong, J.H., Smith, J., Chopik, W.J., Chen, Y., VanderWeele, T.J., & Kim, E.S. (2022). Associations between satisfaction with aging and health and well-being outcomes among older US adults. *JAMA Network Open, 5*(2), e2147797. https://doi.org/10.1001/jamanetworkopen.2021.47797

National Cancer Institute. (n.d.). *Statistics and graphs*. Division of Cancer Control and Population Sciences. U.S. Department of Health and Human Services. https://cancercontrol.cancer.gov/ocs/statistics

National Cancer Institute. (2021, March 5). *Age and cancer risk*. https://www.cancer.gov/about-cancer/causes-prevention/risk/age

Ness, K.K., Armstrong, G.T., Kundu, M., Wilson, C.L., Tchkonia, T., & Kirkland, J.L. (2014). Frailty in childhood cancer survivors. *Cancer, 121*(10), 1540–1547. https://doi.org/10.1002/cncr.29211

Ness, K.K., & Wogksch, M.D. (2020). Frailty and aging in cancer survivors. *Translational Research, 221*, 65–82. https://doi.org/10.1016/j.trsl.2020.03.013

Nightingale, G., Battisti, N.M.L., Loh, K.P., Puts, M., Kenis, C., Goldberg, A., ... Pergolotti, M. (2021). Perspectives on functional status in older adults with cancer: an interprofessional report from the International Society of Geriatric Oncology (SIOG) nursing and allied health interest group and young SIOG. *Journal of Geriatric Oncology, 12*(4), 658–665. https://doi.org/10.1016/j.jgo.2020.10.018

Nogueira, L.M., Crane, T.E., Ortiz, A.P., D'Angelo, H., & Neta, G. (2023). Climate change and cancer. *Cancer Epidemiology, Biomarkers and Prevention, 32*(7), 869–875. https://doi.org/10.1158/1055-9965.EPI-22-1234

O'Donovan, A., & Leech, M. (2020). Personalised treatment for older adults with cancer: The role of frailty assessment. *Technical Innovations and Patient Support in Radiation Oncology, 16*, 30–38. https://doi.org/10.1016/j.tipsro.2020.09.001

Oberoi, S., Garland, A., Yan, A.P., Lambert, P., Xue, L., Decker, K., ... Mahar, A.L. (2024). Mental disorders among adolescents and young adults with cancer: A Canadian population–based and sibling cohort study. *Journal of Clinical Oncology, 42*(13), 1509–1519. https://doi.org/10.1200/jco.23.01615

Olson, L.M., Zonsius, M.C., Rodriguez-Morales, G., & Emery-Tiburcio, E.E. (2022). Promoting safe mobility. *American Journal of Nursing, 122*(7), 46–52. https://doi.org/10.1097/01.Naj.0000842256.48499.47

Overcash, J.A., Beckstead, J., Extermann, M., & Cobb, S. (2005). The abbreviated comprehensive geriatric assessment (aCGA): A retrospective analysis. *Critical Reviews in Oncology/Hematology, 54*(2), 129–136. https://doi.org/10.1016/j.critrevonc.2004.12.002

Overcash, J.A., Beckstead, J., Moody, L., Extermann, M., & Cobb, S. (2006). The abbreviated comprehensive geriatric assessment (aCGA) for use in the older cancer patient as a prescreen: Scoring and interpretation. *Critical Reviews in Oncology/Hematology, 59*(3), 205–210. https://doi.org/10.1016/j.critrevonc.2006.04.003

Pilotto, A., Custodero, C., Maggi, S., Polidori, M.C., Veronese, N., & Ferrucci, L. (2020). A multidimensional approach to frailty in older people. *Ageing Research Reviews, 60*, 101047. https://doi.org/10.1016/j.arr.2020.101047

Powell, D.S., Oh, E.S., Lin, F.R., & Deal, J.A. (2021). Hearing impairment and cognition in an aging world. *Journal of the Association for Research in Otolaryngology, 22*(4), 387–403. https://doi.org/10.1007/s10162-021-00799-y

Sahar, L., Nogueira, L.M., Ashkenazi, I., Jemal, A., Yabroff, K.R., & Lichtenfeld, J.L. (2020). When disaster strikes: The role of disaster planning and management in cancer care delivery. *Cancer, 126*(15), 3388–3392. https://doi.org/10.1002/cncr.32920

Sattar, S., Haase, K., Kuster, S., Puts, M., Spoelstra, S., Bradley, C., ... Alibhai, S. (2021). Falls in older adults with cancer: An updated systematic review of prevalence, injurious falls, and impact on cancer treatment. *Supportive Care in Cancer, 29*(1), 21–33. https://doi.org/10.1007/s00520-020-05619-2

Schwartz, L.F., Dhaduk, R., Howell, C.R., Brinkman, T.M., Ehrhardt, M.J., Delaney, A., ... Henderson, T.O. (2023). The association of neighborhood characteristics and frailty in childhood cancer survivors: A report from the St. Jude Lifetime Cohort Study. *Cancer Epidemiology, Biomarkers and Prevention, 32*(8), 1021–1029. https://doi.org/10.1158/1055-9965.EPI-22-1322

Seiler, A., Blum, D., Deuel, J.W., Hertler, C., Schettle, M., Zipser, C.M., ... Boettger, S. (2021). Delirium is associated with an increased morbidity and in-hospital mortality in cancer patients: Results from a prospective cohort study. *Palliative and Supportive Care, 19*(3), 294–303. https://doi.org/10.1017/S147895152000139X

Siegel, R.L., Miller, K.D., Wagle, N.S., & Jemal, A. (2023). Cancer statistics, 2023. *CA: A Cancer Journal for Clinicians, 73*(1),17–48. https://doi.org/10.3322/caac.21763

Stewart, C.C., Yu, L., Glover, C.M., Mottola, G., Bennett, D.A., Wilson, R.S., & Boyle, P.A. (2020). Loneliness interacts with cognition in relation to healthcare and financial decision making among community-dwelling older adults. *Gerontologist, 60*(8), 1476–1484. https://doi.org/10.1093/geront/gnaa078

Sun, V., Puts, M., Haase, K., Pilleron, S., Hannan, M., Sattar, S., & Strohschein, F.J. (2021). The role of family caregivers in the care of older adults with cancer. *Seminars in Oncology Nursing, 37*(6). https://doi.org/10.1016/j.soncn.2021.151232

Tao, J., Seier, K., Marasigan-Stone, C.B., Simondac, J.-S.S., Pascual, A.V., Kostelecky, N.T., ... Voigt, L.P. (2023). Delirium as a risk factor for mortality in critically ill patients with cancer. *JCO Oncology Practice, 19*(6), e838–e847. https://doi.org/10.1200/OP.22.00395

Turner, J.P., Kantilal, K., Holmes, H., & Koczwara, B. (2020). Optimising medications for patients with cancer and multimorbidity: The case for deprescribing. *Clinical Oncology, 32*(9), 609–617. https://doi.org/10.1016/j.clon.2020.05.015

Williams, G.R., Dunne, R.F., Giri, S., Shachar, S.S., & Caan, B.J. (2021). Sarcopenia in the older adult with cancer. *Journal of Clinical Oncology, 39*(19), 2068–2078. https://doi.org/10.1200/JCO.21.00102

Williams, G.R., Hopkins, J.O., Klepin, H.D., Lowenstein, L.M., Mackenzie, A., Mohile, S.G., ... Dale, W. (2023). Practical assessment and management of vulnerabilities in older patients receiving systemic cancer therapy: ASCO guideline questions and answers. *JCO Oncology Practice, 19*(9), 718–723. https://doi.org/10.1200/OP.23.00263

Williams, G.R., Weaver, K.E., Lesser, G.J., Dressler, E., Winkfield, K.M., Neuman, H.B., ... Klepin, H.D. (2020). Capacity to provide geriatric specialty care for older adults in community oncology practices. *Oncologist, 25*(12), 1032–1038. https://doi.org/10.1634/theoncologist.2020-0189

Young, A.M., Charalambous, A., Owen, R.I., Njodzeka, B., Oldenmenger, W.H., Alqudimat, M.R., & So, W.K.W. (2020). Essential oncology nursing care along the cancer continuum. *Lancet Oncology, 21*(12), e555–e563. https://doi.org/10.1016/S1470-2045(20)30612-4

Yu, M., Hazelton, W.D., Luebeck, G.E., & Grady, W.M. (2020). Epigenetic aging: More than just a clock when it comes to cancer. *Cancer Research, 80*(3), 367–374. https://doi.org/10.1158/0008-5472.CAN-19-0924

Zonsius, M.C., Myftari, K., Newman, M., & Emery-Tiburcio, E.E. (2022). Optimizing older adults' medication use. *American Journal of Nursing, 122*(3), 38–43. https://doi.org/10.1097/01.NAJ.0000822976.96210.5d

CHAPTER 17

Pediatrics, Adolescents, and Young Adults

Lauren V. Ghazal, PhD, FNP-BC, and Marybeth Tetlow, MSN, RN, BMTCN®, OCN®

> **KEY TOPICS**
> practical and psychosocial issues, fertility preservation, financial hardship, health insurance, navigation

Overview

Pediatric, adolescent, and young adult (AYA) cancer survivors are those who received their initial cancer diagnosis from birth to age 39 years (National Cancer Institute [NCI], 2023). The role of the oncology nurse navigator (ONN) is critical for these patients and their families as they continue in the cancer survivorship continuum for longer periods than ever before. Although this chapter will focus on both pediatric and AYA cancer survivors in the United States, more consideration is given to the AYA population because of the lack of literature available on pediatric nurse navigation.

In the United States, pediatric and AYA cancers are rare, accounting for 5.5% of all cases. In 2023, about 17,000 pediatric and 86,000 AYA patients were diagnosed (American Cancer Society, 2020; NCI, 2023). Prevalent cancers vary by age, with leukemias occurring in children and breast, thyroid, and melanoma in young adults (Miller et al., 2020; NCI, 2023, 2024).

This chapter will cover the unique challenges and supportive care approaches for pediatric and AYA patients throughout all stages of the cancer care continuum (Docherty et al., 2015; Jones et al., 2020; Smith et al., 2023). It will examine these topics within the broader context of health care, including medical care and the challenges of age disparities on informing about care, healthcare systems, psychological–spiritual issues, relationship issues, and other practical concerns involving pediatric and AYA patients. This chapter will also review tested psychosocial interventions and offers a quick reference guide to supportive care resources. ONNs will gain insights into clinical care strategies and resources for these young patient groups.

Trends, Transitions, and the Role of the Oncology Nurse Navigator

AYA cancer survival rates are rising because of better care and treatment, with sustained improvement seen when excluding the impact of HIV/AIDS (Bleyer, 2023; Koh et al., 2023; Liu et al., 2018; Siegel et al., 2024). Despite overall progress, osteosarcoma and male breast cancers do not show an increase in survival rates, and cervical and female bladder cancers have declining survival rates (Keegan et al., 2023). Males and non-Hispanic Black AYAs face worse outcomes (Liu et al., 2018). This AYA patient population encounters significant challenges, including low enrollment in clinical trials, disparities in health and healthcare access, and less favorable psychosocial outcomes compared to other age groups (Anderson et al., 2019; Beauchemin et al., 2024; Roth et al., 2020; Siembida, Loomans-Kropp, Tirvedi, O'Mara, et al., 2020).

Despite the urgent need for effective treatments, AYAs have limited access to cancer clinical trials because of the rarity of cancer in this age group, a lack of trials tailored to their specific needs, and a higher likelihood of receiving treatment outside of specialized research centers (Siembida, Loomans-Kropp, Tirvedi, O'Mara, et al., 2020). Additionally, both physicians and patients often lack awareness of applicable trials and eligibility criteria, resulting in insufficient patient–provider communication about cancer clinical trials. A systematic review highlighted the necessity for targeted inventions to enhance the recruitment and engagement of AYA patients in clinical research (Siembida, Loomans-Kropp, Tirvedi, O'Mara, et al., 2020). Key strategies for improvement included increasing awareness of trial availability and strengthening the communication between patients and healthcare providers.

ONNs can relieve challenges and barriers experienced by patients throughout the care continuum (Fox et al., 2022; Kirk et al., 2022; Pannier et al., 2019). Navigation also addresses disparities in clinical care and health and psychosocial outcomes by facilitating timely access for all to quality care in a culturally sensitive manner (Kirk et al., 2022). ONNs caring for AYA patients can work to strengthen patient–provider communication by providing education, referring to centers with clinical trials, and encouraging dialogue among providers (Roth et al., 2020; Siembida et al., 2021). Initiatives within NCI's National Clinical Trials Network aim to bolster the accrual of AYA patients to clinical trials, thus advancing treatment options for this demographic (Roth et al., 2020).

Findings regarding improved survival rates among AYAs are encouraging; however, this population continues to face unique psychosocial challenges when navigating a diagnosis of cancer and its subsequent treatment during formative developmental years. Distinct challenges that AYA patients encounter throughout cancer survivorship include the following (Berkman, Mittal, et al., 2023; McLoone et al., 2023; Smith et al., 2023):
- Identity and sexual development
- Struggles for autonomy
- Fertility preservation
- Neurocognitive effects

- Disruptions in schooling or work
- Isolation from peer or family support networks

The distress caused by a life-threatening illness exacerbates the psychological risk factors of young adulthood, which can manifest in anxiety and depression (Adjei Boakye et al., 2022; Osmani et al., 2023; Zebrack et al., 2016). AYAs experience several transitions across the cancer care continuum: from a state of general health (prediagnosis) to a diagnosis of a life-threatening condition, from diagnosis to treatment, and from treatment to survivorship care or end of life (Jones et al., 2020). In addition to transitioning through their oncologic journey, they are also transitioning in life. This may result in patients swinging from establishing independence in adulthood back to having childhood dependence, disassociating from peers without cancer, connecting with peers with cancer, and having an inability to connect with older adult patients with cancer (Marshall et al., 2018).

Responsibilities and roles of AYA-specific ONNs include coordinating care, providing emotional support, advocating, knowing the internal and external resources, assisting with insurance and financial concerns, and being the point person for these patients (LaRosa et al., 2017, 2019). In-person connection to a navigator (rather than via phone, email, or text) may be more desired in this population to address needs related to insurance, finances, or other information, but these specific needs and questions vary by the developmental level of patients at the time of diagnosis (Pannier et al., 2019).

Challenges Faced by Adolescents and Young Adults With Cancer

Healthcare System

In the United States, cancer care delivery occurs across a range of healthcare settings, which include academic institutions, NCI-designated cancer centers, freestanding community cancer programs, ambulatory care clinics (e.g., radiation clinics, chemotherapy infusion units), individual (or private) practices, and pediatric and medical oncology groups (Beauchemin et al., 2024; Beauchemin, Ji, et al., 2023; Haines et al., 2022; Roth et al., 2020). Within cancer care delivery across all age groups, research has found that AYAs are the least likely to be treated at comprehensive cancer centers (Isenalumhe et al., 2016). In the diagnostic phase, patient navigation has the potential to positively affect the timeliness of diagnostic testing, the patient experience, and preparation for decision-making regarding treatment options (Fox et al., 2022; LaRosa et al., 2019; Pannier et al., 2019).

Among the top barriers to optimal cancer care, AYAs identified a lack of cancer care providers specializing in their care, a lack of connection to an AYA patient community, and their inability to navigate the health system (Cheung & Zebrack, 2017; Siembida et al., 2021). In a study by Fox et al. (2022), a large midwestern cancer center and affiliated children's hospital implemented an AYA-specific patient navigator. In this setting, the navigator was charged with conducting biopsychosocial assessments, connecting patients to supportive services, and coordinating monthly peer support groups, as it had been found that these groups can be very helpful in decreasing distress. The implementation of an AYA navigator increased attendance at and satisfaction with the peer support group. With additional feedback from the peer support group, program organizers were able to expand the program to start another support group for patients to bring a caregiver. This enabled program organizers to tailor the speakers to relevant topics for the audience (Fox et al., 2022, 2024).

Historically, AYA patients with cancer have been caught between the worlds of pediatric and adult medical oncology (Janardan & Wechsler, 2021). When treated in the adult setting, AYAs tend to feel isolated and in need of facilities that are more inclusive to their age and life circumstances (Marshall et al., 2018; Miller & van der Eijk, 2019). When treated in the pediatric setting, AYAs tend to feel isolated with the age gap of being too old for specific supportive services. Most AYA patients who receive their treatment in community settings tend not to have access to key resources for cancer care, including fertility preservation, financial navigation, and other survivorship services (Beauchemin, Ji, et al., 2023). There is a growing awareness, however, of the need for integrated strategies that allow AYAs to benefit from the combined expertise of pediatric and adult oncology clinicians in systems that identify the complex disease-related and psychosocial issues that affect this population (Barr et al., 2016; Levin et al., 2019; Smith et al., 2023).

Patient-, provider-, and system-level characteristics all appear to influence AYAs' perceptions of medical care (Kaal et al., 2018; Siembida, Loomans-Kropp, Tirvedi, O'Mara, et al., 2020). They reported dissatisfaction with their care, the lack of information about treatments and follow-up care, poor communication with healthcare providers, and delays in diagnosis as contributing factors. AYAs' satisfaction with care tends to be associated with being disease-free or free from debilitating side effects. Symptom management and health promotion during and after treatment are critical in fostering mental health and satisfaction with cancer care (Bradford & Chan, 2017; Dorfman et al., 2023; Mitchell et al., 2018). Healthcare providers can benefit from communicating information directly and honestly, without condescension or patronization—all with an awareness of the developing cognitive capacities and limitations of AYA patients.

ONNs are uniquely positioned to help identify and address these barriers to follow-up care (Fox et al., 2022). A randomized controlled trial highlighted how AYAs who received non-clinical peer navigation or text messaging interventions had increased survivorship care self-efficacy or knowledge and increased awareness about seeking survivorship care (Casillas et al., 2019). ONNs can conduct routine comprehensive assessments to identify which barriers their patients are facing and refer them to appropriate resources. For example, ONNs can help patients access financial assistance resources, such as the Expect Miracles Foundation, Triage Cancer, Patient Advocate Foundation, RxAssist, and Cancer for College. Additionally, ONNs can help connect patients with age-appropriate supportive care resources through organizations such as Stupid Cancer and Ulman Foundation. Similarly, non-clinical navigators have been used in pediatric and AYA navigation, including St. Jude Children's Research Hospital (Cox et al., 2021).

A 2022 study in different regions of Canada highlighted very similar needs of Canadian AYAs with cancer; about 7,600 AYAs are diagnosed each year in Canada. This study revealed that these patients needed information about specific health risks with anticipatory guidance and checklists, timely and appropriate supportive care (e.g., check-in visits, navigation support), and increased connections and access to information (Avery et al., 2022).

Medical Care: Side Effects and Symptoms

AYAs with cancer face more intense treatments, higher symptom burden, and poorer treatment outcomes than younger peers (Daniel et al., 2017; Smith et al., 2018). Cancer-related fatigue is the most prevalent and distressing symptom experienced by AYAs and is an independent predictor of quality of life (Nowe et al., 2017; Spathis et al., 2017). It persists beyond cancer treatment and is perceived by patients as being worse one year after the end of treatment when compared to fatigue experienced in the first year following cessation of treatment (Spathis et al., 2017). Cancer-related fatigue is a neglected symptom in AYAs, with no interventional studies focusing on its management (Nowe et al., 2017; Spathis et al., 2017). Promising approaches include exercise and psychosocial interventions, such as education and treatment of concurrent symptoms.

Fear of cancer recurrence is a common and distressing problem among patients. Cancer survivors face an increased risk of second primary malignancies, cardiac toxicity, and infertility (Sung et al., 2022; van der Meer et al., 2024). The overall relative risk of second primary cancers is much higher in patients aged 0–39 years compared with those older than 40 years, likely because of the increased intensity of initial treatment in childhood protocols and longer life expectancies (Sung et al., 2022; van der Meer et al., 2024). AYA patients with a high fear of cancer recurrence report worse functioning in psychological and social domains, as well as lower overall health-related quality of life compared to those with low levels of fear of cancer recurrence (Thewes et al., 2018).

Cardiac toxicity is one of the most feared side effects of anticancer agents (Leerink & Feijen, 2024; Stafford et al., 2024; Tolani et al., 2023; Wong-Siegel et al., 2023). Mortality risk increases because of cardiac problems, such as heart failure, myocardial ischemia, arrhythmias, hypertension, and thromboembolism. The incidence of cardiac toxicity depends on multiple factors, including the following (Stafford et al., 2024):
- Oncologic therapies: type of drug, dose administered during each cycle, cumulative dose, schedule of administration, route of administration, combination of other cardiotoxic drugs, association with radiation therapy
- Patient-specific characteristics: age, presence of cardiovascular risk factors, previous cardiovascular disease, prior mediastinal radiation therapy

Long-term follow-up care recommendations include yearly physical examination and history, risk modification, avoidance of heavy isometric exercise in higher-risk patients, periodic echocardiograms (including corrected QTc intervals), and early cardiology referrals for any detected abnormalities (Adams et al., 2021; Ehrhardt et al., 2023; Hudson et al., 2021).

The risk of infertility from cancer treatments is particularly devastating for young adult patients with cancer. Localized treatments, such as surgery and radiation therapy, may affect fertility by removing or damaging reproductive organs. Systemic therapies, such as chemotherapy, can be toxic to ovaries and testicles, affecting fertility or endocrine function (Hudson et al., 2017; Poorvu et al., 2019). Fertility preservation options are more routinely discussed with male patients than with females (Moss et al., 2016; Poorvu et al., 2019). For interested patients, fertility preservation must be completed before treatment begins. Strategies include removing and freezing gametes (eggs for females and sperm for males) and taking steps to reduce the reproductive impact of cancer treatment. When treatment is completed, patients often are anxious to learn about the status of their fertility, making subsequent fertility testing a common practice for both males and females.

Healthcare teams should be aware of, and sensitive to, the medical and social differences between male and female patients when discussing fertility preservation options (Moravek et al., 2023). Advancements in assisted reproductive technologies, such as cryopreservation of gametes prior to the administration of cancer treatment, provide an opportunity for AYA patients with cancer to potentially preserve their fertility (Hudson et al., 2017; Moravek et al., 2019; Quinn et al., 2016); however, fertility preservation is not covered by most insurance companies, making ongoing advocacy efforts critically important.

In a study presented at the 47th Annual ONS Congress®, Bell et al. (2022) detailed fertility preservation barriers encountered at a large care center, including delayed treatment, no time for preservation, lack of provider and clinician knowledge, cost, and lack of fertility network. They worked to have fertility discussions with all AYA patients, implemented a navigator, developed a collaboration with an endocrinologist and fertility specialist, established a consulting service for urgent needs, secured funding and negotiated costs for patients, and developed a best practice alert in the electronic health record for fertility discussions upon entering a new treatment plan (Bell et al., 2022). AYA navigators can implement strategies to help increase fertility preservation for these patients.

ONNs should routinely discuss symptom management strategies with their patients and facilitate referrals to specialized resources as needed (Naz et al., 2023). With the fear of cancer recurrence, ONNs can collaborate with social work and psychology colleagues in providing strategies for managing anxiety, identifying triggers, and accessing complementary therapies (Jones et al., 2020). Connecting with peer support, either online or in person, can help to provide a safe space to discuss fears and shared experiences. For cancer-related fatigue, survivors can participate in free or low-cost customized exercise regimens catered to their individual needs from certified fitness instructors through Livestrong at the YMCA (Kelly et al., 2022). Facilitating referral to a fertility specialist is needed before treatment begins. ONNs can help connect patients with tools to access fertility preservation services in their area, such as the Alliance for Fertility Preservation.

Psychological–Spiritual Aspects

The diagnosis of cancer during adolescence and young adulthood exacerbates an already uncertain developmental period filled with transitions, such as finding employment, dating, and establishing independence. Physiologically, the AYA population is neurologically underdeveloped in several areas, specifically those that control impulses, anticipate consequences, and reconcile emotional responses to environmental stressors (Bradford et al., 2022; Janssen et al., 2023; Turgeman & West, 2023). Psychologically, mental health disorders are most prevalent in young adulthood (Friend et al., 2018; Kaul et al., 2016). Anxiety and depression can affect the quality of life and survival outcomes for AYAs with cancer, such as nonadherence to treatment, increase in physical pain, and higher disease morbidity (Friend et al., 2018; Li et al., 2022).

AYA patients with cancer experience multiple losses, both socially and physically (McLoone et al., 2023; Murphy et al., 2023; Smith et al., 2018):
- Loss of hair
- Loss of muscle mass
- Loss of reproductive capacity
- Changes in relationships with their peers
- Loss of employment
- Difficulties returning to school or employment

AYAs often juxtapose their lives before and after their cancer diagnosis. They describe changes in their identity as they work to develop their "new normal." They identify benefits, such as enhanced meaning, purpose, and gratitude in their lives, and burdens, such as physical distress (Darabos & Ford, 2020). Over time, AYAs tend to focus less on physical manifestations and more on life purpose and personal strengths (Husson et al., 2017; Straehla et al., 2017).

Longitudinal research with AYA patients with cancer suggests they usually experience high levels of distress at the time of diagnosis and at the time of transition to off-treatment survivorship (Beauchemin, Roth, et al., 2023; Kaul et al., 2016). Additionally, it has been noted that this population is at an increased risk of psychiatric conditions, such as anxiety, depression, substance misuse, and suicide, and that implementation of specialized ONNs has been shown to increase connections to psychological support from a social worker, psychologist, or pastor (Kirk et al., 2022). The identified time frames of diagnosis and transitioning to survivorship can be helpful clinical markers for ONNs to offer assistance and support, particularly as AYA patients transition into an off-treatment survivorship phase. Maintenance of school or work during treatment (i.e., to the extent possible when given treatment effects) can help foster normalcy and social reintegration after treatment (Altherr et al., 2023; Ghazal, Merriman, et al., 2021). Building rapport with AYAs early and often in the care trajectory is critical in identifying and addressing mental health and supportive care needs as they may arise, especially prior to transitions in care.

Spirituality is expressed in varying ways depending on cultural practices and religious beliefs. It has the potential to help foster well-being through hope-derived meaning, courageous coping, or self-transcendence (Mack et al., 2023; McNeil, 2016; Taylor et al., 2015). However, spirituality remains understudied among AYAs with cancer, and no AYA-sensitive instruments to measure spirituality exist (Gürsu et al., 2023; Murphy et al., 2023). When supporting AYAs with spiritual or existential questions and struggles, ONNs are recommended to follow therapeutic communication strategies, such as being nondirective, using spiritual perspective terminology, and keeping responses short and focused on the core spiritual perspective theme expressed by patients. Although it is essential to recognize that spirituality is not important to all AYA survivors, both spiritual well-being and struggle have notable associations with adjustment and coping and warrant clinical attention (Park & Cho, 2017).

Relationships

Difficulty in maintaining or forming new social relationships is often highlighted as one of the most important long-term challenges for AYA cancer survivors. Cancer treatment can lead to isolation from friends and family, particularly for AYAs in treatment during their formative developmental years (Cooper et al., 2017; Howden et al., 2022; Poudel et al., 2021). Being socially isolated because of separation from peers and reduced involvement with social activities has been correlated with adverse health and psychological outcomes, including increased sensitivity to everyday stressors, poor physiologic functioning, and a greater propensity for hypertension (Fox et al., 2023). Cancer survivors who consistently scored low on measures of social functioning reported more physical symptoms and higher levels of psychological distress (Husson et al., 2017). Social functioning improvements usually occur within the first year after diagnosis, and, on average, no significant additional improvements occur between 12 and 24 months (Husson et al., 2017).

Connecting with a cancer peer support group may be helpful for some patients because it can afford opportunities to meet peers who also have a cancer diagnosis, thus decreasing loneliness. It may also allow patients to openly share their struggles and cope emotionally with their diagnosis, help others, relate to peers who share similar circumstances, and learn about opportunities for AYAs with cancer (Miller & van der Eijk, 2019; Olsson et al., 2024; Pennant et al., 2019). However, the diversity of ages and social needs across the population creates challenges with the design, recruitment, group composition, and sustainability of peer support services (Brock et al., 2024; Hotchkiss et al., 2023; McDonnell et al., 2020). A Canadian study found that AYAs want peer support and programs that meet their unique needs; however, barriers exist to these wants, including having inconvenient in-person meetups, finding another patient with whom one can connect, and finding specific support programs. Peers could be matched by their type of cancer, specific concerns, and age (Bender et al., 2022). The study found that AYAs are very interested in digital peer support applications, and many also want to give back by becoming trained peer navigators

(Bender et al., 2022). ONNs could assist in developing a recommended application or program and connect patients to it as either a patient or peer navigator.

AYAs worry about how to disclose and discuss their cancer diagnosis. Research examining cancer-related communication among patients with family and peers suggests that communication occurs on a spectrum, with variation in whom information is shared, as well as differences in the frequency of information sharing and the amount and type of information shared (Iannarino, 2018; Janin et al., 2018). Peer reactions and fear of stigma hindered participants' willingness to disclose. Social skills training focusing on communication in close relationships could potentially assist survivors with these issues.

Practical Issues

Patients face a range of practical issues during and after cancer treatment, such as financial hardship (financial toxicity), gaps in health insurance coverage, engagement in health-risk behaviors, and disruptions in school or work that can hinder their daily functioning and worsen their health and psychosocial outcomes (Bashore & Breyer, 2017; Dahl et al., 2019; Ghazal, Gormley, et al., 2021; Salsman et al., 2019). AYAs may even turn to medical crowdfunding to help fund the direct and indirect costs of cancer treatment (Ghazal et al., 2023). A 2021 report contextualized the economic and human costs of cancer in AYAs to be $23.5 billion overall, translating to roughly $259,324 per patient over their lifetime (Parsons et al., 2023). The Adolescent and Young Adult Health Outcomes and Patient Experience (AYA HOPE) study found that 25% of cancer survivors were uninsured at some point in the first 35 months after their diagnosis (Parsons et al., 2014). When compared with insured AYA cancer survivors, those who are uninsured report having limited access to health care and a greater risk of skipping medical care because of cost (Kirchhoff et al., 2016).

Cancer care is expensive at any age or in any phase of life, and health insurance can be complex and confusing to understand and use. However, insurance is critical on a cancer journey, and the responsibility of navigating it often falls on patients, who are also learning to live with and manage their new diagnosis. In general, this population exhibits low health insurance literacy, defined as "the knowledge and application of health insurance concepts" (Waters et al., 2022, p. 4457). AYAs have limited experience with insurance and the healthcare system, as they are often healthy prior to their diagnosis. Health insurance is often a benefit of full-time employment, and these patients may just be starting their careers, limiting their knowledge and experience of what plan to select. Insurance selections and costs can, therefore, cause emotional distress. Most patients have minimal understanding of their health insurance, leading to uncertainty about what is covered and out-of-pocket costs. They are learning through trial and error, and this can negatively influence their ability to navigate the system (Kirchhoff, van Thiel Berghuijs, et al., 2023; Kirchhoff, Waters, et al., 2023; Waters et al., 2022).

Mann et al. (2022) discussed a promising clinical trial to assess the feasibility and acceptability of a navigator providing AYAs with virtual education on health insurance, laws and processes in health care, and how to control costs. An additional aim of their study was to assess the program participants' satisfaction and hopeful improvement in health insurance literacy, thus decreasing the financial burdens and toxicities of cancer treatment. ONNs can assess the financial hardship and health insurance literacy of patients and families and assist them through available education and resources at the institutional or community level.

Returning to work or school and maintaining career and educational goals can be highly challenging for AYA cancer survivors during and after treatment. A diagnosis of cancer during young adulthood can derail career development and future growth opportunities. Risk factors identified for not returning to full-time employment or school after cancer treatment are being uninsured and quitting work completely after diagnosis (Ghazal, Merriman, et al., 2021; Parsons et al., 2012). Important risk factors contributing to beliefs that cancer negatively impacts employment or education plans are higher treatment intensity and not working after being diagnosed (Altherr et al., 2023; Devine et al., 2022). Patients returning to college may struggle with social integration and maintaining cognitive focus. Among career service staff at colleges and universities, most reported that they do not feel adequately trained or aware of the unique needs of AYA cancer survivors (Blanch-Hartigan & Kinel, 2018). ONNs can refer patients needing career and educational (or vocational) support to specialized cancer and career resource agencies, such as Cancer and Careers.

Unhealthy lifestyle behaviors, such as smoking and binge drinking, are common in AYA cancer survivors (Berger, 2018). Several cancer-related factors are essential in identifying survivors at high risk for nonadherence. Female survivors further from diagnosis are more likely to smoke, whereas male survivors may be less physically active over time (Caru et al., 2023). It is critically important to continue providing health behavior support during treatment and throughout survivorship care.

When comparing patient navigation preferences for AYA cancer services by distance to treatment location, more local patients were interested in patient navigation services (95.2%) compared to distant participants (77.8%) (Warner et al., 2018). Fewer local (38.1%) than distant participants (61.1%) reported challenges getting to appointments. Distant patients needed specific financial support for travel (e.g., fuel, lodging). Both local and distant patients desired to connect with ONNs in person at their initial diagnosis and before using another form of communication (Warner et al., 2018).

AYA patients prefer resources that reduce loneliness, create a sense of community or belonging, and provide opportunities to meet other patients (Cheung & Zebrack, 2017). Regarding age-specific patient navigation preferences, all age groups were interested in face-to-face connection with ONNs and using multiple communication platforms (e.g., phone, text, email) for follow-up (Camp et al., 2023; Pannier et al., 2019). Three of the most frequently cited needs were insurance, finances, and information. They differed in support, healthcare, and resource preferences by developmental age; only adolescents preferred educational support (Pannier et al., 2019). Although all groups preferred financial and family support, the specific type of assistance (medical versus living expenses; partner/spouse, child, or parental assistance) varied by age group. All ONNs working with AYAs should be sensitive to and aware of age-specific navigation preferences.

Psychosocial Interventions

Examination of effective transition therapy for AYAs remains limited (Psihogios et al., 2019; Zhang et al., 2022). In an integrative literature review examining effective transition therapy, Masterton and Tariman (2016) identified four studies that empirically examined interventions: dynamic group therapy, an educational cancer retreat, an online cancer forum, and online cognitive behavioral therapy. The five components of potentially successful interventions most referred to across all studies were cancer education, coping, sexual identity, maintaining normalcy, and support. These components should be considered when developing transitional psychosocial programming for AYAs (Masterton & Tariman, 2016; Zhang et al., 2021). ONNs should routinely discuss psychosocial needs and preferences with patients. The intervention components identified should be addressed openly and regularly throughout the care trajectory. ONNs can provide referrals to age-specific and disease-specific supportive care resources for their patients, such as Stupid Cancer, Elephants and Tea, and the Young Survival Coalition (breast cancer in young women).

Adventure programs are another popular supportive care intervention for AYAs. These programs enable patients to rebuild confidence in their bodies, feel empowered, and feel supported by connecting with other cancer survivor peers.
- Young Adult Cancer Camp (https://yacancercamp.org) is a weekend-long adventure camp run by Elephants and Tea and Young Adults Survivors United. It provides the opportunity for a sleepaway-style camp with various indoor and outdoor activities.
- First Descents (www.firstdescents.org), an outdoor adventure program for AYAs aged 18–39 years, has been found to increase self-esteem, improve body image, and reduce alienation and depression (Zebrack et al., 2017). In response to the expressed needs and preferences of AYAs for continued care and support after attending camp programs, First Descents has created local adventure communities (FDtribs) in major cities across the United States to provide opportunities to receive ongoing support and to maintain involvement with survivor peers.
- Camp Koru (www.projectkoru.org/camp-koru) is a multiday adventure camp that enables young adult cancer survivors to find healing and renewal through outdoor experiences in the ocean and mountains.
- Camp Māk-A-Dream (www.campdream.org) was founded in Montana with the mission of providing free experiences in an intimate community setting for individuals and families affected by cancer, as well as children who have a sibling or parent with cancer.

Underrepresented Adolescent and Young Adult Populations

AYAs are an underserved population of cancer survivors, and their vulnerabilities are heightened by additional, or intersectional, identities. Intersectionality helps people to understand how these various intersecting social identities (race, gender, sexuality, disability, class, and others) and systems of oppression shape experiences and cancer care outcomes (Crenshaw, 1991; Damaskos et al., 2018).

Sexual and Gender Minorities

Lesbian, gay, bisexual, transgender, queer, intersex, and asexual (LGBTQIA+, often abbreviated to LGBTQ+), referred to in the literature as sexual and gender minorities, frequently face an increased risk of stigma and bias (Berkman, Choi, et al., 2023; Cheung et al., 2023; Levin et al., 2019). Acts of bias reported among LGBTQ+ AYAs in the healthcare system include not being asked directly about their sexual orientation or gender identity; a lack of LGBTQ+-specific brochures, resources, and educational materials; and providers' lack of training and knowledge on LGBTQ+-specific healthcare needs and concerns (Kamen, 2018). Research examining factors related to diagnosis, identity disclosure, and social support among LGBTQ+ patients with cancer suggests that friends are the most common members of their support teams and that disclosure and support factors are associated with better self-reported health among LGBTQ+ patients (Franco-Rocha et al., 2023; Kamen, 2018). ONNs can help ensure the inclusion of diverse support team members in LGBTQ+ patient care and foster safe environments for disclosure (Kamen et al., 2015). ONNs can gather LGBTQ+-specific brochures, resources, and educational materials and make them readily available by displaying them in clinic spaces. In addition, ONNs can facilitate referrals to identity-focused cancer or AYA peer support organizations, such as Escape and the National LGBT Cancer Network.

People of Color

People of color also experience disparities in cancer care and outcomes, including clinical trial enrollment (Roth et al., 2021; Siembida, Loomans-Kropp, Trivedi, Bleyer, et al., 2020). Promising interventions tailored to engaging the specific needs of this population include fotonovela interventions in Latino AYA cancer survivors (Casillas et al., 2021). Emerging evidence shows the significant impact of gender and culture on people of color, with worse depressive symptoms in Latino males and worse quality of life in Latino patients (Ritt-Olson et al., 2018). Researchers, clinicians, and patient advocates have made a powerful call for antiracist patient engagement to prevent the tokenization of underrepresented voices and experiences in the AYA oncology space (Cheung et al., 2021, 2024).

Adolescents and Young Adults With Disabilities

A 2021 systematic review of the educational and psychosocial needs of AYA patients with intellectual disabilities who have cancer and their family members found the literature lacking (Ní Shé et al., 2021). Family and paid caretakers were found to serve as enablers and gatekeepers for AYA patients with intellectual disabilities in connecting them to support and screening programs. Family members are also vital in supporting patients during procedures, assisting with reporting symptoms, and communicating with the healthcare team; however, patients with intellectual disabilities must also be empowered and involved. Additionally, healthcare workers should be educated on the importance of providing screening, supporting patients during the screening process, and optimally caring for patients in this population. They should also work to decrease anxiety around the processes and optimize the experience. Evidence of specific necessary support for AYA patients with intellectual disabilities is currently lacking. More attention is needed on this population regarding their cancer experience and survivorship, caregiver support, education and collaboration of healthcare workers, and ethical pathways for information disclosures (Ní Shé et al., 2021).

Recommended Supportive Care Resources

Table 17-1 provides AYA-specific supportive care resources that can be used as a starting point to learn more about what is available and where ONNs can refer patients based on the types of assistance and support needed. The resources have

TABLE 17-1. Recommended Supportive Care Resources for Adolescents and Young Adults With Cancer

Resource	Website	Type of Support
Alliance for Fertility Preservation	www.allianceforfertilitypreservation.org	General information, financial assistance
American Cancer Society	www.cancer.org/cancer/types/cancer-in-young-adults.html	General information, financial assistance, emotional support; provides 24/7 phone hotline with cancer information specialists: 800-227-2345
Cactus Cancer Society (previously Lacuna Loft)	www.cactuscancer.org	Psychosocial support (writing groups and creative arts)
Cancer and Careers	www.cancerandcareers.org	General information (work-related resources)
CancerCare	www.cancercare.org	General information, financial assistance, emotional support
Elephants and Tea	www.elephantsandtea.com	Psychosocial support (writing workshops)
Escape	www.escapeayac.org	Psychosocial support (resources for LGBTQ+ adolescent and young adult cancer survivors)

(Continued on next page)

TABLE 17-1. Recommended Supportive Care Resources for Adolescents and Young Adults With Cancer *(Continued)*

Resource	Website	Type of Support
Expect Miracles Foundation (previously The Samfund)	www.expectmiraclesfoundation.org	General information, financial assistance
First Descents	www.firstdescents.org	Emotional support
Leukemia and Lymphoma Society	www.lls.org	General information, financial assistance, psychosocial support
Livestrong at the YMCA	www.livestrong.org/how-we-help/livestrong-at-the-ymca	Emotional support, psychosocial support
Livestrong Fertility	www.livestrong.org/what-we-do/program/fertility	General information, financial assistance
Livestrong Guidebook	www.livestrong.org/livestrong-guidebook	General information
Livestrong Resources	www.livestrong.org/resources	General information, financial assistance, emotional support
National Cancer Institute	www.cancer.gov/types/aya	General information, financial assistance, emotional support
National LGBT Cancer Network	www.cancer-network.org	General information, emotional support, psychosocial support LGBTQ+ adolescent and young adults with cancer
Patient Advocate Foundation	www.copays.org	General information, financial assistance
Stupid Cancer	www.stupidcancer.org	General information, financial assistance, emotional support
Triage Cancer	www.triagecancer.org	General information, financial assistance (legal and financial navigation), emotional support (by location and topic)
Ulman Foundation	www.ulmanfoundation.org	General information, financial assistance, emotional support
Young Adults Survivors United	www.yasurvivors.org	General information, financial assistance, emotional support, psychosocial support
Young Survival Coalition (for young adults with breast cancer)	www.youngsurvival.org	General information, emotional support, psychosocial support

been tagged with the top four patient navigation needs identified by AYAs: general information, financial assistance, emotional support, and psychosocial support. As resources change frequently and new resources are always becoming available, agencies should be contacted directly for case-specific assistance and questions.

Summary

Pediatric and AYA patients with cancer face unique issues across the key domains of cancer survivorship, including medical care, side effects and symptoms, psychological and spiritual aspects, relationships, and practical issues. ONNs must be familiar with these issues and routinely discuss supportive care needs and symptom management strategies with their patients. ONNs can conduct routine comprehensive assessments to identify their patients' barriers and help facilitate referral to age-appropriate resources. They can be integral in supporting AYA patients and families throughout the care trajectory.

The authors would like to acknowledge Casey Walsh, PhD, LICSW, and Bradley Zebrack, PhD, MSW, MPH, FAPOS, for their contribution to this chapter that remains unchanged from the previous edition of this book.

References

Adams, S.C., Herman, J., Lega, I.C., Mitchell, L., Hodgson, D., Edelstein, K., ... Gupta, A.A. (2021). Young adult cancer survivorship: Recommendations for patient follow-up, exercise therapy, and research. *JNCI Cancer Spectrum, 5*(1), pkaa099. https://doi.org/10.1093/jncics/pkaa099

Adjei Boakye, E., Polednik, K.M., Deshields, T.L., Sharma, A., Molina, Y., Schapira, L., ... Osazuwa-Peters, N. (2022). Emotional distress among survivors of adolescent and young adult cancer or adult cancer. *Annals of Epidemiology, 72*, 48–56. https://doi.org/10.1016/j.annepidem.2022.03.014

Altherr, A., Bolliger, C., Kaufmann, M., Dyntar, D., Scheinemann, K., Michel, G., ... Roser, K. (2023). Education, employment, and financial outcomes in adolescent and young adult cancer survivors— A systematic review. *Current Oncology, 30*(10), 8720–8762. https://doi.org/10.3390/curroncol 30100631

American Cancer Society. (2020). *Cancer facts and figures 2020.* https://www.cancer.org/content/dam /cancer-org/research/cancer-facts-and-statistics/annual-cancer-facts-and-figures/2020/cancer-facts -and-figures-2020.pdf

Anderson, C., Smitherman, A.B., Meernik, C., Edwards, T.P., Deal, A.M., Cannizzaro, N., ... Nichols, H.B. (2019). Patient/provider discussions about clinical trial participation and reasons for nonparticipation among adolescent and young adult women with cancer. *Journal of Adolescent and Young Adult Oncology, 9*(1), 41–46. https://doi.org/10.1089/jayao.2019.0078

Avery, J., Wong, E., Harris, C., Chapman, S., Uppal, S., Shanawaz, S., ... Gupta, A.A. (2022). The transformation of adolescent and young adult oncological and supportive care in Canada: A mixed methods study. *Current Oncology, 29*(7), 5126–5138. https://doi.org/10.3390/curroncol29070406

Barr, R.D., Ferrari, A., Ries, L., Whelan, J., & Bleyer, W.A. (2016). Cancer in adolescents and young adults: A narrative review of the current status and a view of the future. *JAMA Pediatrics, 170*(5), 495–501. https://doi.org/10.1001/jamapediatrics.2015.4689

Bashore, L., & Breyer, E. (2017). Educational and career goal attainments in young adult childhood cancer survivors. *Journal for Specialists in Pediatric Nursing, 22*(2), e12180. https://doi.org/10.1111/jspn.12180

Beauchemin, M.P., Ji, L., Williams, A., Nightingale, C.L., Wolfson, J.A., Salsman, J.M., ... Parsons, S.K. (2023). Comprehensive cancer-related resources for adolescents and young adults (AYAs) treated in the community setting: 2022 landscape survey results. *JCO Oncology Practice, 19*(11, Suppl.), 151. https://doi.org/10.1200/OP.2023.19.11_suppl.151

Beauchemin, M.P., Ji, L., Williams, A.M., Nightingale, C.L., Dressler, E.V., Salsman, J.M., ... Parsons, S.K. (2024). Defining practice capacity for cancer care delivery to adolescents and young adults in the community setting: 2022 Landscape assessment results. *Journal of Adolescent and Young Adult Oncology, 13*(3), 557–563. https://doi.org/10.1089/jayao.2023.0177

Beauchemin, M.P., Roth, M.E., & Parsons, S.K. (2023). Reducing adolescent and young adult cancer outcome disparities through optimized care delivery: A blueprint from the Children's Oncology Group. *Journal of Adolescent and Young Adult Oncology, 12*(3), 314–323. https://doi.org/10.1089/jayao.2022.0136

Bell, D.H., McKenzie, L., Yarbrough, A., Harris, J., Zwhalen, M., Roth, M., ... Livingston, J. (2022, April 27–May 1). Eliminating barriers to fertility discussions in AYA oncology [Conference presentation]. Oncology Nursing Society 47th Congress, Anaheim, CA, United States. https://ons.confex.com/ons/2022/meetingapp.cgi/Paper/10964

Bender, J.L., Puri, N., Salih, S., D'Agostino, N.M., Tsimicalis, A., Howard, A.F., ... Gupta, A.A. (2022). Peer support needs and preferences for digital peer navigation among adolescent and young adults with cancer: A Canadian cross-sectional survey. *Current Oncology, 29*(2), 1163–1175. https://doi.org/10.3390/curroncol29020099

Berger, N.A. (2018). Young adult cancer: Influence of the obesity pandemic. *Obesity, 26*(4), 641–650. https://doi.org/10.1002/oby.22137

Berkman, A.M., Choi, E., Cheung, C.K., Salsman, J.M., Peterson, S.K., Andersen, C.R., ... Roth, M.E. (2023). Risk of chronic health conditions in lesbian, gay, and bisexual survivors of adolescent and young adult cancers. *Cancer, 130*(4), 553–562. https://doi.org/10.1002/cncr.35015

Berkman, A.M., Mittal, N., & Roth, M.E. (2023). Adolescent and young adult cancers: Unmet needs and closing the gaps. *Current Opinion in Pediatrics, 35*(1), 84–90. https://doi.org/10.1097/MOP.0000000000001200

Blanch-Hartigan, D., & Kinel, J. (2018). Addressing career-related needs in adolescent and young adult cancer survivors: University career service professionals' experience and resources. *Journal of Adolescent and Young Adult Oncology, 7*(2), 245–248. https://doi.org/10.1089/jayao.2017.0064

Bleyer, A. (2023). Increasing cancer in adolescents and young adults: Cancer types and causation implications. *Journal of Adolescent and Young Adult Oncology, 12*(3), 285–296. https://doi.org/10.1089/jayao.2022.0134

Bradford, N.K., & Chan, R.J. (2017). Health promotion and psychological interventions for adolescent and young adult cancer survivors: A systematic literature review. *Cancer Treatment Reviews, 55*, 57–70. https://doi.org/10.1016/j.ctrv.2017.02.011

Bradford, N.K., McDonald, F.E.J., Bibby, H., Kok, C., & Patterson, P. (2022). Psychological, functional and social outcomes in adolescent and young adult cancer survivors over time: A systematic review of longitudinal studies. *Psycho-Oncology, 31*(9), 1448–1458. https://doi.org/10.1002/pon.5987

Brock, H., Dwinger, S., Bergelt, C., Sender, A., Geue, K., Mehnert-Theuerkauf, A., & Richter, D. (2024). Peer2Me—Evaluation of a peer supported program for adolescent and young adult (AYA) cancer patients: Study protocol of a randomised trial using a comprehensive cohort design. *BMC Cancer, 24*(1), 788. https://doi.org/10.1186/s12885-024-12547-5

Camp, L., Coffman, E., Chinthapatla, J., Boey, K.A., Lux, L., Smitherman, A., ... Valle, C.G. (2023). Active treatment to survivorship care: A mixed-methods study exploring resource needs and preferences of young adult cancer survivors in transition. *Journal of Adolescent and Young Adult Oncology, 12*(5), 735–743. https://doi.org/10.1089/jayao.2022.0095

Caru, M., Wurz, A., Brunet, J., Barb, E.D., Adams, S.C., Roth, M.E., ... Schmitz, K.H. (2023). Physical activity and physical fitness assessments in adolescents and young adults diagnosed with cancer: A scoping review. *Supportive Care in Cancer, 31*(10), 569. https://doi.org/10.1007/s00520-023-08008-7

Casillas, J.N., Schwartz, L.F., Crespi, C.M., Ganz, P.A., Kahn, K.L., Stuber, M.L., ... Estrin, D.L. (2019). The use of mobile technology and peer navigation to promote adolescent and young adult (AYA) cancer survivorship care: Results of a randomized controlled trial. *Journal of Cancer Survivorship, 13*(4), 580–592. https://doi.org/10.1007/s11764-019-00777-7

Casillas, J.N., Schwartz, L.F., Gildner, J.L., Crespi, C.M., Ganz, P.A., Kahn, K.L., ... Barboa, E. (2021). Engaging Latino adolescent and young adult (AYA) cancer survivors in their care: Piloting a photonovela intervention. *Journal of Cancer Education, 36*(5), 971–980. https://doi.org/10.1007/s13187-020-01724-2

Cheung, C.K., Lee, H., Levin, N.J., Choi, E., Ross, V.A., Geng, Y., ... Roth, M.E. (2023). Disparities in cancer care among sexual and gender minority adolescent and young adult patients: A scoping review. *Cancer Medicine, 12*(13), 14674–14693. https://doi.org/10.1002/cam4.6090

Cheung, C.K., Miller, K.A., Goings, T.C., Thomas, B.N., Lee, H., Brandon, R.E., ... Tucker-Seeley, R.D. (2024). BIPOC experiences of (anti-)racist patient engagement in adolescent and young adult oncology research: An electronic Delphi study. *Future Oncology, 20*(9), 547–561. https://doi.org/10.2217/fon-2023-0771

Cheung, C.K., Tucker-Seeley, R., Davies, S., Gilman, M., Miller, K.A., Lopes, G., ... Lewis, M.A. (2021). A call to action: Antiracist patient engagement in adolescent and young adult oncology research and advocacy. *Future Oncology, 17*(28), 3743–3756. https://doi.org/10.2217/fon-2020-1213

Cheung, C.K., & Zebrack, B. (2017). What do adolescents and young adults want from cancer resources? Insights from a Delphi panel of AYA patients. *Supportive Care in Cancer, 25*(1), 119–126. https://doi.org/10.1007/s00520-016-3396-7

Cooper, T.M., Sison, E.A.R., Baker, S.D., Li, L., Ahmed, A., Trippett, T., ... Brown, P.A. (2017). A phase 1 study of the CXCR4 antagonist plerixafor in combination with high-dose cytarabine and etoposide in children with relapsed or refractory acute leukemias or myelodysplastic syndrome: A Pediatric Oncology Experimental Therapeutics Investigators' Consortium study (POE 10-03). *Pediatric Blood and Cancer, 64*(8), e26414. https://doi.org/10.1002/pbc.26414

Cox, K.H, Morgan, J., & Russo, C. (2021). Using a non-clinical patient navigator program in a pediatric oncology network. *Journal of Oncology Navigation and Survivorship, 12*(3). https://www.jons-online.com/issues/2021/march-2021-vol-12-no-3/3646-using-a-nonclinical-patient-navigator-program-in-a-pediatric-oncology-network

Crenshaw, K. (1991). Demarginalizing the intersection of race and sex: A black feminist critique of antidiscrimination doctrine, feminist theory, and antiracist politics. In *University of Chicago Legal Forum* (Vol. 1989, Issue 1, article 8). http://chicagounbound.uchicago.edu/uclf/vol1989/iss1/8

Dahl, A.A., Fosså, S.D., Lie, H.C., Loge, J.H., Reinertsen, K.V., Ruud, E., & Kiserud, C.E. (2019). Employment status and work ability in long-term young adult cancer survivors. *Journal of Adolescent and Young Adult Oncology, 8*(3), 304–311. https://doi.org/10.1089/jayao.2018.0109

Damaskos, P., Amaya, B., Gordon, R., & Walters, C.B. (2018). Intersectionality and the LGBT cancer patient. *Seminars in Oncology Nursing, 34*(1), 30–36. https://doi.org/10.1016/j.soncn.2017.11.004

Daniel, L.C., Aggarwal, R., & Schwartz, L.A. (2017). Sleep in adolescents and young adults in the year after cancer treatment. *Journal of Adolescent and Young Adult Oncology, 6*(4), 560–567. https://doi.org/10.1089/jayao.2017.0006

Darabos, K., & Ford, J.S. (2020). "Basically, you had cancer and now you don't": Exploring the meaning of being a "cancer survivor" among adolescents and young adult cancer survivors. *Journal of Adolescent and Young Adult Oncology, 9*(4), 534–539. https://doi.org/10.1089/jayao.2019.0176

Devine, K.A., Christen, S., Mulder, R.L., Brown, M.C., Ingerski, L.M., Mader, L., ... Schulte, F.S.M. (2022). Recommendations for the surveillance of education and employment outcomes in survivors of childhood, adolescent, and young adult cancer: A report from the International Late Effects of Childhood

Cancer Guideline Harmonization Group. *Cancer, 128*(13), 2405–2419. https://doi.org/10.1002/cncr.34215

Docherty, S.L., Kayle, M., Maslow, G.R., & Santacroce, S.J. (2015). The adolescent and young adult with cancer: A developmental life course perspective. *Seminars in Oncology Nursing, 31*(3), 186–196. https://doi.org/10.1016/j.soncn.2015.05.006

Dorfman, C.S., Shelby, R.A., Stalls, J.M., Somers, T.J., Keefe, F.J., Vilardaga, J.P., ... Oeffinger, K.C. (2023). Improving symptom management for survivors of young adult cancer: Development of a novel intervention. *Journal of Adolescent and Young Adult Oncology, 12*(4), 472–487. https://doi.org/10.1089/jayao.2022.0100

Ehrhardt, M.J., Leerink, J.M., Mulder, R.L., Mavinkurve-Groothuis, A., Kok, W., Nohria, A., ... Armenian, S.H. (2023). Systematic review and updated recommendations for cardiomyopathy surveillance for survivors of childhood, adolescent, and young adult cancer from the International Late Effects of Childhood Cancer Guideline Harmonization Group. *Lancet Oncology, 24*(3), E108–E120. https://doi.org/10.1016/S1470-2045(23)00012-8

Fox, R.S., Armstrong, G.E., Gaumond, J.S., Vigoureux, T.F.D., Miller, C.H., Sanford, S.D., ... Oswald, L.B. (2023). Social isolation and social connectedness among young adult cancer survivors: A systematic review. *Cancer, 129*(19), 2946–2965. https://doi.org/10.1002/cncr.34934

Fox, R.S., Fowler, B., Carrera, J.B., Reichek, J., & Sanford, S.D. (2022). Increasing access to psychosocial care for adolescents and young adults with cancer by integrating targeted navigation services. *Psycho-Oncology, 31*(5), 856–859. https://doi.org/10.1002/pon.5916

Fox, R.S., Torres, T.K., Badger, T.A., Katsanis, E., Yang, D., Sanford, S.D., ... Oswald. L.B. (2024). Delivering a group-based quality of life intervention to young adult cancer survivors via a web platform: Feasibility trial. *JMIR Cancer, 10,* e58014. https://doi.org/10.2196/58014

Franco-Rocha, O.Y., Wheldon, C.W., Osier, N., Lett, E., Kesler, S.R., Henneghan, A.M., & Suárez-Baquero, D.F.M. (2023). Cisheteronormativity and its influence on the psychosocial experience of LGBTQ+ people with cancer: A qualitative systematic review. *Psycho-Oncology, 32*(6), 834–845. https://doi.org/10.1002/pon.6133

Friend, A.J., Feltbower, R.G., Hughes, E.J., Dye, K.P., & Glaser, A.W. (2018). Mental health of long-term survivors of childhood and young adult cancer: A systematic review. *International Journal of Cancer, 143*(6), 1279–1286. https://doi.org/10.1002/ijc.31337

Ghazal, L.V., Gormley, M., Merriman, J.D., & Santacroce, S.J. (2021). Financial toxicity in adolescents and young adults with cancer: A concept analysis. *Cancer Nursing, 44*(6), E636–E651. https://doi.org/10.1097/NCC.0000000000000972

Ghazal, L.V., Merriman, J., Santacroce, S.J., & Dickson, V.V. (2021). Survivors' dilemma: Young adult cancer survivors' perspectives of work-related goals. *Workplace Health and Safety, 69*(11), 506–516. https://doi.org/10.1177/21650799211012675

Ghazal, L.V., Watson, S.E., Gentry, B., & Santacroce, S.J. (2023). "Both a life saver and totally shameful": Young adult cancer survivors' perceptions of medical crowdfunding. *Journal of Cancer Survivorship, 17*(2), 332–341. https://doi.org/10.1007/s11764-022-01188-x

Gürsu, O., Gürcan, M., & Turan, S.A. (2023). Rebuilding and guiding the self with spirituality: A grounded theory of experiences of adolescents and young adults with cancer. *Oncology Nursing Forum, 50*(4), 487–497. https://doi.org/10.1188/23.ONF.487-497

Haines, E., Asad, S., Lux, L., Gan, H., Noskoff, K., Kumar, B., ... Birken, S. (2022). Guidance to support the implementation of specialized adolescent and young adult cancer care: A qualitative analysis of cancer programs. *JCO Oncology Practice, 18*(9), e1513–e1521. https://doi.org/10.1200/OP.22.00063

Hotchkiss, M.E., Ahmad, Z.N., & Ford, J.S. (2023). Cancer–peer connection in the context of adolescent and young adult cancer: A qualitative exploration. *Journal of Adolescent and Young Adult Oncology, 12*(1), 83–92. https://doi.org/10.1089/jayao.2021.0170

Howden, K., Yan, A.P., Glidden, C., Romanescu, R.G., Scott, I., Deleemans, J.M., ... Oberoi, S. (2022). Loneliness among adolescents and young adults with cancer during the COVID-19 pandemic: A cross-sectional survey. *Supportive Care in Cancer, 30*(3), 2215–2224. https://doi.org/10.1007/s00520-021-06628-5

Hudson, J.N., Stanley, N.B., Nahata, L., Bowman-Curci, M., & Quinn, G.P. (2017). New promising strategies in oncofertility. *Expert Review of Quality of Life in Cancer Care, 2*(2), 67–78. https://doi.org/10.1080/23809000.2017.1308808

Hudson, M.M., Bhatia, S., Casillas, J., & Landier, W. (2021). Long-term follow-up care for childhood, adolescent, and young adult cancer survivors. *Pediatrics, 148*(3), e2021053127. https://doi.org/10.1542/peds.2021-053127

Husson, O., Zebrack, B., Block, R., Embry, L., Aguilar, C., Hayes-Lattin, B., & Cole, S. (2017). Posttraumatic growth and well-being among adolescents and young adults (AYAs) with cancer: A longitudinal study. *Supportive Care in Cancer, 25*(9), 2881–2890. https://doi.org/10.1007/s00520-017-3707-7

Iannarino, N.T. (2018). "It's my job now, I guess": Biographical disruption and communication work in supporters of young adult cancer survivors. *Communication Monographs, 85*(4), 491–514. https://doi.org/10.1080/03637751.2018.1468916

Isenalumhe, L.L., Fridgen, O., Beaupin, L.K., Quinn, G.P., & Reed, D.R. (2016). Disparities in adolescents and young adults with cancer. *Cancer Control, 23*(4), 424–433. https://doi.org/10.1177/107327481602300414

Janardan, S.K., & Wechsler, D.S. (2021). Caught in the in-between: Challenges in treating adolescents and young adults with cancer. *JCO Oncology Practice, 17*(6), 299–301. https://doi.org/10.1200/OP.21.00178

Janin, M.M.H., Ellis, S.J., Wakefield, C.E., & Fardell, J.E. (2018). Talking about cancer among adolescent and young adult cancer patients and survivors: A systematic review. *Journal of Adolescent and Young Adult Oncology, 7*(5), 515–524. https://doi.org/10.1089/jayao.2017.0131

Janssen, S.H.M., Vlooswijk, C., Manten-Horst, E., Sleeman, S.H.E., Bijlsma, R.M., Kaal, S.E.J., ... Husson, O. (2023). Learning from long-term adolescent and young adult (AYA) cancer survivors regarding their age-specific care needs to improve current AYA care programs. *Cancer Medicine, 12*(12), 13712–13731. https://doi.org/10.1002/cam4.6001

Jones, J.M., Fitch, M., Bongard, J., Maganti, M., Gupta, A., D'Agostino, N., & Korenblum, C. (2020). The needs and experiences of post-treatment adolescent and young adult cancer survivors. *Journal of Clinical Medicine, 9*(5), 1444. https://doi.org/10.3390/jcm9051444

Kaal, S.E.J., Prins, J.B., Jansen, R., Manten-Horst, E., Servaes, P., van der Graaf, W.T.A., & Husson, O. (2018). Health-related quality of life priorities in adolescents and young adults (AYA) with cancer: Discrepancies with health care professionals' perceptions. *Annals of Oncology, 29*(Suppl. 8), viii630. https://doi.org/10.1093/annonc/mdy300.085

Kamen, C. (2018). Lesbian, gay, bisexual, and transgender (LGBT) survivorship. *Seminars in Oncology Nursing, 34*(1), 52–59. https://doi.org/10.1016/j.soncn.2017.12.002

Kamen, C.S., Smith-Stoner, M., Heckler, C.E., Flannery, M., & Margolies, L. (2015). Social support, self-rated health, and lesbian, gay, bisexual, and transgender identity disclosure to cancer care providers. *Oncology Nursing Forum, 42*(1), 44–51. https://doi.org/10.1188/15.ONF.44-51

Kaul, S., Avila, J.C., Mutambudzi, M., Russell, H., Kirchhoff, A.C., & Schwartz, C.L. (2016). Mental distress and health care use among survivors of adolescent and young adult cancer: A cross-sectional analysis of the National Health Interview Survey. *Cancer, 123*(5), 869–878. https://doi.org/10.1002/cncr.30417

Keegan, T.H.M., Abrahão, R., & Alvarez, E.M. (2023). Survival trends among adolescents and young adults diagnosed with cancer in the United States: Comparisons with children and older adults. *Journal of Clinical Oncology, 42*(6), 630–641. https://doi.org/10.1200/JCO.23.01367

Kelly, D., Campbell, P., Torrens, B., Charalambous, A., Ostlund, U., Eicher, M., ... Wells, M. (2022). The effectiveness of nurse-led interventions for cancer symptom management 2000–2018: A systematic review and meta-analysis. *Health Sciences Review, 4,* 100052. https://doi.org/10.1016/j.hsr.2022.100052

Kirchhoff, A.C., Kaul, S., Fluchel, M., Parmeter, C.F., & Spraker, H.L. (2016). Healthcare utilization and quality among survivors of adolescent and young adult cancer [Abstract]. *Journal of Clinical Oncology, 34*(3, Suppl.), 21. https://doi.org/10.1200/jco.2016.34.3_suppl.21

Kirchhoff, A.C., van Thiel Berghuijs, K.M., Waters, A.R., Kaddas, H.K., Warner, E.L., Vaca Lopez, P.L., ... Park, E.R. (2023). Health insurance literacy improvements among recently diagnosed adolescents and young adults with cancer: Results from a pilot randomized controlled trial. *JCO Oncology Practice, 20*(1), 93–101. https://doi.org/10.1200/OP.23.00171

Kirchhoff, A.C., Waters, A.R., Chevrier, A., & Wolfson, J.A. (2023). Access to care for adolescent and young adults with cancer in the United States: State of the literature. *Journal of Clinical Oncology, 42*(6), 642–652. https://doi.org/10.1200/JCO.23.01027

Kirk, J., Jespersen, J., & McKillop, S. (2022). Early psychosocial contact for adolescents and young adults (AYAs) with cancer: The impact of the AYA oncology navigator. *Journal of Adolescent and Young Adult Oncology, 11*(2), 240–244. https://doi.org/10.1089/jayao.2021.0036

Koh, B., Tan, D.J.H., Ng, C.H., Fu, C.E., Lim, W.H., Zeng, R.W., ... Huang, D.Q. (2023). Patterns in cancer incidence among people younger than 50 years in the US, 2010 to 2019. *JAMA Network Open, 6*(8), e2328171. https://doi.org/10.1001/jamanetworkopen.2023.28171

LaRosa, K.N., Stern, M., Bleck, J., Lynn, C., Hudson, J., Reed, D.R., ... Donovan, K.A. (2017). Adolescent and young adult patients with cancer: Perceptions of care. *Journal of Adolescent and Young Adult Oncology, 6*(4), 512–518. https://doi.org/10.1089/jayao.2017.0012

LaRosa, K.N., Stern, M., Lynn, C., Hudson, J., Reed, D.R., Donovan, K.A., & Quinn, G.P. (2019). Provider perceptions' of a patient navigator for adolescents and young adults with cancer. *Supportive Care in Cancer, 27*(11), 4091–4098. https://doi.org/10.1007/s00520-019-04687-3

Leerink, J.M., & Feijen, E.A.M. (2024). Secondary prevention of anthracycline cardiotoxicity in childhood cancer survivors. *Lancet Oncology, 25*(2), 154–156. https://doi.org/10.1016/S1470-2045(24)00001-9

Levin, N.J., Zebrack, B., & Cole, S.W. (2019). Psychosocial issues for adolescent and young adult cancer patients in a global context: A forward-looking approach. *Pediatric Blood and Cancer, 66*(8), e27789. https://doi.org/10.1001/jamapediatrics.2015.4689

Li, W., Xu, Y., Luo, X., Wen, Y., Ding, K., Xu, W., ... Sun, H. (2022). Alleviating excessive worries improves co-occurring depression and pain in adolescent and young adult cancer patients: A network approach. *Neuropsychiatric Disease and Treatment, 18,* 1843–1854. https://doi.org/10.2147/NDT.S376408

Liu, L., Moke, D.J., Tsai, K.-Y., Hwang, A., Freyer, D.R., Hamilton, A.S., ... Deapen, D. (2018). A reappraisal of sex-specific cancer survival trends among adolescents and young adults in the United States. *Journal of the National Cancer Institute, 111*(5), 509–518. https://doi.org/10.1093/jnci/djy140

Mack, J.W., Cernik, C., Uno, H., Laurent, C.A., Fisher, L., Xu, L., ... Kushi, L. (2023). Quality of end-of-life care among adolescents and young adults with cancer. *Journal of Clinical Oncology, 14*(6), 621–629. https://doi.org/10.1200/JCO.23.01272

Mann, K., Waters, A.R., Park, E.R., Perez, G.K., Vaca Lopez, P.L., Kaddas, H.K., ... Kirchhoff, A.C. (2022). HIAYA CHAT study protocol: A randomized controlled trial of a health insurance education intervention for newly diagnosed adolescent and young adult cancer patients. *Trials, 23*(1), 682. https://doi.org/10.1186/s13063-022-06590-5

Marshall, S., Grinyer, A., & Limmer, M. (2018). The experience of adolescents and young adults treated for cancer in an adult setting: A review of the literature. *Journal of Adolescent and Young Adult Oncology, 7*(3), 283–291. https://doi.org/10.1089/jayao.2017.0123

Masterton, K.J., & Tariman, J.D. (2016). Effective transitional therapy for adolescent and young adult patients with cancer: An integrative literature review. *Clinical Journal of Oncology Nursing, 20*(4), 391–396. https://doi.org/10.1188/16.CJON.391-396

McDonnell, G.A., Shuk, E., & Ford, J.S. (2020). A qualitative study of adolescent and young adult cancer survivors' perceptions of family and peer support. *Journal of Health Psychology, 25*(5), 713–726. https://doi.org/10.1177/1359105318769366

McLoone, J.K., Sansom-Daly, U.M., Paglia, A., Chia, J., Larsen, H.B., Fern, L.A., ... Signorelli, C. (2023). A scoping review exploring access to survivorship care for childhood, adolescent, and young adult cancer survivors: How can we optimize care pathways? *Adolescent Health, Medicine and Therapeutics, 14,* 153–174. https://doi.org/10.2147/AHMT.S428215

McNeil, S.B. (2016). Spirituality in adolescents and young adults with cancer: A review of literature. *Journal of Pediatric Hematology/Oncology Nursing, 33*(1), 55–63. https://doi.org/10.1177/1043454214564397

Miller, C., & van der Eijk, M. (2019). The benefits of peer connection for adolescent and young adult oncology patients. *Journal of Oncology Navigation and Survivorship, 10*(11). https://www.jons-online.com/issues/2019/november-2019-vol-10-no-11/2635-the-benefits-of-peer-connection-for-adolescent-and-young-adult-oncology-patients

Miller, K.D., Fidler-Benaoudia, M., Keegan, T.H., Hipp, H.S., Jemal, A., & Siegel, R.L. (2020). Cancer statistics for adolescents and young adults, 2020. *CA: A Cancer Journal for Clinicians, 70*(6), 443–459. https://doi.org/10.3322/caac.21637

Mitchell, L., Tam, S., Lewin, J., Srikanthan, A., Heck, C., Hodgson, D., ... Gupta, A. (2018). Measuring the impact of an adolescent and young adult program on addressing patient care needs. *Journal of Adolescent and Young Adult Oncology, 7*(5), 612–617. https://doi.org/10.1089/jayao.2018.0015

Moravek, M.B., Appiah, L.C., Anazodo, A., Burns, K.C., Gomez-Lobo, V., Hoefgen, H.R., ... Nahata, L. (2019). Development of a pediatric fertility preservation program: A report from the Pediatric Initiative Network of the Oncofertility Consortium. *Journal of Adolescent Health, 64*(5), 563–573. https://doi.org/10.1016/j.jadohealth.2018.10.297

Moravek, M.B., Pavone, M.E., Burns, K., Kashanian, J.A., Anderson, R.A., Klosky, J.L., ... Meacham, L.R. (2023). Fertility assessment and treatment in adolescent and young adult cancer survivors. *Pediatric Blood and Cancer, 70*(Suppl. 5), e28854. https://doi.org/10.1002/pbc.28854

Moss, J.L., Choi, A.W., Keeter, M.K.F., & Brannigan, R.E. (2016). Male adolescent fertility preservation. *Fertility and Sterility, 105*(2), 267–273. https://doi.org/10.1016/j.fertnstert.2015.12.002

Murphy, K.M., Siembida, E., Lau, N., Berkman, A., Roth, M., & Salsman, J.M. (2023). A systematic review of health-related quality of life outcomes in psychosocial intervention trials for adolescent and young adult cancer survivors. *Critical Reviews in Oncology/Hematology, 188*, 104045. https://doi.org/10.1016/j.critrevonc.2023.104045

National Cancer Institute. (2023). *Cancer stat facts: Cancer among adolescents and young adults (AYAs) (ages 15–39)*. https://seer.cancer.gov/statfacts/html/aya.html

National Cancer Institute. (2024). *Adolescents and young adults with cancer*. https://www.cancer.gov/types/ayaSpacing

Naz, H., Apesoa-Varano, E.C., Romero, C., Keegan, T., Malogolowkin, M., Callas, C., ... Alvarez, E. (2023). How do adolescent and young adult patients with cancer manage their chemotherapy-related symptoms at home? *Journal of Adolescent and Young Adult Oncology, 12*(6), 923–928. https://doi.org/10.1089/jayao.2022.0153

Ní Shé, É., McDonald, F.E.J., Mimmo, L., Ross, X.S., Newman, B., Patterson, P., & Harrison, R. (2021). What are the psycho-social and information needs of adolescents and young adults cancer care consumers with intellectual disability? A systematic review of evidence with recommendations for future research and practice. *Children, 8*(12), 1118. https://doi.org/10.3390/children8121118

Nowe, E., Stöbel-Richter, Y., Sender, A., Leuteritz, K., Friedrich, M., & Geue, K. (2017). Cancer-related fatigue in adolescents and young adults: A systematic review of the literature. *Critical Reviews in Oncology/Hematology, 118*, 63–69. https://doi.org/10.1016/j.critrevonc.2017.08.004

Olsson, M., Eliasson, I., Kautsky, S., Hård af Segerstad, Y., & Nilsson, S. (2024). Co-creation of a digital platform for peer support in a community of adolescent and young adult patients during and after cancer. *European Journal of Oncology Nursing, 70*, 102589. https://doi.org/10.1016/j.ejon.2024.102589

Osmani, V., Hörner, L., Klug, S.J., & Tanaka, L.F. (2023). Prevalence and risk of psychological distress, anxiety and depression in adolescent and young adult (AYA) cancer survivors: A systematic review and meta-analysis. *Cancer Medicine, 12*(17), 18354–18367. https://doi.org/10.1002/cam4.6435

Pannier, S.T., Warner, E.L., Fowler, B., Fair, D., Salmon, S.K., & Kirchhoff, A.C. (2019). Age-specific patient navigation preferences among adolescents and young adults with cancer. *Journal of Cancer Education, 34*(2), 242–251. https://doi.org/10.1007/s13187-017-1294-4

Park, C.L., & Cho, D. (2017). Spiritual well-being and spiritual distress predict adjustment in adolescent and young adult cancer survivors. *Psycho-Oncology, 26*(9), 1293–1300. https://doi.org/10.1002/pon.4145

Parsons, H.M., Harlan, L.C., Lynch, C.F., Hamilton, A.S., Wu, X.-C., Kato, I., ... Keegan, T.H.M. (2012). Impact of cancer on work and education among adolescent and young adult cancer survivors. *Journal of Clinical Oncology, 30*(19), 2393–2400. https://doi.org/10.1200/JCO.2011.39.6333

Parsons, H.M., Schmidt, S., Harlan, L.C., Kent, E.E., Lynch, C.F., Smith, A.W., & Keegan, T.H.M. (2014). Young and uninsured: Insurance patterns of recently diagnosed adolescent and young adult cancer survivors in the AYA HOPE study. *Cancer, 120*(15), 2352–2360. https://doi.org/10.1002/cncr.28685

Parsons, S.K., Keegan, T.H.M., Kirchhoff, A.C., Parsons, H.M., Yabroff, K.R., & Davies, S.J. (2023). Cost of cancer in adolescents and young adults in the United States: Results of the 2021 report by Deloitte Access Economics, commissioned by Teen Cancer America. *Journal of Clinical Oncology, 41*(17), 3260–3268. https://doi.org/10.1200/JCO.22.01985

Pennant, S., Lee, S.C., Holm, S., Triplett, K.N., Howe-Martin, L., Campbell, R., & Germann, J. (2019). The role of social support in adolescent/young adults coping with cancer treatment. *Children, 7*(1), 2. https://doi.org/10.3390/children7010002

Poorvu, P.D., Frazier, A.L., Feraco, A.M., Manley, P.E., Ginsburg, E.S., Laufer, M.R., ... Partridge, A.H. (2019). Cancer treatment-related infertility: A critical review of the evidence. *JNCI Cancer Spectrum, 3*(1), pkz008. https://doi.org/10.1093/jncics/pkz008

Poudel, P.G., Bauer, H.E., Srivastava, D.K., Krull, K.R., Hudson, M.M., Robison, L.L., ... Huang, I.-C. (2021). Online platform to assess complex social relationships and patient-reported outcomes among adolescent and young adult cancer survivors. *JCO Clinical Cancer Informatics, 5*, 859–871. https://doi.org/10.1200/CCI.21.00044

Psihogios, A.M., Schwartz, L.A., Deatrick, J.A., Ver Hoeve, E.S., Anderson, L.M., Wartman, E.C., & Szalda, D. (2019). Preferences for cancer survivorship care among adolescents and young adults who experienced healthcare transitions and their parents. *Journal of Cancer Survivorship, 13*(4), 620–631. https://doi.org/10.1007/s11764-019-00781-x

Quinn, G.P., Woodruff, T.K., Knapp, C.A., Bowman, M.L., Reinecke, J., & Vadaparampil, S.T. (2016). Expanding the oncofertility workforce: Training allied health professionals to improve health outcomes for adolescents and young adults. *Journal of Adolescent and Young Adult Oncology, 5*(3), 292–296. https://doi.org/10.1089/jayao.2016.0003

Ritt-Olson, A., Miller, K., Baezconde-Garbanati, L., Freyer, D., Ramirez, C., Hamilton, A., & Milam, J. (2018). Depressive symptoms and quality of life among adolescent and young adult cancer survivors: Impact of gender and Latino culture. *Journal of Adolescent and Young Adult Oncology, 7*(3), 384–388. https://doi.org/10.1089/jayao.2017.0078

Roth, M., Beauchemin, M., Kahn, J.M., & Bleyer, A. (2021). Patterns of National Cancer Institute-sponsored clinical trial enrollment in Black adolescents and young adults. *Cancer Medicine, 10*(21), 7620–7628. https://doi.org/10.1002/cam4.4292

Roth, M., Mittal, N., Saha, A., & Freyer, D.R. (2020). The Children's Oncology Group Adolescent and Young Adult Responsible Investigator Network: A new model for addressing site-level factors impacting clinical trial enrollment. *Journal of Adolescent and Young Adult Oncology, 9*(4), 522–527. https://doi.org/10.1089/jayao.2019.0139

Salsman, J.M., Bingen, K., Barr, R.D., & Freyer, D.R. (2019). Understanding, measuring, and addressing the financial impact of cancer on adolescents and young adults. *Pediatric Blood and Cancer, 66*(7), e27660. https://doi.org/10.1002/pbc.27660

Siegel, R.L., Giaquinto, A.N., & Jemal, A. (2024). Cancer statistics, 2024. *CA: A Cancer Journal for Clinicians, 74*(1), 12–49. https://doi.org/10.3322/caac.21820

Siembida, E., Loomans-Kropp, H.A., Trivedi, N., Bleyer, A., & Roth, M. (2020). Racial disparities in adolescent and young adult cancer clinical trial enrollment. *Journal of Clinical Oncology, 38*(29, Suppl.), 91. https://doi.org/10.1200/JCO.2020.38.29_suppl.91

Siembida, E.J., Loomans-Kropp, H.A., Trivedi, N., O'Mara, A., Sung, L., Tami-Maury, I., ... Roth, M. (2020). Systematic review of barriers and facilitators to clinical trial enrollment among adolescents and young adults with cancer: Identifying opportunities for intervention. *Cancer, 126*(5), 949–957. https://doi.org/10.1002/cncr.32675

Siembida, E.J., Reeve, B.B, Zebrack, B.J., Snyder, M.A., & Salsman, J.M. (2021). Measuring health-related quality of life in adolescent and young adult cancer survivors with the National Institutes of Health Patient-Reported Outcomes Measurement Information System: Comparing adolescent, emerging adult, and young adult survivor perspectives. *Psycho-Oncology, 30*(3), 303–311. https://doi.org/10.1002/pon.5577

Smith, A.W., Keegan, T., Hamilton, A., Lynch, C., Wu, X.-C., Schwartz, S.M., ... AYA HOPE Study Collaborative Group. (2018). Understanding care and outcomes in adolescents and young adult with cancer: A review of the AYA HOPE study. *Pediatric Blood and Cancer, 66*(1), e27486. https://doi.org/10.1002/pbc.27486

Smith, M., Korenblum, C., Mosher, P.J., Gupta, A.A., & Avery, J. (2023). The future of adolescent and young adult supportive care: Looking beyond the COVID-19 pandemic. *Journal of Adolescent and Young Adult Oncology, 13*(2), 239–241. https://doi.org/10.1089/jayao.2023.0039

Spathis, A., Hatcher, H., Booth, S., Gibson, F., Stone, P., Abbas, L., ... Barclay, S. (2017). Cancer-related fatigue in adolescents and young adults after cancer treatment: Persistent and poorly managed. *Journal of Adolescent and Young Adult Oncology, 6*(3), 489–493. https://doi.org/10.1089/jayao.2017.0037

Stafford, L.K., Tang, X., Brandt, A., Ma, J., Banchs, J., Livingston, J.A., ... Hildebrandt, M.A.T. (2024). Risk of anthracycline-induced cardiac dysfunction in adolescent and young adult (AYA) cancer survivors: Role of genetic susceptibility loci. *Pharmacogenomics Journal, 24*(21), 1–7. https://doi.org/10.1038/s41397-024-00343-0

Straehla, J.P., Barton, K.S., Yi-Frazier, J.P., Wharton, C., Baker, K.S., Bona, K., ... Rosenberg, A.R. (2017). The benefits and burdens of cancer: A prospective longitudinal cohort study of adolescents and young adults. *Journal of Palliative Medicine, 20*(5), 494–501. https://doi.org/10.1089/jpm.2016.0369

Sung, H., Siegel, R.L., Hyun, N., Miller, K.D., Yabroff, K.R., & Jemal, A. (2022). Subsequent primary cancer risk among 5-year survivors of adolescent and young adult cancers. *Journal of the National Cancer Institute, 114*(8), 1095–1108. https://doi.org/10.1093/jnci/djac091

Taylor, E.J., Petersen, C., Oyedele, O., & Haase, J. (2015). Spirituality and spiritual care of adolescents and young adults with cancer. *Seminars in Oncology Nursing, 31*(3), 227–241. https://doi.org/10.1016/j.soncn.2015.06.002

Thewes, B., Kaal, S.E.J., Custers, J.A.E., Manten-Horst, E., Jansen, R., Servaes, P., ... Husson, O. (2018). Prevalence and correlates of high fear of cancer recurrence in late adolescents and young adults consulting a specialist adolescent and young adult (AYA) cancer service. *Supportive Care in Cancer, 26*(5), 1479–1487. https://doi.org/10.1007/s00520-017-3975-2

Tolani, D., Wilcox, J., Shyam, S., & Bansal, N. (2023). Cardio-oncology for pediatric and adolescent/young adult patients. *Current Treatment Options in Oncology, 24*(8), 1052–1070. https://doi.org/10.1007/s11864-023-01100-4

Turgeman, I., & West, H. (2023). Adolescents and young adults with cancer. *JAMA Oncology, 9*(3), 440. https://doi.org/10.1001/jamaoncol.2022.6132

van der Meer, D.J., van der Graaf, W.T.A., van de Wal, D., Karim-Kos, H.E., & Husson, O. (2024). Long-term second primary cancer risk in adolescent and young adult (15-39 years) cancer survivors: A population-based study in the Netherlands between 1989 and 2018. *ESMO Open, 9*(1). https://doi.org/10.1016/j.esmoop.2023.102203

Warner, E.L., Fowler, B., Pannier, S.T., Salmon, S.K., Fair, D., Spraker-Perlman, H., ... Kirchhoff, A.C. (2018). Patient navigation preferences for adolescent and young adult cancer services by distance to treatment location. *Journal of Adolescent and Young Adult Oncology, 7*(4), 438–444. https://doi.org/10.1089/jayao.2017.0124

Waters, A.R., Mann, K., Warner, E.L., Vaca Lopez, P.L., Kaddas, H.K., Ray, N., ... Kirchhoff, A.C. (2022). "I thought there would be more I understood": Health insurance literacy among adolescent and young adult cancer survivors. *Supportive Care in Cancer, 30*(5), 4457–4464. https://doi.org/10.1007/s00520-022-06873-2

Wong-Siegel, J.R., Hayashi, R.J., Foraker, R., & Mitchell, J.D. (2023). Cardiovascular toxicities after anthracycline and VEGF-targeted therapies in adolescent and young adult cancer survivors. *Cardio-Oncology, 9*(1), 30. https://doi.org/10.1186/s40959-023-00181-2

Zebrack, B., Kwak, M., & Sundstrom, L. (2017). First Descents, an adventure program for young adults with cancer: Who benefits? *Supportive Care in Cancer, 25*(12), 3665–3673. https://doi.org/10.1007/s00520-017-3792-7

Zebrack, B., Santacroce, S., Patterson, P., & Gubin, A. (2016). Adolescents and young adults with cancer: A biopsychosocial approach. In A. Abrams, A. Muriel, & L. Weiner (Eds.), *Pediatric psychosocial oncology: Textbook for multidisciplinary care* (pp. 199–217). Springer. https://doi.org/10.1007/978-3-319-21374-3_12

Zhang, A., Wang, K., Zebrack, B., Tan, C.Y., Walling, E., & Chugh, R. (2021). Psychosocial, behavioral, and supportive interventions for pediatric, adolescent, and young adult cancer survivors: A systematic review and meta-analysis. *Critical Reviews in Oncology/Hematology, 160*, 103291. https://doi.org/10.1016/j.critrevonc.2021.103291

Zhang, A., Zebrack, B., Acquati, C., Roth, M., Levin, N.J., Wang, K., & Schwartz, S. (2022). Technology-assisted psychosocial interventions for childhood, adolescent, and young adult cancer survivors: A systematic review and meta-analysis. *Journal of Adolescent and Young Adult Oncology, 11*(1), 6–16. https://doi.org/10.1089/jayao.2021.0012

CHAPTER 18

Navigation Resources

Note. Some resources are listed within specific chapters (e.g., adolescent and young adult resources)

Patient and Caregiver Resources

General Cancer Education and Support

American Cancer Society
800-227-2345
www.cancer.org

American Institute for Cancer Research
800-843-8114
www.aicr.org

CancerCare
800-813-4673
www.cancercare.org

Cancer Support Community
888-793-9355
www.cancersupportcommunity.org

National Cancer Institute
800-422-6237
www.cancer.gov

National Comprehensive Cancer Network
215-690-0300
- Guidelines for Patients
  www.nccn.org/patientresources/patient-resources/guidelines-for-patients
- Resources for Patients and Caregivers
  www.nccn.org/patientresources/patient-resources/resources-for-patients-caregivers

Diagnosis-Specific Education and Support

Blood Cancer

Leukemia and Lymphoma Society
800-955-4572
www.lls.org

Lymphoma Research Foundation
800-500-9976
www.lymphoma.org

Brain Cancer

Brain Tumor Network
844-286-6110
www.braintumornetwork.org

National Brain Tumor Society
617-924-9997
www.braintumor.org

Breast Cancer

BreastCancer.org
610-642-6550
www.breastcancer.org

Susan G. Komen
877-465-6636
www.komen.org

Colorectal Cancer

Colorectal Cancer Alliance
877-422-2030
www.colorectalcancer.org

Fight Colorectal Cancer
888-793-9355
www.fightcolorectalcancer.org

Head and Neck Cancer

Head and Neck Cancer Alliance
866-792-4622
www.headandneck.org

HNC Living Foundation
913-402-6028
www.hncliving.org/for-patients

Kidney Cancer

KidneyCAN
info@kidneycan.org
www.kidneycan.org

Kidney Cancer Association
800-850-9132
www.kidneycancer.org

Lung Cancer

American Lung Association
800-586-4872
www.lung.org

LUNGevity
833-797-5800
www.lungevity.org

Melanoma

Melanoma Research Alliance
202-336-8935
www.curemelanoma.org/patient-eng

Melanoma Research Foundation
202-347-9675
www.melanoma.org/patients-caregivers

Ovarian Cancer

Ovarian Cancer Research Alliance
212-268-1002
www.ocrahope.org

Pancreatic Cancer

National Pancreatic Cancer Foundation
800-859-6723
www.npcf.us

Pancreatic Cancer Action Network
877-272-6226
www.pancan.org

Pediatric and Young Adults

National Children's Cancer Society
314-241-1600
www.thenccs.org

Stupid Cancer
212-619-1040
www.stupidcancer.org

Prostate Cancer

Prostate Cancer Foundation
800-757-2873
www.pcf.org/patient-resources

ZERO Prostate Cancer
202-463-9455
www.zerocancer.org

Rare Cancers

Rare Cancer Alliance
www.rare-cancer.org

TargetCancer Foundation
617-765-4881
www.targetcancer.org

Sarcoma

Sarcoma Alliance
415-381-7236
www.sarcomaalliance.org

Sarcoma Foundation of America
301-253-8687
www.curesarcoma.org/sarcoma-resources

Financial Assistance

GoodRx (discount prescriptions)
www.goodrx.com

Patient Advocate Foundation
800-532-5274
www.patientadvocate.org

Legal and Practical Issues

Cancer and Careers
646-929-8032
www.cancerandcareers.org

Triage Cancer
424-258-4628
www.triagecancer.org

Miscellaneous

Cleaning for a Reason
info@cleaningforareason.org
www.cleaningforareason.org

Meals on Wheels America
888-998-6325
www.mealsonwheelsamerica.org

Funeral Consumers Alliance
802-865-8300
www.funerals.org

Nutrition Education Services Center
877-467-1936
www.llsnutrition.org

Navigator Resources

Certification Programs

Foundation for Learning (clinical and non-clinical navigation certifications)
844-586-8446
www.aonnffl.org

Oncology Nursing Certification Corporation (clinical nursing certification)
877-769-6622
www.oncc.org/get-certified

Communication

Motivational Interviewing
www.ncbi.nlm.nih.gov/books/NBK64964

Plain Language Guidelines
www.plainlanguage.gov/guidelines

General Education and Guidelines

Association of Cancer Care Centers
301-984-9496
www.accc-cancer.org

National Comprehensive Cancer Network Guidelines by Cancer Type
215-690-0300
www.nccn.org/guidelines/category_1

Professional Organizations	
Academy of Oncology Nurse and Patient Navigators 844-586-8446 www.aonnonline.org	Oncology Nursing Society 866-257-4667 www.ons.org

Professional Publications	
Clinical Journal of Oncology Nursing www.ons.org/publications-research/cjon	*Oncology Nurse Advisor* www.oncologynurseadvisor.com
Journal of Oncology Navigation and Survivorship www.jons-online.com	*Oncology Nursing Forum* www.ons.org/publications-research/onf

Training Programs	
American Cancer Society Leadership in Oncology Navigation (ACS LION) https://cancer.catalog.instructure.com/courses/acslion	George Washington University Oncology Patient Navigator Training: The Fundamentals https://cme.smhs.gwu.edu/gw-cancer-center-/content/oncology-patient-navigator-training-fundamentals#group-tabs-node-course-default1

Transportation	
American Cancer Society Road to Recovery 800-227-2345 www.cancer.org/support-programs-and-services/road-to-recovery.html	Modivacre www.modivcare.com

Index

The letter *f* after a page number indicates that relevant content appears in a figure; the letter *t*, in a table

A

AARP Home and Family Caregiving Resource Center, 252*t*
Abbreviated Comprehensive Geriatric Assessment (aCGA), 246, 246*t*, 247
abemaciclib, 160*t*–161*t*
abiraterone acetate, 161*t*
Abramson Cancer Center, 180
ABT-263, 160*t*
ABT-737, 160*t*
Academy of Oncology Nurse and Patient Navigators (AONN+), 8*t*, 10, 12, 68, 78, 288
  Knowledge Domains, 78, 79*t*
  metrics toolkit, 78, 81–82, 84, 84*t*, 140
Accessia Health, 99*t*
access to care. *See* barriers to care
Accountable Health Communities Health-Related Social Needs Screening Tool, 60–61
accreditation, 10, 54, 59–61
addiction, 226. *See also* substance misuse
adherence, to treatment, 87, 133–135
Adolescent and Young Adult Health Outcomes and Patient Experience (AYA HOPE), 269
adolescent patients, 122–123, 261
  barriers faced by, 262–267
  communication needs of, 122–123
  financial/insurance concerns, 269–270
  ONN roles with, 262–263
  psychological/spiritual needs, 267–268
  resources for, 273–275, 273*t*–274*t*, 286
  social relationship needs, 268–270
  underrepresented populations in, 271–273
adult patients, communication needs of, 123–124
advance directives, 121, 137, 139
advanced disease, 137–138, 190, 203*f*
Advanced Practice Nurse Retreat Project Team, 77
adventure programs, 271
Affordable Care Act. *See* Patient Protection and Affordable Care Act

age-friendly healthcare, 241–246, 244*f*, 248–251
  resources for, 252*t*–253*t*
Age-Friendly Health Systems, 252*t*
Age-Friendly Health Systems initiatives, 244, 244*f*
ageism, 242–243
agonists, 159
Alliance for Fertility Preservation, 267, 273*t*
Alliance of Nurses for Healthy Environments, 252*t*
alternative payment models (APMs), 37, 80–81
American Association for the Treatment of Opioid Dependence, 233*t*
American Cancer Society (ACS), 273*t*, 285
  basic needs program, 98
  on cancer care disparities, 59
  data collection by, 62–63
  Hope Lodge, 134
  Leadership in Oncology Navigation (LION) program, 12–13, 288
  metrics, 82
  National Navigation Roundtable, 8*t*, 78, 79*t*
  in navigation history, 5, 8*t*–9*t*
  patient navigation app, 14
  Road to Recovery, 134, 288
  on survivorship care, 194*t*
American College of Surgeons Commission on Cancer (ACoS CoC), 8*t*, 10, 30, 54, 56
  accreditation standards of, 60, 78–79
  data collection by, 63
  on mental health screening, 212
  on survivorship care, 205
American Foundation for Suicide Prevention, 233*t*
American Geriatrics Society, 252*t*
American Hospital Association, 233*t*
American Institute for Cancer Research, 285
American Journal of Nursing, 252*t*
American Lung Association, 286
American Nurses Association, 77
American Psychiatric Association, 213, 233*t*

American Psychological Association, 233*t*
American Psychosocial Oncology Society, 212, 233*t*
American Red Cross, 252*t*
American Rescue Plan, 106, 107*t*
American Society of Clinical Oncology
  biomarker testing guidelines, 158
  Patient-Centered Oncology Payment model, 80–81
  on survivorship care, 194*t*, 205–206
amivantamab, 162
analytic patients, 64
angiogenesis pathway, 161*t*
antagonists, 159
antibody-drug conjugates (ADCs), 162
antigen-presenting cell vaccines, 163
anxiety, 199, 214–217, 229. *See also* panic attacks
  in adolescent/young adult patients, 263, 267
  in older adults, 250
Anxiety and Depression Association of America, 233*t*
apoptosis pathway, 161*t*
artificial intelligence (AI)
  in mental health care, 213
  in navigation, 14–15
asparaginase, 161*t*
The Assistance Fund, 99*t*, 100
Association for Behavioral and Cognitive Therapies, 233*t*
Association of Cancer Care Centers, 95, 287
Association of Oncology Social Work (AOSW), 8*t*, 10, 43, 79*t*
Association of Pediatric Hematology/Oncology Nurses, 10
atezolizumab, 161*t*
azacitidine, 161*t*

B

barriers to care, 19–23, 20*t*, 145–146, 179
  analysis of, 30
  assessment of, 45, 59–60, 64–65, 66*f*
  early identification of, 6–7, 8*t*–9*t*, 130
  spiritual, 176
  tracking of, 85
  treatment timeliness as metric of, 70–71
basic needs programs, 98
BATHE mnemonic, 218, 219*f*
belinostat, 161*t*
BETTER communication model, 200
"Better Society Gumbo," 183–184
bevacizumab, 156, 160*t*–161*t*
Biden, Joe, 6, 12
binge drinking, in survivorship phase, 270

biomarker testing, 132–133, 150, 156
  case studies on, 165*f*–166*f*
  challenges in, 164
  guidelines for, 158, 164
  techniques for, 157–158, 157*t*
bispecific antibodies, 162
blended ONN staffing models, 51
blinatumomab, 162
blood cancer, resources on, 285. *See also* Leukemia and Lymphoma Society
bortezomib, 161*t*
brain cancer, 99*t*, 285
Brain Tumor Network, 285
breast cancer, 72, 79–80, 136, 152, 285
breast health nurse navigator (BNN), 116
Brown, Brené, 172
burnout, 181–183, 229, 232, 233*t*
Bush, George W., 8*t*, 12
business plans, 33, 34*t*–36*t*, 36*f*
  templates for, 33, 36*f*

C

cabozantinib, 160*t*
Cactus Cancer Society, 273*t*
CAGE-AID questionnaire, 226, 226*f*
Camp Koru, 271
Camp Māk-A-Dream, 271
Cancer and Aging Research Group, 252*t*
Cancer and Careers, 270, 273*t*, 287
CancerCare, 98, 99*t*, 273*t*
Cancer Financial Assistance Coalition, 98
Cancer for College, 264
Cancer Moonshot, 6, 12
Cancer Nursing's Potential to Reduce the Growing Burden of Cancer Across the World (2021), 9
Cancer Prevention and Control Research Network, 130
cancer recurrence
  fear of, 198, 265–266
  navigation during, 118*t*, 119–120, 120*t*, 125, 137–138
cancer registries, 62–63, 62*f*
cancer-related fatigue, 195–196, 249–250, 265–266
Cancer Support Community, 194*t*, 285
cardiovascular toxicity risk, 193, 265
care continuum–specific navigation model, 52, 53*t*, 55*t*, 57, 129. *See also specific phases*
care coordination, 4
care partners, for older adults, 241, 251
carfilzomib, 161*t*
case workers, 43
Catholic sisters, 173

celecoxib, 160*t*
cell cycle pathway, 161*t*
cell therapy, 163
Centers for Disease Control and Prevention, 62, 130
Centers for Medicare and Medicaid Innovation, Enhancing Oncology Model, 37, 60–61, 80, 133
Centers for Medicare and Medicaid Services
　billing codes, 12–13, 37, 78, 81
　navigation reimbursement by, 9*t*, 12–13, 32, 37, 45–46, 78
　Oncology Care Model, 132
certification, 4–5, 5*f*, 8*t*–9*t*, 23, 78, 287
cetuximab, 160*t*
champions/stakeholders, 31, 33, 37, 83–84
chaplains, 178–180
Chartis, 82
chemical coping, 211–212, 224–225. *See also* substance misuse
　communication with patients using, 226–227
　by healthcare professionals, 228
　symptoms of, 225–226, 226*f*
chimeric antigen receptor T-cell therapy, 163, 197
Cleaning for a Reason, 287
clinical champions. *See* champions/stakeholders
clinical dashboards, 87–89
Clinical Journal of Oncology Nursing, 288
clinical navigators, 11–12, 31, 37, 42, 49, 51–52
clinical trials
　adolescents/young adults in, 262
　case studies on, 166*f*
　digital barriers to, 22
　racial diversity in, 71–72, 272
Clinton, Bill, 8*t*
Code of Ethics for Nurses, 173
cognitive changes, 197, 250–251
colon cancer, 65, 165*f*
Colorado Patient Navigator Training Collaborative, 12
colorectal cancer, 150–151, 201–202, 286
Colorectal Cancer Alliance, 286
communication skills, 115–116, 179
　age-related, 121–124
　case studies on, 124–125
　with depression, 218–220, 219*f*
　with family and friends, 269
　on genomics, 164–165
　models for, 118*f*
　during panic attacks, 216–217
　with patients with psychosis, 223–224
　at prediagnosis/diagnosis phase, 116–117, 124–125
　during recurrence, 118*t*, 119–120, 120*t*
　resources on, 287

　and spiritual nursing care, 177
　with substance addiction/misuse, 226–227
　at survivorship phase, 119, 120*t*
　at treatment phase, 117–119
Communication Skills Attitude Scale, 177
community-engaged navigation model, 54–56, 55*t*
community health workers, 42, 49, 50*t*
community needs assessment, 30, 61
　external, 61–64, 62*f*
　goal formation from, 67–68, 68*f*
　internal, 64–67, 66*f*
　template for, 68, 69*t*–70*t*
comorbidities
　with cancer, 147–148
　with mental illness, 212
comparative genomic hybridization (CGH), 157*t*
compassion fatigue, 182, 229, 232
competencies, 4–5, 5*f*, 8*t*–9*t*, 10–11, 11*f*, 43–44, 51
　application to practice, 44–45, 45*f*, 85
　and practice standards, 78–79, 79*t*
complicated grief, 230
Confusion Assessment Method, 250
Connor-Davidson Resilience Scale, 181
Consolidated Omnibus Budget Reconciliation Act (COBRA), 96
co-pay assistance programs, 99–100, 99*t*
Cost Plus, 99
cost-sharing subsidies, 106, 108*t*
coverage gap (donut hole), 100
COVID-19 pandemic, 175, 177, 183
　cancer survivorship care during, 206
　effects on mental health, 211–212, 217, 228–232
crizotinib, 160*t*
cultural humility, 175
Cyprus University of Technology, 9

D

dashboards, 87–89
data collection, 61–64, 62*f*, 85–86
data manipulation, 85
decitabine, 161*t*
delirium, 221, 250
Delirium Observation Screening Scale, 250
Delirium Rating Scale-Revised-98, 250
deliverables, timetable for, 33, 34*t*–36*t*, 36*f*
delusions, 221–222
dementia, 250
demographic data collection, 62
depression, 199, 217–218, 233*t*
　in adolescent/young adult patients, 263, 267
　communication skills for, 218–220, 219*f*

in older adult patients, 250
symptoms of, 218
detox treatment, 226
Developing and Retaining a Robust and Diverse Cancer Workforce (2024), 6
Diagnostic and Statistical Manual of Mental Disorders (DSM-5-TR)
   on depression, 218
   on panic attacks, 214, 216
   on schizophrenia, 222
   on substance misuse, 225
diagnostic navigation/navigators, 42, 53*t*, 55*t*, 116–117, 118*t*, 124–125, 130–133
diagnostic overshadowing, 221
digital divide, 22, 63–64
digital health platforms, 14, 21
disability benefits, 96, 107–108, 134
discovery–delivery disconnect, 7
disease-specific navigation model, 52, 57
disparities. *See* healthcare disparities
distress, 45, 85, 198–199
   in adolescent/young adult patients, 263, 267
   screening for, 212–213
Distress Thermometer, 45, 60, 96, 132
DNA damage response pathway, 159, 161*t*
drug assistance programs, 99
drug-seeking, 226
duloxetine, 196
durvalumab, 161*t*

E

early detection navigation, 53*t*, 55*t*, 130–131
eFrailty, 246–247
electronic health records (EHRs), 82–83, 85–86
Elephants and Tea, 271, 273*t*
Emory Saint Joseph's Hospital, 180
empathy, 218–220, 219*f*, 233*t*
The Empathy Center, 233*t*
enasidenib, 161*t*
end-of-life care
   communication about, 120–121, 121*t*, 138
   navigation in, 138–140
   planning in, 137
   research gap within, 140
endometrial cancer, 65
Engage, 233*t*
Enhancing Oncology Model (EOM), 37, 60–61, 80
enzalutamide, 161*t*
enzymes, 159
EOM 2024 Health Equity Plan Guide, 61
epidemiology, of cancer, 7
epidermal growth factor receptor (EGFR), 162

epigenetic modifier pathways, 161*t*
erlotinib, 160*t*
Escape, 272, 273*t*
European Oncology Nursing Society, 9
European Society for Medical Oncology, 192, 192*f*
evidence-based practice (EBP), 175–177
Evidence-Based Practice Competence Questionnaire, 177
Exercise is Medicine, 194*t*
Expect Miracles Foundation, 264, 274*t*
external barriers, 64, 66*f*. *See also* barriers to care
external data, 61–64, 62*f*
Extra Help (Medicare), 92, 100–102

F

FACT-Breast assessment, 136
FACT-General assessment, 136
FACT spiritual health assessment, 178
faith community nursing, 180
fall risk, in older adult patients, 245, 249–250
Family and Medical Leave Act, 107–108, 134
Family Reach, 98
fatigue, 195–196, 249–250, 265–266
fertility issues, 199–200, 266, 274*t*
fertility preservation, 266–267
FICA spiritual health assessment, 178
Fight Colorectal Cancer, 286
Financial Advocacy Bootcamp, 95
Financial Advocacy model, 93–94
financial burden/distress, 54, 96. *See also* financial toxicity
Financial Navigation model, 93–95
financial navigation/navigators, 42–43, 49, 50*t*, 53–54, 57, 93–95
financial plan, for navigation program, 32
financial resources, 97–100, 99*t*, 264, 287
financial toxicity, 54, 91, 134, 200
   for adolescents/young adults, 269–270
   assessment of, 96–97, 97*f*, 134
   early intervention for, 95
   educational trainings on, 95
   impact of, 91–92, 93*f*
   during survivorship, 135
   technological interventions for, 95–96
First Descents, 271, 274*t*
fluorescence in situ hybridization (FISH), 157*t*
focus groups, 66–67
FOLFOX chemotherapy, 201
folinic acid, 201
Foundation for Learning, 287
Foundations in Faith Community Nursing course, 180

four-tiered process for patient-centered care and communication (PC4), 139
frailty, 242–243, 245
frailty screening, 245–247, 246t, 250
Freeman, Harold, 4, 6–7, 8t
fulvestrant, 161t
Functional Assessment of Cancer Therapy questionnaires, 136
Fund Finder, 100
funding, for navigation programs, 12–13, 29, 32
Funeral Consumers Alliance, 287

G

G-codes, 81. See also Centers for Medicare and Medicaid Services
generalist navigation model, 51–52, 57
genetic testing, 148–150
Genomics Advisory Board (GAB), 164
Genomics and Precision Oncology Learning Library, 156, 164, 166
George Washington Cancer Center, Patient Navigation Core Competencies, 78, 79t
George Washington University
  National Cancer Survivorship Resource Center, 194t, 206
  Oncology Patient Navigator Training, 288
  School of Medicine and Health Sciences, 12
Geriatric 8 (G8) assessment, 246, 246t, 247
geriatric oncology, 242–243. See also age-friendly healthcare
GeriatricsCareOnline.org, 253t
geriatric syndromes, 245, 247
Gerontological Advanced Practice Nurses Association, 253t
gero-oncology perspective, 241–243, 252t–253t. See also age-friendly healthcare
Global Consortium on Climate and Health Education, 243–244, 252t
Global Navigation Program (ACS) (2017), 9t
Good Day's Chronic Disease Fund, 99t
GoodRx, 99, 287
grief, 230
Groningen Frailty Indicator (GFI), 246, 246t

H

hallucinations, 221–223
Harold P. Freeman Patient Navigation Institute, 8t. See also Freeman, Harold
Hartford Institute for Geriatric Nursing, 253t
head and neck cancer, 65, 286
Head and Neck Cancer Alliance, 286

HealthCare Chaplaincy Network, 178
healthcare chaplains, 178–180
healthcare disparities, 19, 59, 65, 130. See also barriers to care
  financial toxicity with, 92
  in mental illness, 221
health insurance
  access to, 22–23
  for adolescents/young adults, 269–270
  coverage denial, 166f
  optimization of, 100–108
  patient understanding of, 92, 134, 269–271
Health Insurance Marketplace, 106. See also Marketplace insurance
Health Insurance Portability and Accountability Act (HIPAA), 85
health literacy, 117–118
HealthWell Foundation, 99t
Healthy People 2030, 22
high-risk clinical phenomena, 247–248
high-speed internet, 21–22. See also technology
HNC Living Foundation, 286
holistic nursing care, 173–176
homelessness, navigation support with, 71, 150–151
Honesty and Ethics poll (2023), 130
Hope Lodge program, 134
HOPE spiritual health assessment, 178
hormone pathway, 159, 161t
hospice, communication about, 120–121, 121t, 125, 140. See also end-of-life care
hub-and-spoke model, of cancer clinics, 56
human gene therapy, 163

I

imetelstat, 160t
immune checkpoint inhibitors, 156, 162–163, 197
immune checkpoints pathways, 161t
immunohistochemistry, 157t
immunomodulatory therapy, 161–163
incarceration, navigation during/after, 150–151
infertility. See fertility issues
Inflation Reduction Act (2022), 106
information seekers vs. avoiders, 124
Institute for Healthcare Improvement, 244–245, 244f
insurance. See health insurance
insurance optimization, 100–108
integrative therapies, 180
intellectual disabilities, 272–273
internal barriers, 64–65, 66f. See also barriers to care
internal data, 64
International Society of Nurses in Cancer Care, 7, 9

internet access, 21–22, 63–64
Interprofessional Spiritual Care Education Curriculum, 177–178
ipilimumab, 160t–161t, 197
ivosidenib, 161t

J

James Cancer Hospital, 56
Jefferson Scale of Empathy, 177
job descriptions, creation of, 31
Joint Position on the Role of Oncology Nursing and Oncology Social Work in Patient Navigation (2010), 8t
Journal of Oncology Navigation and Survivorship, 288

K

KidneyCAN, 286
kidney cancer, 286
Kidney Cancer Association, 286
kinase pathways, 159
KRAS G12V variant, 166f

L

language barriers, to care access, 23, 146–147
languishing, 229, 232
legal resources, 287
Leukemia and Lymphoma Society, 98, 99t, 274t, 285
LGBTQ+ patient navigation, 148–150, 272, 274t
lifestyle behaviors, in survivorship, 270
limited English proficiency (LEP), 23, 146–147
Livestrong, 266, 274t
loneliness
  in adolescents/young adults, 268, 270
  in healthcare professionals, 229–230, 232
  in older adults, 251
longitudinal navigation model, 52–53, 57
Low Income Subsidy, 92, 100–101
lung cancer, 160t, 164, 286
LUNGevity, 286
Lymphoma Research Foundation, 285
Lynch syndrome, 148

M

marketing plan, for navigation program, 32–33
Marketplace insurance, 92, 96, 106–107, 106t–108t
market share and competitor analysis, for navigation program, 32

Maslach Burnout Inventory (MBI), 182–183
maximum out-of-pocket (MOOP) responsibilities, 92, 101–102, 106
Meals on Wheels America, 287
Medicaid expansion, 22, 104
Medicare Advantage plans, 92, 103
Medicare Part D, 100–102
Medicare Parts A and B, 102
Medicare Plan Finder Tool, 103
Medicare Prescription Payment Plan, 101–102
Medicare Savings Program (MSP), 92, 102
Medicare Supplement plans, 103–104, 105t
melanoma, 286
Melanoma Research Alliance, 286
Melanoma Research Foundation, 286
Memorial Delirium Assessment Scale, 250
mental health, 211. *See also* anxiety; depression; psychosis; substance misuse
  affected by COVID-19 pandemic, 211–212, 217, 228–232
  resources for, 233, 233t
  screening for, 212
Mental Status Examination (MSE), 213–214, 215f
mentation. *See* cognitive changes
mentorship programs, 13
Merit-Based Incentive Payment System (MIPS), 37, 80
Merritt, Tyler, 183–184
mesenchymal-epithelial transition (MET), 162
messenger RNA (mRNA), 156
metabolic pathways, 161t
metastatic disease, 137–138, 190, 203f
methotrexate, 161t
metrics, 31, 68, 77–78
  establishment of, 78–81, 79t
  evaluation/implementation of, 83–89, 84t, 88t, 140
  selection/display of, 87–89
microsatellite instability-high (MSI-H), 158
Mika Health mobile app, 213
mismatch repair deficiency (dMMR), 158
mission statement, for navigation program, 30
mobile apps, 14, 213
mobility, in older adult patients, 245, 249–250
Modivacre, 134, 288
monoclonal antibodies (mAbs), 161–162
moral distress, 229, 231–232
moral injury, 229, 232
motivational interviewing (MI), 117, 136, 227, 287
Mullan, Fitzhugh, 190
multicomplexity, in older adult patients, 244–245, 247
Musella Brain Tumor Foundation, 99t

N

Narcotics Anonymous, 226
National Academies of Sciences, Engineering, and Medicine, 20, 20*t*
National Academy of Medicine, 212
National Accreditation Program for Breast Centers (NAPBC), 10, 54, 56, 60, 78–80, 205
National Alliance on Mental Illness, 233*t*
National Association of Social Workers, 8*t*, 79*t*
National Brain Tumor Society, 285
National Cancer Act (1971), 6
National Cancer Database, 62–63
National Cancer Institute, 6, 37, 62, 194*t*, 274*t*, 285
National Cancer Plan (2023), 6
National Cancer Program, 6
National Cancer Survivorship Resource Center, 194*t*
National Children's Cancer Society, 286
National Coalition for Cancer Survivorship, 189, 194*t*–195*t*
National Comprehensive Cancer Network (NCCN), 285, 287
    biomarker testing guidelines, 158, 165*f*–166*f*
    on cancer care disparities, 59
    Distress Thermometer, 45, 60, 96, 132
    on integrative therapies, 180
    on mental health screening, 212
    on survivorship care, 192–193, 192*f*, 194*t*
National Hearings on Cancer and the Poor (ACS), 5, 8*t*
National Institute of Mental Health, 233*t*
National Institute on Aging, 253*t*
National LGBT Cancer Network, 272, 274*t*
National Minority Quality Forum, 59
National Navigation Roundtable Survey, 8*t*, 78, 79*t*, 82–83, 83*f*
National Organization for Rare Disorders, 99*t*
National Pancreatic Cancer Foundation, 286
National Standards for Cancer Survivorship Care, 194*t*
natural disasters, navigation during/after, 152
NaVectis Group, financial navigation training, 95
navigation. *See* oncology nurse navigation
Navigation Metrics Toolkit, 78, 81–82, 84, 84*t*, 140
navigation models, 11, 51–53, 53*t*, 132–133
navigation programs
    evaluation of, 36–37
    goal-setting for, 30–31, 67–68, 68*f*
    marketing plan for, 32–33
    metrics for, 31, 68, 77–81, 79*t*, 83–89, 88*t*, 140
    mission/vision for, 30
    needs assessment for, 30, 61 (*See also* community needs assessment)
    organizational/operational/financial plans for, 31–32
    plan for building, 29–37
    stakeholders/champions for, 31, 33, 37, 83–84, 86
    sustainability of, 37
    timing and deliverables, 33, 34*t*–36*t*, 36*f*
navitoclax, 160*t*
needs assessment. *See* community needs assessment
NeedyMeds, 99
neuropathy, 196
next-generation sequencing (NGS), 157*t*, 158
Nightingale, Florence, 77, 173
niraparib, 160*t*–161*t*
nivolumab, 161*t*
Nixon, Richard, 6
nonanalytic patients, 64
non-clinical navigators, 11–12, 31, 37, 42–43, 49, 51–52
non-kinase pathways, 159
non-small cell lung cancer, 160*t*, 164
Norris Comprehensive Cancer Center, 71–72
NTRK gene fusion, 166*f*
nursing education, 175–176
Nursing Need theory, 174, 179
Nursing Safety and Quality Initiative, 77
nursing-sensitive outcomes, 77–78
Nutrition Education Services Center, 287

O

OARS mnemonic, in motivational interviewing, 227
Obama, Barack, 12
obatoclax, 160*t*
Office of the Surgeon General, 233*t*
olaparib, 160*t*–161*t*
older adults, 241. *See also* age-friendly healthcare; gero-oncology perspective
    communication needs of, 124
    medication issues for, 138–139
OncoLink Survivorship Care Plan, 194*t*, 205
Oncology Care Model, 37, 60
Oncology Navigation Standards of Professional Practice, 57, 129, 140
    ONN education/role delineation in, 12
    publication of, 9*t*, 10, 36–37
    used in competencies assessment, 45
Oncology Nurse Advisor, 288
oncology nurse navigation (ONN), 4–5, 5*f*, 50*t*. *See also* navigation models; navigation programs
    best practices for, 23, 68–72
    case studies on, 146–152

clinical vs. non-clinical, 11–12, 31, 37, 42–43, 49, 51–52 (*See also* role definition/delineation)
competencies in (*See* competencies)
education/credentialing for, 12
funding for, 9t, 12–13
history of, 5–7, 8t–9t
resources on, 285–288
role delineation in (*See* role definition/delineation)
role integration, 13
role integrity, 14
Oncology Nurse Navigation: Delivering Patient-Centered Care Across the Continuum (ONS), 8t–9t
Oncology Nurse Navigation Role Delineation Study (ONS), 8t
Oncology Nurse Navigator, Genomics (ONNG), 133
Oncology Nurse Navigator Competencies, 4, 8t, 146–152
Oncology Nursing Certification Corporation (ONCC), 4–5, 5f, 8t–9t, 23, 287
Oncology Nursing Forum, 288
Oncology Nursing Society (ONS), 41, 288. *See also under* ONS
   on barriers to care, 146
   on competencies, 4–5, 8t–9t, 23, 31, 43–45, 79t
   on end-of-life research gap, 140
   on fertility preservation, 266
   on nurse navigation roles, 4, 8t–9t, 10–11, 31, 51
   on nursing-sensitive outcomes, 77–78
   Oncology Nurse Navigation Role Delineation Study, 8t–9t
   position statements on navigation, 8t, 9, 9t, 14
   on standards of practice, 10, 129
   on survivorship care, 193, 194t
Oncology Patient Navigator Training: The Fundamentals, 12, 288
oncology social workers (OSWs), 42–43, 50t, 180
oncolytic viruses, 163
ONN Certified Generalist exam, 12
ONS Biomarker Database, 165f
ONS Genomics Advisory Board (GAB), 164
ONS Genomics and Precision Oncology Learning Library, 156, 164, 166
ONS Genomics Taxonomy, 164
ONS Navigation Focus Group, 8t
OpenAI, 14. *See also* artificial intelligence
open-ended questions, 117, 136. *See also* motivational interviewing
Open Enrollment Period (OEP), 103, 107–108
opioids, 224–225, 233t
organizational/operational plan, for navigation program, 31–32

outreach navigation, 55t
ovarian cancer, 158, 286
Ovarian Cancer Research Alliance, 286
oxaliplatin, 201

P

pain, 196, 224. *See also* chemical coping
palbociclib, 160t–161t
palliative care, 121, 121t
palliative navigation, 55t
pancreatic cancer, 166f, 286
Pancreatic Cancer Action Network, 286
panic attacks, 214
   communication during, 216–217
   symptoms of, 214–216
panic disorder (PD), 214
panitumumab, 160t
panobinostat, 161t
PARP inhibitors, 158
pathway targets, 159–160, 161t
Patient Access Network Foundation, 100
Patient Advocate Foundation, 98, 264, 274t, 287
patient assistance programs (PAPs), 94, 98–99
patient-centered communication, 119, 139–140
Patient-Centered Oncology Payment model, 80–81
patient-facing AI (PF-AI) apps, 14–15
Patient Health Questionnaire-9 (PHQ-9), 132
Patient Navigation and Community Health Worker Training, 12
Patient Navigation Program in Cancer Care (2005), 8t
Patient Navigator Outreach and Chronic Disease Prevention Act (2005), 8t, 12
Patient Protection and Affordable Care Act (2010), 8t, 22, 104–107, 106t–107t
Patient-Reported Outcomes Measures (PROMIS), 132
patient service areas, 61
pazopanib, 160t
PC4 (four-tiered process for patient-centered care and communication), 139
pediatric patients, 261, 286. *See also* adolescent patients
   communication needs of, 122
   ONN roles with, 262–263
peer navigators, 51
peer support
   for adolescents/young adults, 264, 266
   in the workplace, 231
pembrolizumab, 158, 161t
Penn Medicine, 180

personalized medicine, 155. *See also* precision oncology
PEWTER communication model, 116–117, 118*f*, 124–125, 139
pharmacy assistance programs, 99
Physician Fee Schedule (CMS), 13
Pink Aid, 98
Pink Fund, 98
Plain Language Guidelines, 287
planetary crisis, 243–244, 252*t*
PLISSIT communication model, 199–200
poly (ADP-ribose polymerase) (PARP) inhibitors, 158
polymerase chain reaction (PCR), 157*t*
polypharmacy, 245, 249
potentially inappropriate medications (PIMs), 249
Practical Geriatric Assessment, 246
precision oncology, 132–133, 155–156, 166. *See also* biomarker testing; targeted therapies
  case studies on, 165*f*–166*f*
  challenges in, 163–166, 165*f*–166*f*
prehabilitation, 193
premium assistance programs, 100
President's Cancer Panel, 6
primary care providers, 204–205
primary data collection, 62, 62*f*
Principal Care Management (PCM) reimbursement, 13, 37
Principal Illness Navigation (PIN) reimbursement, 12–13, 37, 78, 81
process mapping, 65–66
process-oriented communication, 139
Professional Oncology Navigation Task Force (PONT), 9*t*, 10, 12, 36, 41–42, 79*t*
professional organizations, 288
professional publications, 288
program design, 11–12
promotores/promotoras de salud, 49, 50*t*
prostate cancer, 148–150, 286
Prostate Cancer Foundation, 286
proteasome pathway, 161*t*
psychological first aid (PFA), 213
psychosis, 220–224. *See also* schizophrenia
psychosocial needs
  in adolescents/young adults, 267–268
  in survivorship, 197–199

Q

Qualified Disabled Working Individual (QDWI), 102
Qualified Individual (QI), 102
Qualified Medicare Beneficiary (QMB), 102

quality of life, 182, 232
Quality Oncology Practice Initiatives (QOPI) certification, 78
Queensland University of Technology, 9

R

Ramachenderan, Jonathan, 175
ramucirumab, 161*t*
Rare Cancer Alliance, 287
rare cancers, 99*t*, 287
real-time quantitative reverse transcription polymerase chain reaction (qRT-PCR), 157*t*, 158
receptors, 159
recurrence
  fear of, 198, 265–266
  navigation during, 118*t*, 119–120, 120*t*, 125, 137–138
Reducing Cancer Care Inequities (2023), 6
reimbursement, for patient navigation services, 9*t*, 12–13, 32, 45–46
religion, 171–173. *See also* spirituality
religiosity, 172
Report to the Nation: Cancer in the Poor (ACS), 5, 8*t*
resilience, 181, 213, 229
resources, for navigation, 285–288
return on investment (ROI), measurement of, 86–87, 88*t*
Rhode Island Hospital, 71
ribociclib, 160*t*–161*t*
Road to Recovery (ACS), 134, 288
role definition/delineation, 4, 8*t*–9*t*, 41–43, 49–51, 50*t*
  in business plans, 31
  and competencies, 10–11, 11*f*
  regular re-evaluation of, 36
role integration, 13
role integrity, 14
Role of the Oncology Nurse Navigator Throughout the Cancer Trajectory (ONS) (2021), 9*t*, 11, 11*f*
romidepsin, 161*t*
RSC spiritual care framework, 178
rucaparib, 161*t*
rural navigation, 56, 152
RxAssist, 264

S

safety plan, for suicidal risk, 220
Sanford Health, 133
Sanger sequencing, 157*t*, 158
sarcoma, 287

Sarcoma Alliance, 287
Sarcoma Foundation of America, 287
schizophrenia, 211, 221–223
Schwartz Center for Compassionate Healthcare, 232
Schwartz Rounds, 232
screening navigation, 53*t*, 55*t*, 130–131
screening tools, 45, 60–61
Seasons of Survival, 190
secondary data collection, 62–63, 62*f*
second primary cancers, risk in younger patients, 265
self-care, 181–183
setting-specific navigation models, 54–56, 55*t*
severe mental illness and impairment (SMII), 211, 232–233. *See also* anxiety; depression; psychosis; substance misuse
sexual health, in survivorship, 199–200
Share a Smile, 98
short-term disability benefits, 107–108
signal transduction pathway, 161*t*
SingleCare, 99
small molecule therapy, 159–160, 160*t*–161*t*
SMART goals, 31
smoking, in survivorship phase, 270
smoothing programs, 101–102
social determinants of health, 19–20, 45, 130, 132, 173, 179. *See also* barriers to care
social isolation, 230, 251, 268
Social Security Administration, 100–101
Social Security Disability Insurance, 96
social workers, 42–43, 50*t*, 180
sonidegib, 161*t*
Special Enrollment Periods (SEPs), 103, 107
Specified Low-Income Medicare Beneficiary (SLMB), 102
SPIKES communication model, 116–117, 118*f*, 124, 139
spiritual care, 171. *See also* spirituality
 for adolescents/young adults, 267–268
 assessment tools/framework, 178–179
 barriers to providing, 176
 components of, 176
 education/training in, 175–176
 for healthcare workers, 181–183
 navigation and, 179–181
Spiritual Care Competency Scale, 176
spiritual distress, 175
spiritual health, 172, 178
Spiritual Health Scale, 176
spiritual intelligence, 177
Spiritual Intelligence Questionnaire, 177
spirituality, 171–175. *See also* spiritual care

Spirituality and Spiritual Care Rating Scale, 177
staffing, of navigator teams, 51
stakeholders, 31, 33, 37, 83–84, 86
standards of practice, 10, 51
St. Elizabeth Healthcare (Kentucky), 52
stem cell transplantation, 163
St. Jude Children's Research Hospital, 264–265
Stupid Cancer, 264, 271, 274*t*, 286
substance misuse, 211, 224–227, 226*f*, 233*t*
 in adolescent/young adult patients, 267
 in healthcare professionals, 228–229
 in older adult patients, 249
suicidal depression, 217–220, 233*t*
suicide risk
 in adolescents/young adults, 267
 with cancer, 217–218
sunitinib, 160*t*
Supportive Care Framework for Cancer Care, 179
surveys, 66
survivorship, 189
 navigation during (*See* survivorship care)
 resources for, 194*t*–195*t*, 204–205, 204*t*
 stages of, 190–191, 191*f*
 treatment effects during, 194*t*–195*t*, 1920193
survivorship care. *See also* survivorship navigation/navigators
 for adolescents/young adults, 264, 267
 case study on, 201–202
 components of, 190–192, 192*f*
 educational resources on, 193, 194*t*–195*t*
 future directions in, 206–207
 models of, 204*t*, 205–206
 ONN role in, 200–202, 203*f*
 program development for, 205–206
survivorship care planning, 132, 135, 194*t*–195*t*
survivorship care plans (SCPs), 202, 205
 templates for, 194*t*, 205
Survivorship Learning Library, 194*t*
survivorship navigation/navigators, 53–54, 53*t*, 55*t*, 57, 119, 120*t*, 135–136. *See also* survivorship care
Susan G. Komen, 12, 285
symptom clusters, 193–195
system-related barriers to care, 65, 66*f*

T

talazoparib, 160*t*
tamoxifen, 161*t*
TargetCancer Foundation, 287
targeted therapies, 156–157, 159–163, 160*t*–161*t*. *See also* biomarker testing
 case studies on, 165*f*–166*f*
task-oriented communication, 139

technology
  availability of, 63–64
  as barrier to care access, 21–22, 82
  in navigation, 14–15
telehealth, 14, 21, 63, 213
Tilburg Frailty Indicator, 246, 246*t*
timeliness of care, 70–71. *See also* barriers to care
timetable, for navigation program, 33, 34*t*–36*t*, 36*f*
time toxicity, 200
tivantinib, 160*t*
Traditional Financial Counseling model, 93–94
transgender patients, 148–150. *See also* LGBTQ+ patient navigation
transportation, 20–21, 146, 250, 288
trastuzumab, 156
trauma, 229
treatment navigation/navigators, 42, 53*t*, 55*t*, 117–119, 133–135
tremelimumab, 160*t*
Triage Cancer, 264, 274*t*, 287
  financial navigation training, 95
  Insurance and Financial Intensive Training for Health Care, 12
Triage Risk Screening Tool (TRST), 246, 246*t*
trilaciclib, 161*t*
tumor microenvironment, 156, 163–164
tumor molecular burden-high (TMB-H), 158

U

Ulman Foundation, 264, 274*t*
Ultra Brief screen and Confusion Assessment Method (UB-CAM), 250
uncertainty, 116, 198
undocumented immigrant status, 146–147
unhoused patients, navigation support for, 71, 150–151
Unitary Caring Science, 174

U.S. Aging, 253*t*
U.S. Census Bureau, 62

V

value-based payment model, 80
venetoclax, 161*t*
vismodegib, 161*t*
Voices of a Broken System: Real People, Real Problems (2001), 6
vorinostat, 161*t*
Vulnerable Elder Survey-13 (VES-13), 246, 246*t*, 247

W

"What's the Meaning of This?" support group, 180
World Health Organization, 182, 218
writing workshops, 180

Y

Young Adult Cancer Camp, 271
young adult patients, 261, 286
  barriers faced by, 262–267
  communication needs of, 122–123
  financial/insurance concerns, 269–270
  ONN roles with, 262–263
  psychological/spiritual needs, 267–268
  resources for, 273–275, 273*t*–274*t*, 286
  social relationship needs, 268–270
  underrepresented populations, 271–273
Young Adults Survivors United, 271, 274*t*
Young Survival Coalition, 271, 274*t*

Z

ZERO Prostate Cancer, 286